MATERIA MEDICA

STU

Volume-1

(For BHMS, DHMS, NIH, Post-graduate students, Research scholars and Homoeopathic physicians)

70 Homoeopathic Medicines

Explained in a lucid & visualised form including questions of last 25 years.

Written & illustrated by

DR. RITU KINRA

B.H.M.S. (Delhi University)

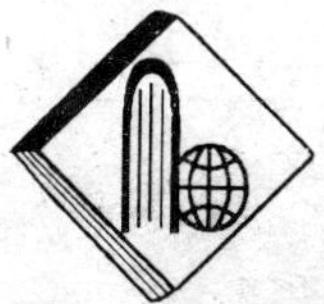

B. Jain Publishers (P) Ltd.

New Delhi.

First edition : 1999
Reprint edition : 2000 2001, 2002, 2003

Price: Rs. 125.00

Published by :
Kuldeep Jain
For
B. Jain publishers (P.) Ltd.
1921, Street No. 10, Chuna Mandi,
Paharganj, New Delhi 110 055 (INDIA)
Phones: 2358 3100, 2358 1300, 2358 0800, 2358 1100
Fax: 011-2358 0471; *Email:* bjain@vsnl.com
Website: **www.bjainbooks.com; www.healthharmonybooks.com**

Printed in India by:
J. J. Offset Printers
522, FIE, Patpar Ganj, Delhi - 110 092

ISBN 81-7021-925-6
BOOK CODE : BK-5380

DEDICATED

TO MY

GRANDPARENTS

AUTHOR'S INTRODUCTION

Dear Friends,

I have written this book especially to help students who join this profession in their first year.

Its an effort to help them to know how homocopathic medicine works, detailed explaination of the medicines in their course, mnemonics to help them visualise better, questions that have been framed on those medicines till date. Also there are viva type of questions that are mostly asked during the examination.

While I was studying I faced some problems and I have made an attempt to help my friends in better understanding of the drugs. I hope that my endeavour should be of help to all my friends, teaching community and all homoeopathic physicians who are so sincerely involved in this profession.

I shall be glad to take any suggestion/criticism for the improvement of this book.

RITU KINRA
(B.H.M.S.)

ACKNOWLEDGEMENT

The book is a mere speck in the vast sands of knowledge. I am grateful to God for allowing me to lift that speck.

In my humble endeavour, there are certain people who have played a particularly important part. First I owe and give my special thanks to my father in the development of this book and ideas in it; to my mother from whom I have learnt a great deal, to my brother who long urged and finally persuaded me to write the book; to all my teachers and friends who gave me inspiration to work harder.

I wish to express my sincere thanks to Dr. P.N. Jain who saw through my keeness, encouraged and provided me the format.

Finally I express my gratitude to Mr. Subhash Saini for his help in bringing out this book in the present form.

To everything there is a season, and a time to every purpose under the heaven;

A time to be born, and a time to die;
A time to plant, and a time to pluck,
A time to suffer and a time to heal

(Ecclessistes iii, 1-8)

RITU KINRA
(BHMS)

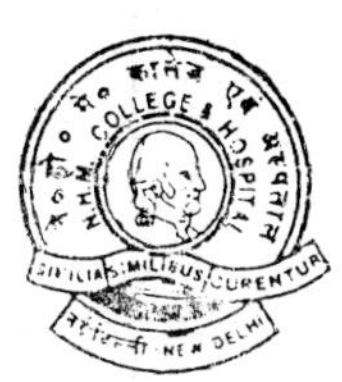

GOVERNMENT OF NATIONAL CAPITAL TERRITORY OF DELHI

Nehru Homoeopathic Medical College & Hospital
(Affiliated to University of Delhi)
B-Block. Defence Colony, New Delhi-110 024 Phone: 4621193

Ref. No. Dated : 20.07.1999

FOREWORD

I am happy to go through this book. I am extremely glad to note that the author has ventured to write the book at such a young age. The contents are comprehensive and have been presented in a very lucid and interesting manner.

The book has been especially designed and written to help the students of first year to overcome the difficulties that they undergo. It starts with an introduction on Organon of Medicine followed by explanation of drugs; sketches for an easy comprehension and viva questions to have a better grasp.

I am sure it will be appreciated by one and all.

20/7/99

Dr. V.K. Khanna
DHMS; MBS; MD.
Principal
Nehru Homoeopathic Medical College
and Hospital, New Delhi-24.

MESSAGE

It gives me great pleasure in writing these words about the first edition of this well-written book on Homoeopathy by Dr. Ritu Kinra a devoted Doctor. The book contains the essence of true knowledge of Homoeopathy. The author has tried her best to cover all the essential points which are very useful to understand the science and medicines. The book gives an easily readable and understandable form of the Homoeopathic treatment for various ailments. It is sincerely hoped that the first edition of this book would prove useful for the students, Doctors and lovers of Homoeopathy and generate further interest in this miracle science.

The greatest Healer is God. I pray to him that this first book of its kind may prove a gem in the Homoeopathic field and the earnest efforts of the author prove fruitful.

DR. R. P. SINGH

D.H.M.S. (Delhi)

Ex. S. Medical Officer Incharge
M.C.D. Homoeo Dispensary

Date : 20th July 1999.

MESSAGE

I had observed the sincerity of Dr. Ritu Kinra while her internship at Lawrence Road dispensary. At such a young age her interest for drawing symptomatic pictures for medicines and thorough observation for the reference of various medicines is highly appreciable. This book would be of immense help to students of homoeopathy and even the physicians.

May God Bless her with success in everything she plans.

DR. JYOTI GOSWAMI

Medical Officer Incharge
Delhi Admn. Dispensary

Date : 20th July 1999.

HOW DOES CURE TAKE PLACE WITH HOMOEOPATHIC MEDICINES

Founder of Homoeopathy – Dr. Samuel Hahnemann (10th Apr. 1755 – 2nd July 1843)

Principle of Homoeopathy – "LIKE CURES LIKE" or Similia Similibus Curantur.

Therapeutic Law of Nature – "A weaker dynamic affection is permenantly extinguished in the living organism by a stronger one, if the latter (whilst differing in kind) is very similar to former in its manifestations."

For example – Measles and whooping cough have very similar type of fever and cough but measles has an eruption on skin while whooping cough does not have it. Bosquillon noticed that in an epidemic where both the diseases prevailed at the same time, many children who had suffered from measles were not attacked by whooping cough.

A Homoeopathic medicine is given to a sick person

↓

It affects the deranged vital force through the medicines on santient faculty of nerves.

↓

A stronger and similar medicinal disease is produced. This stronger and similar medicinal disease extinguishes the original weaker disease (as per therapeutic law of nature).

↓

The vital force is now only affected by medicinal disease.

↓

This medicinal disease is removed in two ways.

↓	↓
Medicinal disease becomes weaker due to minute doses and fixed duration of action of medicines.	**Secondary curative action of vital force.**

The vital force is thus free from both diseased forces and medicinal forces

↓

The free vital force is thus enabled to carry on healthily the vital operations of the organism.

PERFECT HEALTH IS THUS RESTORED.

SUMMARY

Original disease attacked by similar and stronger medicinal disease.

↓

According to Therapeutic Law of Nature, weaker and orginal disease is annihilated and similar and stronger medicinal disease remains.

Stronger medicinal disease acts on vital force.

This medicinal disease disappears as medicine is discontinued or due to secondary action of vital force

HEALTH RESTORED.

What is a Miasm ?

Miasm – An inborn or acquired state peculiar to an individual which predisposes him to a group of diseases or mental condition.

Types :

1. PSORA

2. SYCOSIS

3. SYPHILIS.

PSORA – It is the most important chronic miasm which is the only fundamental cause and produces innumerable forms of disease.

Primary manifestation consists of a peculiar cutaneous eruption, sometimes only a few vesicles accompanied by intolerable voluptious tickling, itching and peculiar odour.

When the primary manifestation is suppressed, it produces various other diseased conditions affecting the functions of diverse tissues and organs coming under different nosological labels.

SYPHILIS – Chronic miasm primarily manifested outwardly by a veneral chancre.

When the allopathic physician destroys the chancre a painful substitute the 'bubo' appears which hastens onwards to suppuration.

When the secondary ailment is also destroyed – the nature develops far more secondary ailments through the out break of chronic syphilis. It *destroys* tissues, organs and bones and produces bone caries and *ulceration*.

SYCOSIS – Sycosis is a chronic miasm which is primarily manifested externally by cauli flower like growth on skin.

Sycosis is a contageous constitutional disease which results from suppression of chronic gonorrhoea. Gonorrhoea is a veneral disease characterised by inflammatory discharge of mucus from urethra. It produces *hypertrophy* of tissues and organs such as *tumors*, rheumatic or gouty conditions.

DIATHESIS – An unusual constitutional susceptibility or predisposition to a peculiar disease.

a) Rheumatic – Predisposition to rheumatism.

b) Heamorrhagic – Predisposition to heamorrhage.

c) Tubercular – Predisposition to tuberculosis.

d) Scrofulous – Predisposition to glandular swelling especially in the neck.

TEMPERAMENT – Ones customary form of natural disposition.

a) Bilious – It is marked by a general pigmentation, high blood pressure, slow pulse, well developed nipple, strong appetite, tenacity of purpose.

b) Choleric – Bilious temperament.

c) Nervous – Subject is mentally or physically alert with rapid pulse excitability but not always having fixity of purpose.

d) Leucophlegmatic – Pallor of skin with slow and shallow respiration, sluggish circulation and a tendency to inflammation of skin and lymphatics.

c) Lymphatic – Same as leucophlegmatic.

f) Sanguine – Fresh complexion; light hair and eyes; a full pulse, good digestion, quick but not lasting temper.

g) Melancholic – One marked by emaciation, irritability and a pessimistic out look to the world.

INDEX

34. COLOCYNTHIS	BITTER CUCURBITACEA
35. DROSERA ROTUNDIFOLIA	SUNDEW
36. DULCAMARA	BITTER SWEET
37. EUPHRASIA	EYEBRIGHT
38. FERRUM PHOSPHORICUM	IRON PHOSPHATE
39. GELSIMIUM NITIDUM	YELLOW JASMINE
40. GRAPHITES	BLACK LEAD
41. HELLEBORUS NIGER	SNOW ROSE
42. HEPAR SULPHURIS	SULPHATE OF LIME
43. HYOSCYAMUS NIGER	HENBANE
44. IGNATIA AMARA	SAINT IGNATIUS BEAN
45. IPECACUANHA	IPECAC
46. KALI BICHROMICUM	POTASSIUM BICHROMATE
47. KALI CARBONICUM	POTASSIUM CARBONATE
48. KALI MURIATICUM	POTASSIUM CHLORIDE
49. KALI PHOSPHORICUM	POTASSIUM PHOSPHATE
50. KALI SULPHURICUM	POTASSIUM SULPHATE
51. LACHESIS MUTA	SURUKUKU SNAKE
52. LEDUM PALUSTRE	MARSH TEA
53. LYCOPODIUM CLAVATUM	CLUB MOSS
54. MAGNESIA PHOSPHORICA	PHOSPHATE OF MAGNESIUM
55. MERCURIUS SOLUBILIS	QUICK SILVER
56. MERCURIUS CORROSIVUS	CORROSIVE SUBLIMATE
57. NATRUM MURIATICUM	COMMON SALT
58. NATRUM PHOSPHORICUM	SODIUM PHOSPHATE
59. NATRUM SULPHURICUM	SODIUM SULPHATE
60. NITRIC ACID	NITRIC ACID
61. NUX VOMICA	POISON NUT
62. PODOPHYLLUM	MAY APPLE
63. PULSATILLA NIGRICANS	ANEMONE (wild flower)
64. RHUS TOXICODENDRON	POISON OAK
65. SECALE CORNUTUM	SPURRED RYE 'fungus'
66. SILICEA	PURE SILICA
67. SULPHUR	FLOWERS OF SULPHUR – BRIMSTONE
68. SPONGIA TOSTA	ROASTED SPONGE
69. THUJA OCCIDENTALIS	ARBOR VITEA; TREE OF LIFE
70. VERATRUM ALBUM	WHITE HELLEBORE

1. ABROTANUM

Cushing Devennter Gatchell

Common Name – Southern wood.
Lady's Love (Compositae).

Miasm – Psora in background.

Constitution – Marasmus most pronounced in the *lower extremities* from malnutrition. Children are emaciated and weak. Face is wrinkled and pale with blue-ring around the eyes. Gnawing hunger and bloated abdomen. Head is so weak that the child cannot hold it up.

Temperament – *Inhuman and cruel.*

Relation with heat and cold – Chilly patient.

Diathesis – Tubercular diathesis.

KEYNOTES

1) ***Marasmus in the lower extremities.***
2) Patient has a *gnawing hunger* despite which he is weak and looses flesh (Nat mur, Tuberculinum, Iodum).
3) ***Emaciation begins in the lower limbs and spreads upwards so that face is the last affected.***
4) *Stools* – contain undigested food particles (lientria).
5) *Alternate diarrhoea and constipation* (Antim crud, Nux vom, Sulphur, Veratrum album, Antim tart, Podophyllum, Chelidonium).
6) Metastasis of *mumps* to the testicle or mammary glands (Carbo veg, Pulsatilla).
7) Rheumatic conditions with lameness and stiffness of joints. Suppressed rheumatism can lead to cardiac symptoms (Ledum, Kalmia, Aurum met). Rheumatism is caused by suddenly checked diarrhoea.
8) *Gout* is present with swelling and inflammation.
9) *Abrotanum has cured pleurisy* after Bryonia and Aconite have failed.
10) *Hydrocele* in boys. Bleeding from navel in infants.

Particulars :

1) MARASMUS
2) PLEURISY
3) RHEUMATISM AND GOUT
4) GASTRO INTESTINAL SYMPTOMS

MARASMUS

- Marasmus in the lower extremities due to malnutrition.
- Ascending emaciation.
- Patient has a gnawing hunger.
- Child is very weak and finds it difficult to hold up his head.
- Stools – contain undigested food particles. Alternate diarrhoea with constipation..
- *Sensation of creeping chills along the convolutions of the brain.*
- Hectic fever is very weakening in marasmus.
- *Skin* – flabby and hangs loose.

In pleurisy Abrotanum can be used after Bryonia and Aconite. A pressing sensation remains in the affected side.

Case – "A woman lying on the bed with dyspnoea, anxiety, cold sweat and pain in the heart was surrounded by friends to see her die."

History – She had suffered from rheumatism and that she had used crutches to get about the house for many months. She had recently been cured by a strong liniment only a few days before this attack.

Cure – Abrotanum cured her promptly.

RHEUMATISM AND GOUT

Cause – Suddenly checked diarrhoea, piles.

Character of pain – Lameness and stiffness of joints.

- Ankle and wrists are affected more.
- Suppressed rheumatism may cause cardiac symptoms.
- Other symptoms – Epistaxis, bloody urine, anxiety, trembling, when there has been a history of suppressed diarrhoea.
- Diarrhoea alternates with rheumatism.

Aggravation – Night/cold.

Amelioration – Motion.

GASTRO INTESTINAL SYMPTOMS (GIT)

- Extirpation of heamorrhoids or checking of diarrhoea may lead to gastric symptoms.
- Frequent desire for stool but passes little at a time.
- Destroys worms – ascarides.
- Contraction of limbs from cramps or following colic. Abrotanum can also be used in itching *chilblains*.

General Modalities :

Aggravation – NIGHT/COLD.

Amelioration – MOTION.

Relations :

Abrotanum is followed well by Bryonia and Baryta carb.

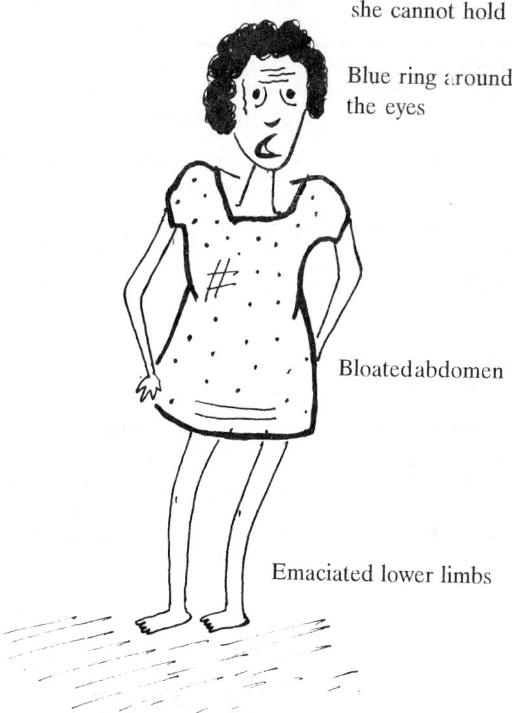
Wrinkled flabby skin.
She is so weak that
she cannot hold her head
Blue ring around
the eyes
Bloatedabdomen
Emaciated lower limbs

ABROTANUM

Important Questions ?

Q.1. Describe Abrotanum child. [1973, Supp]
Q.2. Describe Abrotanum in marasmus. [1975, 76 Supp, 79, 81, 82]
Q.3. Write down the chracteristic symptoms of Abrotanum. [1982]
Q.4. Describe Abrotanum in heart diseases. [1976]
Q.5. Compare picture of Abrotanum and Iodum child.

ABROTANUM	IODUM
• Chilly patient.	• Hot patient.
• Diathesis – Tubercular.	• Diathesis – Tubercular, Scrofulous.
• Emaciation – Ascending type. Child is very weak and is unable to hold up head.	• Emaciation – Emaciation of the whole body with hypertrophy and induration of all glands.
• Eats well but looses flesh.	• Eats well but looses flesh.
• Other symptoms – • Rheumatic conditions with heart irritation. • Patient is cruel and ill natured. • Skin is flabby and hangs loose in folds.	• Other symptoms • Desires cold things. • Acrid and corossive discharges. • Child is very restless. • Pulsations all over the body. • Constriction and squeezing in the heart.

2. ACONITUM NAPELLUS

Hahnemann

Common Name – Monkshood (Ranunculacea)

[called Monkshood because of the shape of the flowers which turn over and give the appearance of a hood.]

Aconite is one of the deadliest and most rapidly acting poison.

Aconite is the acute of Sulphur.

(Both Aconite and Sulphur are used in acute inflammatory conditions.)

Miasm – Psora in the background.

Constitution – Aconite is a short acting remedy. It is used in acute cases in Plethoric/Sanguine persons. Strong robust people who lead a sedentry life. Aconite is a remedy for rosy, chubby and plethoric persons.

Temperament – Sanguine temperament.

Relation with heat and cold – Warm blooded patient. *Aconite is a short acting remedy.*

KEYNOTES

1) Aconite is the remedy for ***cold dry weather.***
2) Aconite is indicated in ***first stage of inflammation.***
3) Everything starts ***suddenly and violently*** like a storm and passes away in the same manner.
4) Patient *predicts the time of death*. There is fear of death. Aconite patient calls for the doctor due to fear of death. He wants to call the doctor immediately. Face of Aconite expresses fear. Ailments caused due to fright (mental/physical).
5) Trio of restlessness – Aconite, Arsenic album, Rhus tox.
   Aconite patient has a lot of strength and wants to keep constantly moving.
6) *Trio of pain* – Aconite, Chamomilla, Coffea.
   Pain is intolerable in Aconite patient. Pain is associated with numbness, *pricking and tingling* in the extremities and even complete aneasthesia.
7) Easy *bleeding* of pure bright red blood attended by great fear of death.
8) *Fever* – Sthenic type of fever.
   - Dry heat of skin with full hard bounding pulse.
   - Sensation of numbness, pricking and tickling in the extremities and even complete aneasthesia.

- Later warm and profuse sweat follows with relief.
- Unquenchable thirst for large quanties of cold water.
- Plethoric or red face becomes pale on rising.

9) *Unquenchable thirst* for large quantities of cold water.

MIND

- *Fear* is the keynote. Great fear, anxiety and worry, fear of dark, fear of people, fear of death, fear of ghosts.

Fear of death is so much so that the patient predicts the date and time of death. An Aconite patient wants to call the doctor immediately.

Fear of death may be so much that cases have been found where people have actually killed themselves.

- *Tension* in the arteries, emotional, physical and mental tension.
- *Intolerance of music* – Can bear no sound. So sensitive are the ears.
- *Restlessness* – Tossing about. Aconite patient is strong and robust and hence moves frequently.
- *Pains are intolerable.* They drive him crazy.
- Patient imagines that his *body is deformed*. Lips are too thick and features are distorted.
- Imagines that he does all the thinking from the stomach.

Particulars :

1) FEVER
2) PARALYSIS
3) NEURALGIA
4) HEAD
5) EYES
6) EAR
7) RESPIRATORY SYSTEM
8) GIT
9) URINARY SYMPTOMS
10) FEMALE GENITAL SYMPTOMS
11) MEASLES.

FEVER

Aconite produces sthenic or continuous fever.

Cause – Cold dry air, exposure to cold air after overheating, fright, shock, sweating.

Onset – Sudden and violent and comes down as quickly.

Symptoms – (i) Dry heat of the skin.
(ii) Full hard and bounding pulse.
(iii) Anxiety, restlessness, fear of death.
(iv) Unquenchable thirst.

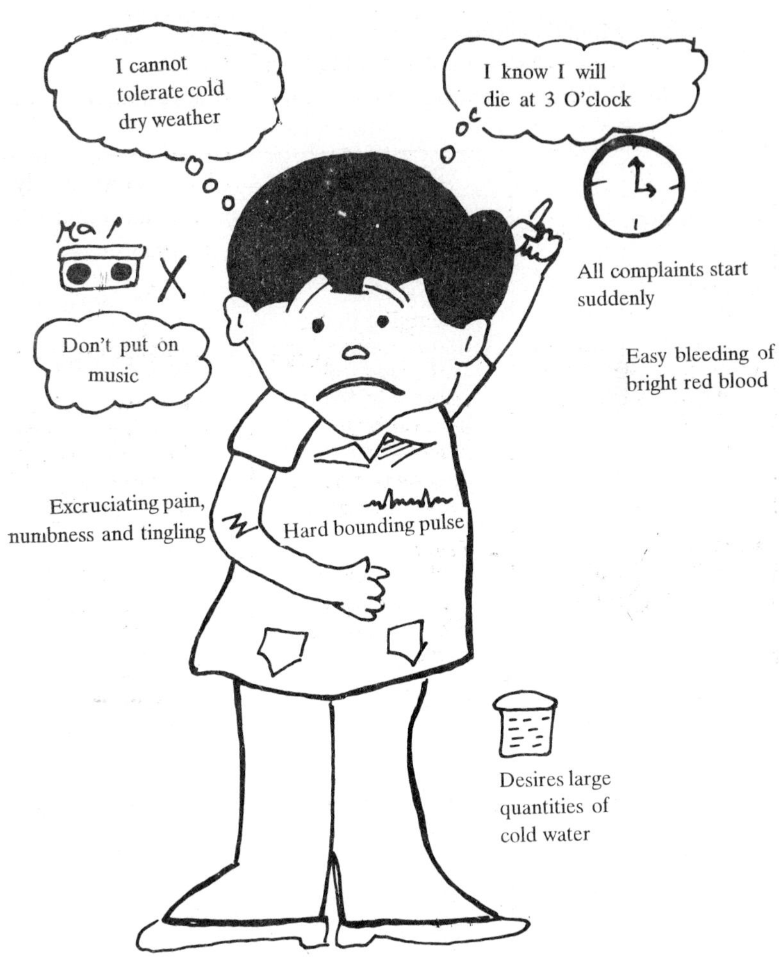

ACONITE NAPELLUS

on rising.

(vi) High rise of temperature.

These symptoms are later followed by profuse critical sweat with relief.

Mind – Mental calmness contraindicates the use of Aconite.

- Intolerance of music with fear and anxiety.

Dr. Farrington has given the following comparison in fever :

ACONITE	GELSIMIUM	APIS
• Continuous fever.	• Intermittent or remittent fever.	• Intermittent or typhoid fever.
• Chill followed by dry hot skin and full hard bounding pulse. Later warm sweat brings relief.	• Partial chill beginning in the hands running up and down the spine followed by general heat. *Sweat* is gradual and moderate but always brings relief.	• Burning heat in some places. Coolness in others. Heat is particularly felt in the abdomen. Skin is hot and dry or alternately dry and moist.
• *Pulse* Full hard and bounding pulse.	• *Pulse* Full and flowing but not hard pulse. 'Water hammer pulse.'	• Pulse Accelerated full strong wiry and frequent.
• *Blood* Not qualitatively altered.	• *Blood* Change in favour of depression.	• Blood Tends towards toxemia with a typhoid type.

• *Fever* Sthenic type. Indicated in bilious fever in initial stages. It is indicated in full blooded robust individuals who readily suffer from sudden active congestions.	• Fever Fever develops under circumstances which favour paresis of motor nerves of both voluntary and involuntary muscles. It corresponds to that stage in which blood vessels are dilated and full but lack the firmness and resistance of a fully developed sthenic inflammation.	• *Fever* Apis has a hot skin and strong pulse but the tendency of Apis is towards typhoid and effusions (Meningitis, pleuritis, rheumatism, typhoid, diptheria) There is a tendency to defibrination of blood and lastly decomposition of fluids.
• Aconite bears no relation to intermittent fever.		
• Aconite is not indicated when there is appearance of effusion.	Fever is accompained by muscular weakness, desire for absolute rest and drowsiness.	
• *Mind* • Anguish • Despair • Restlessness. Tossing about during fever. Fears that he will die. Throws off the clothes.	• Mind Irritable and sensitive children sometimes wakeful, nervous, even threatened with convulsions. Eyelids are heavy and looks as if intoxicated. Wants to remain perfectly quiet.	• *Mind* • Fidgety, restless. • Wants to sleep but he is so nervous that he cannot sleep. • Low muttering delirium. • Chill begins in knees or abdomen at 3 P.M. • Heat with dry skin – occasional transient spells of sweating.

- Belladonna follows Aconite well but is given where there is presence of brain symptoms.

A – Aconite causes Turmoil in Circulation.

B – Belladonna causes Turmoil in Brain.

C – Chamomilla causes Turmoil in Temperament.

- When sthenic fever fails to yield to Aconite, its chronic Sulphur may be given.

FERRUM PHOS	ACONITE
• 1) IInd stage of inflammation producing dilatation of blood vessels.	• 1) Ist stage of inflammation or congestive stage.
• 2) Pulse – Full and soft. Indicated in congestion of any part of the body when the discharges are blood streaked (dysentry, heamoptysis).	• 2) Pulse – Full, hard and throbbing.

PARALYSIS

- Aconite produces motor paralysis accompanied by coldness, numbess, tingling in affected parts.
- Icy coldness of extremities.

NEURALGIA

Cause – Exposure to dry cold winds.

Symptoms – Violent congestion of the affected part which is usually the face. Face is red and swollen. Pains drive the patient to despair; there is neuralgia in the affected part. Tingling in the affected part.

SPIGELIA	COLCHICUM
• Left sided prosopalgia. Burning and sticking pains. Intense excitement with intolerance of pains.	• Left sided prosopalgia. Paralytic weakness of muscles Lacks the severity of Spigelia.

HEADACHE

Cause – Cold dry wind, fright, cooling suddenly when warm.

Location – Frontal region.

Symptoms – Fullness and heaviness in the head. Burning headache as if brain were agitated by boiling water; throbbing in the head. Vertigo and nausea from sitting and rising.

Aggravation – Night, evening, warm room.

Amelioration – Open air.

EYES

Eyes take on sudden inflammation.

Cause – Dry cold winds.

Appearance of eye – Eyes take on great swelling without any discharge or with watery mucus. In inflammation with thick mucus Aconite should never be prescribed.

EARACHE

Cause – Dry cold winds.

Pain – Intense throbbing pain in ear. Music is intolerable.

RESPIRATORY SYSTEM

Coryza :

Cause – Exposure to cold air, checked sweat.

Symptoms – Coryza associated with throbbing headache. Nasal mucous membrane may be dry and hot or may be fluent and hot with frequent sneezing. Muscles all over the body feel sore so that sneezing forces him to support his chest.

Concomitant – Intense restlessness.

Modalities – Amelioration – Open air.

Cough

Cause – Exposure to cold air, checked sweat.

Character of cough – Sudden and violent. It may be croupy. Cough is dry, hoarse, suffocating, loud and rough.

Aggravation – Evening, night.

Amelioration – Open air.

Heart :

- Congestion of the heart with syncope.
- Palpitation of the heart is worse on walking.
- Attacks of intense pain start from the heart down the left arm and are associated with numbness and tingling of the fingers.
- Hypertrophy associated with numbness and tingling of fingers.

Pneumonia

Stage – Ist stage of pneumonia.

Symptoms – • Congestion of lungs.

- Engorgement of the lungs.
- Cough – Hard, dry and painful.
- Expectoration – Serous watery and a little blood streaked. (never thick and blood streaked.)

Mind – Patient is full of restlessness, anxiety and fear.

(Bryonia takes the place of Aconite when hepatisation has commenced.)

Cough – Hard and painful and is associated with thicker expectoration.

Aggravation – Motion.

Amelioration – Keeping still, pressure.

Pleurisy :

Stage – Early stages.

Cause – Checked perspiration, cold dry air.

Sensation – Sharp stitches on either side of the chest with chill followed by febrile action.

Croup :

ACONITE	SPONGIA
• Croup caused due to cold.	• Less inflammation.
• Violent croup with inflammation of larynx.	• Inflammation grows with spasms
• Intense febrile excitement.	
• Little watery discharge.	• Discharge is entirely dry.

Heamoptysis :

ACONITE	MILLEFOLIUM	LEDUM PAL	CACTUS G.
• Bright red blood.	• Profuse flow of bright red blood.	• Heamoptysis of drunkards or persons of rheumatic origin.	• Heamoptysis with strong throbbing of heart.
• Anxiety, restlessness and fever.	• No fever		• Constriction or band around the chest.

GASTRO INTESTINAL SYSTEM

Cause – Complaints are caused by taking cold, exposure to very hot summer.

Symptoms – Gastric catarrah.

- Acute sharp inflammation of stomach.
- Retching, vomiting of bile, vomiting of food.
- Burning and tearing pains.
- Anxiety and restlessness.

Mind – Anxiety, restlessness, fearful.

Dysentry :

Cause – Autumn season when warm days are followed by cold nights.

Symptoms – Tenesmus + pure bright red blood + mucus is passed along with stools.

Mind – Restlessness, anxiety, anguish.

Constitution – Rosy chubby infants with summer troubles.

GENITO URINARY SYMPTOMS

Cause – Fear, cold dry winds.

Symptoms – Scanty and suppressed urine. Inflammation of bladder with cutting and tearing pains. Orchitis may also be caused.

Character of urine – Hot, dry, clear or bloody.

FEMALE GENITAL ORGANS

Ovaries and uterus become inflamed due to fright.

Menses – Suppression of menses caused due to fright.

Dysmenorrhoea is caused by thickening of peritoneum over the ovaries and suppression of menses.

Pregnancy – Administered in mental symptoms like fear of death which may cause abortion.

Parturition – After a tedious parturition there are violent after pains, fever,uterine heamorrhages with bright red blood accompanied with fear of death.

Lochia :

Symptoms – Suppressed lochia, high fever, violent thirst, lax mammae, oversensitiveness.

Cause – Violent emotions.

Puerperal fever may be caused due to exposure to cold air or water after confinement.

MEASLES

Stage – Early stage.

Symptoms – High fever, red conjunctiva, dry barking cough, restlessness and itching, burning of skin.

General Modalities :

Aggravation – EVENING AND NIGHT
(Pains are insupportable)
WARM ROOM
RISING FROM BED
LYING ON AFFECTED SIDE.

Amelioration – OPEN AIR.

Relations :

Complementry to – Coffee: fever, sleeplessness, intolerance of pain.

Arnica – Traumatism.

Sulphur – All cases.

Antidotes – Bell, Cham, Coffea, Nux vom, Sepia, Spongia, Sulph.

Antidoted by – Acetic acid, Alcohol.

Important Questions ?

Q.1. Write down indications of Aconite in following :

1) Mental symptoms [DMSInter 1972, 76]
2) Fever [1975, 76, 77, 95, 96]
3) Acute tonsillitis [1975, 76, 1976 (Supp)]
4) Cough and Cold [1976, 76 (Supp)]
5) Cardiac symptoms [1977]
6) Restlessness [1973 Supp, 75, 76, DMS. Inter 1981, DMS Final 1976]
7) Diarrhoea, Bacillary dysentry [DSM 1976, (Final 1979)]
8) Eye symptoms [1977]
9) Convulsions
10) Delirium [1991 Final]
11) Urinary Symptoms [1988 Final]
12) Nerve injury [1996]

Q.2. Compare restlessness of Aconite, Arsenic album, Rhus tox.

ACONITE	ARSENIC ALBUM	RHUS TOX.
• Patient is strong and robust.	• Mental restlessness accompanied with great exhaustion and prostration.	• Patient is very restless on account of great pain, rigidity and stiffness.
• Mental and physical restlessness is marked.	• Patient tries to move himself in the bed.	• Pain, rigidity and stiffness are *ameliorated* by constant motion. Continued motion exhausts the Rhus patient.

• Due to increased physical strength the Aconite patient moves frequently.	• Restlessness becomes so marked that he is able to move only his limbs until at last hc becomes so weak that he is not able to move and lies in perfect quietness due to extreme prostration.	
• There is great fear and anxiety.		• *Aggravation* – Night, cold damp weather, perspiration.
• He cannot bear pains or fever without constantly tossing about in the bed.	• Patient is full of suicidal tendency.	• *Amelioration* – Motion, warm application.

3. AESCULUS HIPPOCASTANUM

Cooly

Common Name – Horse chestnut (Sapindacea).
[Used in chest complaints of horses.]

Constitution – Used for persons with heamorrhoidal tendency and who suffer with gastric, bilious and catarrhal troubles. Plethoric people with *vascular fullness* which affects the extremities and the whole body.

Temperament – Irritable and confused patient.

Relation with heat and cold – Superficial pains are ameliorated by heat. Deeper pains are ameliorated by cold.

KEYNOTES

1) ***Fullness*** in various parts caused by general ***venous stasis.***
2) *Despondent*, gloomy, very irritable, looses temper easily and gains control slowly.
3) *Mucous membranes of mouth, throat, rectum are swollen, burn, feel raw and dry.*
4) Frequent inclination to *swallow* with burning, pricking, stinging and dry constricted fauces.
5) Rectum – feels hot and dry. Sensation – as if *full of sticks*.
6) ***Heamorrhoids—Blind, painful, burning, purplish.***
7) *Constipation* – Hard dry stools, difficult to pass with dryness and heat in rectum.
8) ***Severe lumbo-sacral backache with lameness and heaviness.***
9) *Prolapse of uterus* and *acrid, dark leucorrhoea* with lumbo sacral backache, great fatigue from walking.
10) *Paralytic feeling in limbs.*

Particulars :

1) MIND
2) HEAD
3) EYES
4) CORYZA
5) THROAT
6) VENOUS CONGESTION
7) GIT
8) BACKACHE
9) FEMALE SYMPTOMS
10) RHEUMATISM

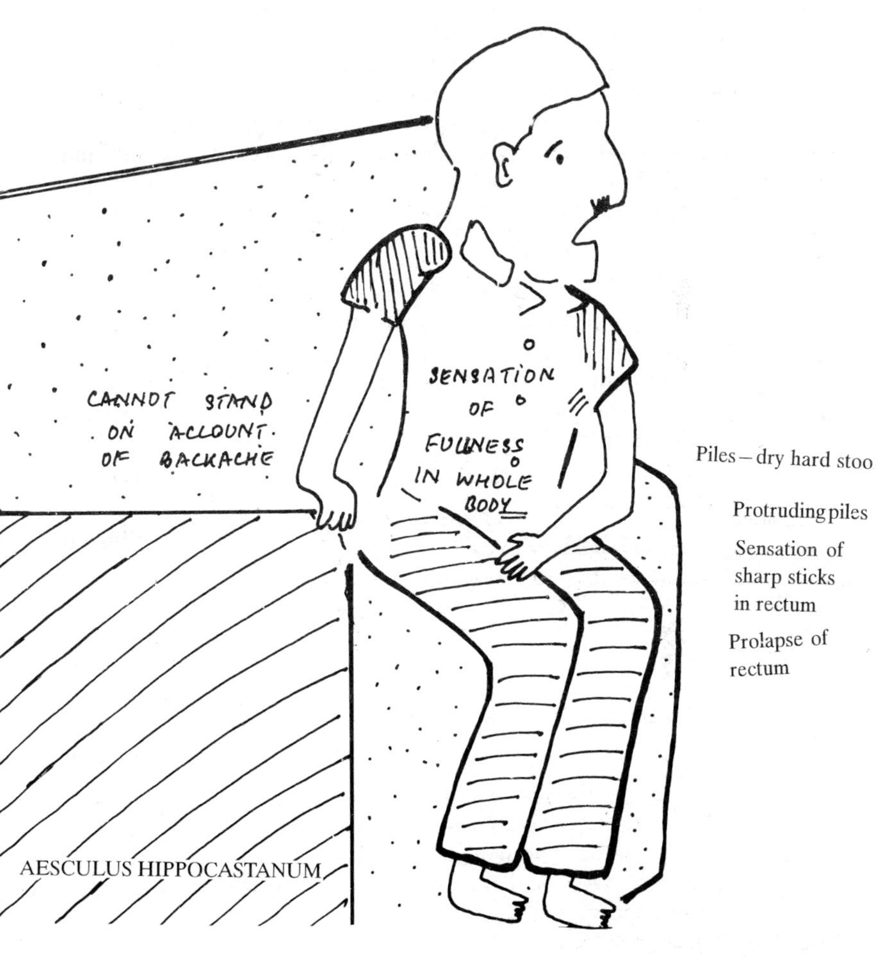
CANNOT STAND ON ACCOUNT OF BACKACHE
SENSATION OF FULLNESS IN WHOLE BODY
Piles – dry hard stoo
Protruding piles
Sensation of sharp sticks in rectum
Prolapse of rectum
AESCULUS HIPPOCASTANUM

MIND

- Condition of Aesculus is worse during sleep hence symptoms are observed on waking.
- Patient wakes up with confusion of mind, looks all around the room in confusion and is bewildered.
- Sad, irritable, loss of memory and aversion to work.
- Aggravation of mental symptoms is caused when there is general venous stasis. Venous stasis is aggravated by sleep, lying down. Ameliorated by – bodily exertion.
- Patient resents something done against his wish and he becomes irritated. Patient is never irritable if his wishes are complied to.
- Confusion of mind and vertigo.

HEADACHE

Location – Back of the head. Dull frontal headache.

Sensation – As if head would be crushed.

- Violent aching pains with *fullness of brain.*
- Pressure in the forehead with nausea followed by stitches in the right hypochondrium.
- Neuralgic stitches from right to left in forehead followed by flying pains in epigastrium.

EYES

- Eyes have 'heamorrhoids' i.e. enlarged blood vessels.
- Redness, burning, lachrymation with enlarged blood vessels.
- Fullness in the eyes.

CORYZA

- Thin watery coryza with sensation of rawness and dryness.
- Patient is sensitive to inhaled cold air.

THROAT

- Rawness and dryness in acute and chronic forms of pharyngitis. Dryness of posterior nares and throat with sneezing followed by acute coryza. Stinging and burning in the posterior nares and throat. Dark and congested fauces with feeling of fullness. Catarrhal laryngitis.

VENOUS CONGESTION

- Engorged and full veins which may be bursting.
- Tendency to produce varicose veins, ulceration and round about these is present duskiness.
- Varicose veins produce a purplish areola around them.
- Tendency to develop an inflammatory state which is sluggish and passive.

GIT

- Engorged veins left in the throat after sore throat disappears.
- Varicose veins in the eyes after eye troubles have disappeared.

Stomach :

- Congestion and ulceration of stomach.
- Constant distress and burning in the stomach.
- As soon as the patient has swallowed food or a little later it becomes sour and he eructates it till the stomach becomes empty of its contents. (Phos, Ferrum, Arsenicum alb)

Liver :

- Congestion of liver accompanied with piles.
- Aching and pinching pains in the right hypochondrium.

  Aggravation – Walking.

  Amelioraton – Rest.

Rectum :

- Digestion is slow, bowels are constipated and there is protrusion of the rectum when at stool.
- Heamorrhoids with fullness in right hypochondrium.
- Rectal complaints caused after eating. Eating causes – distress, sticking, burning.
- Rectum feels full of sticks.
- Blind heamorrhoids. Heamorrhoidal veins are all distended and ulcerate.
- Stools become jammed into the rectum against the distended heamorrhoidal veins and the ulceration takes place with bleeding and great suffering.
- **Constipation** – dry, hard, knotty stools which are white.

Rectal complaints :

AESCULUS H	NITRIC ACID
• Full of sticks.	• Splinter pricking sharply during passage of stools.
• Pains come on hours after stool.	• Endures agonies during and after stool for hours.
• Large purple protruding piles with sawing knife pain that does not permit standing, sitting, lying. Person can only kneel down.	• Fissures and bleeding piles. Tendency to ulceration with acrid and offensive discharge. General weakness and debility.

AESC. H	COLLINSONIA
• Sense of fullness in the rectum. Rectum feels full of sticks.	• Sense of weight and constriction in the rectum.
• Blind piles. Pain soreness and aching in the back.	• Bleeding piles.
• May or may not be accompanied by constipation.	• Greatly constipated with colic. (Piles + Colic + Constipation – 3 Keynotes.)

BACKACHE

Pain in the back attend the rectal symptoms.

Location – Pain low down in the back through the sacrum and the hips.

Sensation :

- Patients suffering from heamorrhoids generally complain of backache, pain in the back of the neck, basilar headaches.
- Walking aggravates the complaints and pain from the sacrum goes to the hips.
- Dull backache makes walking impossible.
- Backache aggravated on attempting to rise or walk after sitting.
- Patient has to make painful efforts before he succeeds in walking.

Case :

"A nurse had attended a cold humid funeral with the result that she did not know how she was to go on duty because of the awful pain in the lower part of the back. A pain that would not let her stoop or rise from stooping."

Aesc. H cured her.

FEMALE SYMPTOMS

- Dragging pains in the pelvis with copious leucorrhoea and pressing pains in the hips when walking.
- Uterus feels engorged.
- Lower part of the abdomen feels full before and during menses.
- Uterine soreness with throbbing in the hypogastrium.
- Leucorrhoea with discharge – dark yellow thick and sticky leucorrhoea.

- Leucorrhoea with lameness in the back across the sacroiliac articulation. Back gives out when walking.

RHEUMATISM

Tyler—"People carry horse chest nut in their clothing to cure rheumatism."

- Gouty rheumatic affections in elbows of the hands/forearm.
- Flying type of pains.

General Modalities :

Aggravation – STOOPING
INHALING COLD AIR
WALKING
MOVEMENT OF BOWELS.

Amelioration – REST.

- Venous stasis is ameliorated by motion.
- Superficial stinging pains are ameliorated by heat.
- Deeper affections are ameliorated by cold.

Relations :

- Useful after Nux vom and Sulphur have improved but failed to cure piles.
- After Collinsonia has improved piles Aesculus cures.

Antidotes – Nux vomica.

Important Questions ?

Q.1. Give indications of Aesculus in :
1) Rectal Symptoms [1992 Final]
2) Heamorrhoids [1986 Final]

Q.2. Give difference between :
Aesculus/Nitric Acid in Rectal symptoms. [1988 Final]
Aesculus/Collinsonia in Rectal symptoms. [1989 Final]

4. AETHUSA CYNAPIUM

Nenning

Common Name – Fools Parsley (Umbelliferea).
Miasm – Touches all 3 Miasms – Psora, Sycosis, Syphilis in acute state.
Constitution – *Sunken condition.*

- The child appears dying with a pale hippocratic face.
- Whitish blue pallor around the lips.
- Eyes are sunken and there is a sunken condition around the nose.
- *Well marked linea nasalis.*
- Child is so weak that he cannot hold up his head.

Temperament – Idiocy may alternate with furor and irritability

Relation with heat and cold – Hot patient.

KEYNOTES

1) Complaints are caused due to *dentition and hot summer weather.*
2) ***Child cannot bear milk.*** (Magnesia carb) Child takes milk and almost before it has time to coagulate,the milk comes up partly in curds and partly in liquid. Accompanying the vomiting there is a thin yellowish, greenish stool.
3) ***Milk is vomited in large curds as soon as taken.***
4) Complete *absence of thirst* (Apis/Pulsatilla).
5) Regurgitation of food an hour or so after eating. Copious greenish vomiting.
6) Child is too *weak* to stand and even when held up, their heads droop down. (Abrotanum)
7) Great *prostration and sleepiness* after vomiting, stool or spasm. Patient has an anxious, pain stricken and drawn look.
8) ***Well marked linea nasalis.***
9) *Idiotic* child with incapacity to think and fix attention. Patient is very confused.
10) *Herpetic eruptions* on the end of the nose.
11) *Epileptic spasms* with a red face, clenched thumbs, eyes turned downwards, pupils fixed and dilated, foam at the corners of mouth, locked jaws.

Pulse – Small, hard and quick.

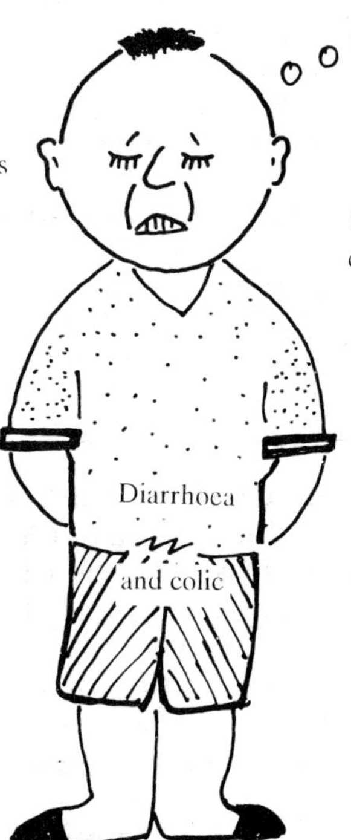
I can't take milk. Whenever I drink milk it gives me diarrhoea and vomiting.
Greatprostration sleepiness, eyes turneddownwards
Linea nasalis
Herpes on nose
Dentition causes complaints
Vomiting of curdled milk, white frothy matter
regurgitation of food an hour after eating
Diarrhoea
and colic

AETHUSA CYNAPIUM

Particulars :

1) MIND
2) CHILD
3) STOMACH
4) CONVULSIONS/EPILEPSY.

MIND

- Restless, anxious and crying child.
- Person sees rats, cats, dogs etc running around.
- Inability to think or fix attention.
- Dr. Clarke recommends it highly in patients suffering from want of power and concentration. "Aethusa helped a young undergraduate in bringing back his long lost power of concentration."
- Aethusa is a very good drug for examination funk (fear of exams).
- Child is very sleepy and prostrated.
- Child has an anxious and pain stricken drawn look.

CHILD

Cause of complaints – Dentition, hot summer weather, bad hygiene, brain touble in hot weather.

- Child cannot bear *milk* in any form. There is gastric irritation frequently met with in children during dentition.
- As soon as the person drinks milk it is *vomited* out in large quantities.
- If the milk is kept down for a little while it is vomited out in large *greenish curds*.
- Great *prostration and sleepiness* after vomiting.
- Child is too *weak* to stand and even when held up, his head droops down.
- After vomiting the child goes to sleep due to prostration and on waking there is violent hunger to eat or drink milk and to vomit again.
- Vomiting is often complicated with *diarrhoea* which is light yellow, bilious in colour. *Stools* are preceded with colic tenesmus, convulsions and followed by exhaustion, drowsiness.
- If not checked on time grave complications like – cholera infantum, hydrocephalus may take palce.

Concomitants :

1) Complete absence of thirst.
2) Great weakness and prostration.
3) Idiocy and incapacity to think.
4) Well marked linea nasalis.
5) Herpetic eruptions on the end of nose.

STOMACH

- Aethusa suits improperly fed babies.
- Digestion becomes absolutely ceased from brain troubles and excitement.
- Dyspepsia caused due to constant feeding in nibblers or hungry fellows. A time comes when the stomach ceases to act.
- There is vomiting, exhaustion, sweat and long sleep.
- Gastric catarrah – cannot tolerate milk in any form.

CONVULSION/EPILEPSY

[Sometimes brain troubles do not affect the stomach but the child goes into convulsions.]

- Brain troubles caused due to hot summer weather. Cold and clammy hands with deathly countenance, sweat, exhaustion and sleep.
- Convulsions with great weakness, prostration and sleepiness.
- Child doses off after vomiting and after stool with convulsion.
- Idiocy in children with confusion.
- Convulsions with a red face, clenched thumbs, eyes turned downwards, pupils fixed and dilated, foam at the mouth, locked jaw, pulse – small, hard and quick.
- Well marked linea nasalis.

General Modalities :

Aggravation – EATING
DRINKING
VOMITING
SUMMER WEATHER
DENTITION, 3-4 A.M.

Amelioration – OPEN AIR
COVERING
TIGHT BANDAGE ON HEAD

Relations :

Complementry to – Calcarea carbonicun.

Antidoted by – Vegetable Acids.

Resembles – Antim crudum, Natrum mur, Silicea, Sulphur.

Important Questions ?

Q.1. Give symptoms of Aethusa in :

a) Vomiting [1978-S, 72, 76, 77, 93]
b) GIT [1974, 81, 82]
c) Epilepsy [1975, 76, 81, 86]
d) Child [1995-S]

e) Compare child of Aethusa/Calcarea carb/Cina/Chamomilla [1995-S]

AETHUSA	CALCAREA CARB.
• Sunken condition hippocratic face with a well marked linea nasalis.	• With chalky complexion goes – Fatness without fitness. – Sweating without heat. – Bones without strength – Tissues of plus quantity and minus quality. – Mere flabby, bulky with weakness and weariness.
• Intolerance of milk. Vomiting of large curds as soon as taken in with yellowish greens stools. • Complete absence of thirst. • Great weakness and prostration.	• Great sensitiveness to take cold.
• **Mind** – Idiotic and confused.	• **Mind** – Desire for eggs, great apprehension, obstinate and self willed.
• Epileptic spasms.	• Sour sweat especially on the back of the head. Sour discharges 'sour smelling child'.
• Herpetic eruptions around the nose.	• Large head with open fontanelles. • Weak bones, disposed to fracture, delayed dentition.

CINA 'touchiness'	CHAMOMILLA 'cannot bear it'
• Dark rings around the eyes with emaciation.	• One cheek red hot and the other pale cold.
• Worm troubles – Nocturnal enuresis. – Grinds teeth.Boring nose. – Diarrhoea of white undigested food particles. – Canine hunger.	• Complaints caused due to dentition.

• **Desire** – Sweets, undigested food particles.	• Diarrhoea – Greenish copious with rotten egg smell. Stools are hot and offensive. • Wants to be carried.
• **Mind** – Irritable child. Does not want to be touched.	• **Mind** – Irritable child, refuses things when offered. Anger may even lead to convulsions.
• Yawning brings complaints.	• Numbness.
• Canine hunger with clean tongue.	• Oversensitive child.
• Turbid urine when passed but turns milky on standing.	
• Child sleeps in knee elbow position.	
Aggravation – Sweets, undigestible things, overeating.	**Aggravation** – Open air, heat, anger.
Amelioration – Lying on abdomen, boring nose in pillow.	**Amelioration** – Carrying, fasting, warm wet weather.

5. ALLIUM CEPA

Hering

Common Name – Raw Onion.

Miasm – Psora is in the background.

Constitution – Allium cepa is used for catarrhal inflammation of mucous membrane. It is used for acute stage of disease.

Relation with heat and cold – Hot patient.

KEYNOTES

1) Complaints are caused due to *warm room and evening.*

2) Acute catarrhal *inflammation* of mucous membranes with increased secretion. Complaints start from *left and go to right.*

3) ***Coryza : Profuse, watery and acrid.***

Lachrymation : Bland and excessive.

4) *Catarrhal dull headache with coryza.*

Aggravation – Evening, warm room

Amelioration – Open air.

5) Neuralgic *long thread like pains* in face, head, neck, chest.

6) In coryza inflammation may spread to the ear, throat and larynx.

Earache – Violent earache. Pain goes from the throat towards the eustachian tube. Long thread like pains, deep from the forehead.

Larynx – Catarrhal laryngitis. Cough compels the patient to grasp the larynx. It seems as if it would *tear and split* the larynx.

7) ***Colic*** :Cause – Cold, getting feet wet, salads, cucumbers, heamorrhoids. Aggravation – Sitting.

Amelioration – Moving about, doubling up

8) ***Traumatic chronic neuritis*** – Neuralgia of stump after amputation with burning and stinging pains.

9) *Sore and raw* spots on feet, especially heel, from friction. Efficatious when *feet* are *rubbed sore*.

10) Strong craving for raw onions

Particulars :

1) HEADACHE

2) EYES

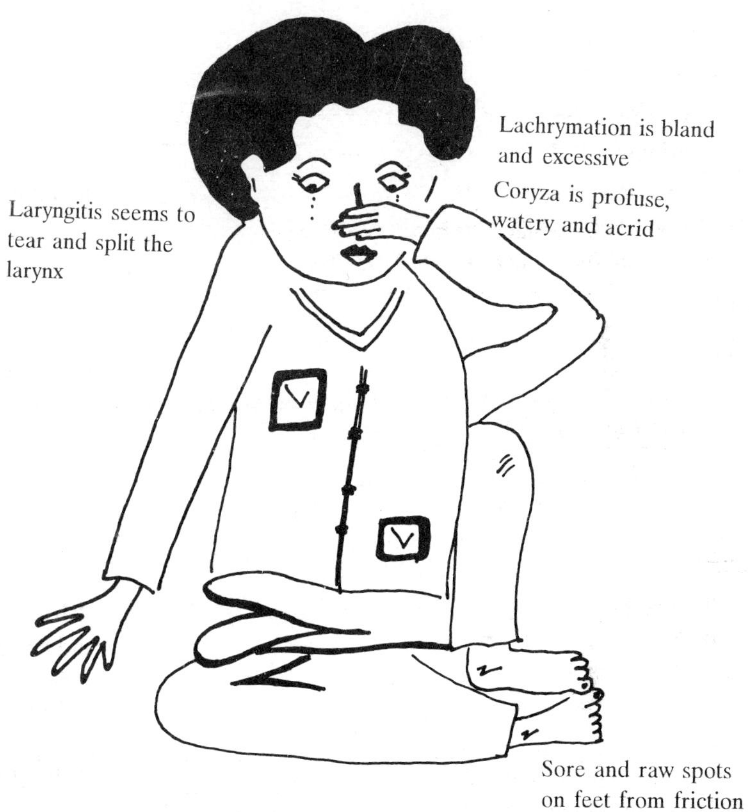
Lachrymation is bland
and excessive
Coryza is profuse,
watery and acrid
Laryngitis seems to
tear and split the
larynx
Sore and raw spots
on feet from friction

ALLIUM CEPA

3) NOSE

4) EARACHE

5) LARYNGITIS

6) WHOOPING COUGH

7) COLIC

8) NEURITIS

9) PHLEBITIS

HEAD

- Dull and congestive headache associated with coryza.
- Headache may become bursting and throbbing later with photophobia. Aggravation – Evening.
  Amelioration – Warm Room.

EYES

- *Bland, excessive* discharge from the eyes. Tears do not excoriate as they flow down over the cheek.
- Eyes burn and smart as from smoke in the eyes.
- Eyes are watery, suffused; capillaries injected; excessive lachrymation. Cause of lachrymation – Evening, warm room

NOSE

a) Coryza

b) Nasal polyps.

Coryza **:**

- Sneezing comes up with increasing frequency.
- *Acrid and excoriating* discharge drips from the nose constantly.
- Discharge burns like fire and excoriates the upper lip and wings of the nose till there is redness and rawness.
- Patient has a sensation of *fullness* in the nose with throbbing and burning. There may also be nose bleed.
- *Thread like pain* may extend through the jaws, in face and extending into the head.
- Acrid discharge and stuffing of nose takes place first in the left nose and then goes to the right nose.
- *Hay Fever* is caused in august every year with morning coryza, violent sneezing. Person is very sensitive to odour of flowers and skin of peaches.

Aggravation – Evening, indoors, warm room.

Amelioration – Open air.

Allium Cepa **(Raw Onion)**	*Euphrasia* **(Eye Bright)**
• Nasal discharge – (Coryza) – Acrid and Excoriating • Lachrymation – Bland	• Nasal discharge – (Coryza) bland • Lachrymation – Acrid and excoriating

Nasal Polyps – Allium cepa is used for treating nasal polyps. [Mar V., Sang nit, Psorinum]

EARACHE

- In coryza inflammation may spread to the ear causing violent earache.
- Jerking pain from the throat radiates towards the eustachian tube.
- Violent earache even to discharge of pus from the ear.
- Thread like pain radiating towards the ear from the forehead.

[*Pulsatilla* – Earache in sensitive children who cry pitifully.

Chamomilla – Snappish children with earache. Children who throw away something they ask for.]

LARYNGITIS

- Hoarse harsh ringing spasmodic cough excited by constant tickling in the larynx.
- Cough produces a raw *splitting pain* in the larynx.
- Pain is so acute and severe that it compels the patient to crouch from suffering and to make every *effort to suppress cough*.
- Patient feels as if cough would *tear and split* the larynx. Cough compels the patient to *grasp the larynx*.
- Cold may extend down the bronchial tubes with much coughing and rattling of mucus.

Aggravation – Evening, warm room.

Amelioration – Open air, cold room.

WHOOPING COUGH

[Allium Cepa is excellent for whooping cough].

Child shudders and dreads the cough because of teasing pain in the larynx.

Concomitants – Indigestion, vomiting, flatulence – offensive flatus, child doubles up with colic.

COLIC

[Onion is a flatulent vegetable]

Cause of colic – Cold, getting feet wet, overeating – cucumbers, salads (Colic of children)

Symptoms :

- Cutting, rending, teasing pains drawing the child double.
- Colicky pains begin in the abdomen and spread over whole abdomen.
- Indigestion, vomiting, offensive flatus and the child doubles up with colic.

  Aggravation – Sitting

  Amelioration – Motion.

NEURITIS

- Traumatic chronic neuritis – neuralgia of the stump after amputation.
- Sore and raw spots on the feet, especially heel from friction. "Efficatious when feet are rubbed and sore."

PHLEBITIS

Puerperal phlebitis after forceps delivery.

Panaritia – Red streaks up the arms. Pains (Whitlow) drive the child to despair when he is in bed.

General Modalities :

Aggravation – EVENING
WARM ROOM
Amelioration – COLD ROOM
OPEN AIR

Relations :

Complementry to – Phosphorus, Pulsatilla, Sarsaparilla, Thuja
Remedies that follow well – Calcarea carb, Silicea

Inimicals – Aloes S, Allium sativum

Antidotes – Arnica, Chamomilla, Nux, Thuja, Veratrum album.

Important Questions ?

Q.1. Write symptoms of Allium cepa in
Coryza [1972-s, 86-s, 95]
Neuralgia [1976, 82]

Q. 2. Give difference between Allium cepa and Euphrasia in Coryza.

6. ALOE SOCOTRINA

Helbio

Common Name – Socotrina Aloes (Liliacea)

Miasm – Psora in the backround

Constitution – Adapted to indolent "weary" persons averse to either mental or physical labour. Extreme prostration with perspiration.

Temperament – Bilious temperament.

Relation with heat and cold – *Hot* patient

KEYNOTES

1) Complaints are *aggravated* by *heat and relieved* by *cold application*.
2) ***Itching and burning of anus***. Itching appears every year as winter approaches.
3) Production of mucus in *jelly like lumps* from throat or rectum. (Kali bich)
4) Weakness and loss of power of sphincter ani causes *'insecurity of rectum'*. There is *want of confidence in sphincter ani*.
5) Constipation precedes diarrhoea. Solid, marble like stool and masses of jelly like mucus pass involuntarily.
6) ***Fullness*** in the region of liver, abdomen, rectum, intestines.
7) Morning diarrhoea – Patient has to hurry to the closet immediately after eating or drinking. *Colic* before and during stool followed by weakness.
8) *Offensive, burning and copious flatus is passed with small amount of stool.*
9) **Heamorrhoids** – *bleeding, blue* like a bunch of grapes (Muriatic acid). *Sore, bleeding and tender* heamorrhoids relieved by application of cold water.

Particulars :

1) HEAD
2) MENTALS
3) GIT
4) FEMALE

HEADACHE

Headache is associated with bowel disturbance.

Location – Headache across the forehead.

Sensation –

Head feels hot and the patient wants something cool upon it.

- Skin is hot and dry and the patient wants to be uncovered at night in bed.
- Heaviness in eyes with nausea.

Concomitants – Headache alternates with lumbago

Aggravation – Heat

Amelioration – Cold application

MENTALS

- Disinclined to move
- Life seems to be a burden – Colicky flatulent pains in the abdomen drive the patient to despair. Hates people, repels every one.

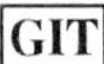

GIT

Liver :

- There is portal congestion
- Pain and burning in right hypochondrium
- Fullness, distension with stitching pains in the liver region
- Dry and hot skin without fever

Constipation :

- Constipation precedes diarrhoea
- Great *fullness* with urging to go to stool. Only copious hot flatus passes giving relief but urging soon returns.
- Patient feels several times in a day that they must go for stool but only a little *wind passes*.
- *Hard lumps* mingled with *jelly like mucus*.
- These *marble* like nodules may escape unconciously.
- There is entire *loss of sensation* in the anus, aneasthesia and no feeling during passage of stool.

Diarrhoea :

Cause – Eating and drinking, after each meal.

Time – Early morning diarrhoea. Great urging for stool and even before he reaches the bathroom he spoils his clothes.

Sensation – Weakness and loss of sensation in the sphincter ani – this causes an insecurity of rectum.

- Offensive burning and copious *flatus*. Patient is afraid to pass flatus for the fear that stool would escape.
- Sensation as if rectum is *full of feacal* matter which would fall out if not for extreme caution.

Character of Stool – Yellow offensive excoriating which burns like fire with sore anus.

Before Stool – Colicky pains before stool. Pains present in lower portion of abdomen.

- Rumbling, violent, sudden urging to stool.
- Heaviness in rectum.

During Stool – Colicky pains

- Stool gurgles out with noisy rumbling of flatus.
- Passage of jelly like mucus with stools.
- Patient feels hungry during diarrhoea.

After Stool – Colicky pains are relieved

- *Profuse sweating and extreme weakness*. Weakness is sometimes so great that the patient is compelled to go to the bed with diarrhoea.

"Little ones soon after they begin to walk will drop yellow drops of mucus and feaces. They cannot hold the stool and it passes out involuntarily. Every mouthful of food or drink hurries the child to stool.

In constipation – hard round marble like stools and mucus may be passed. "Aloes is the cure thus".

DIARRHOEA :

ALOES S	PODOPHYLLUM
• Worse – Hot weather	• Worse – Hot weather dentition
• Morning diarrhoea	• Morning diarrhoea
• Yellow feaces, transparent jelly like mucus which drops out of the rectum unnoticed. Want of confidence in sphincter ani. Passage may be involuntary when expelling flatus or passing urine.	• Painless, profuse, putrid, Polychromatic(Multicoloured), prolapse ani with stool which gushes out Stool – Chalk like; jelly like undigested with yellow meal like sediment
• Fullness in the rectum	• Weakness and sinking in rectum

Dysentry :

- Jelly like mucus + yellowish offensive feaces + blood

Before Stool – Rumbling and gurgling in rectum with copious flatus and colicky pains.

During Stool – Colicky pains, involuntary stools, passage of much *flatus*

After stools – Weakness and prostration

Heamorrhoids :

- Piles – *Bleeding, blue bunch of grapes.*
- Itching and smarting (burning) in the anus prevents sleep

- Patient has to constantly bore his finger into the anus to relieve *itching*.
- Heamorrhoids are bleeding, sore and tender.

Amelioration – Cold water

Aggravation – Heat, after applying any ointment.

PILES :

ALOES S	MURIATIC ACID
• Blue heamorrhoids	• Blue heamorrhoids which prolapse while urinating
• Intensly *itching*	• Intensly sore and sensitive to touch of even bed clothes.
• Relief – Cold water	• Relief – Hot application

FEMALE SYMPTOMS

Prolapse of uterus associated with

- Fullness
- Heat of body surface
- Tendency to morning diarrhoea
- Dragging down of uterus
- Sensation of plug wedged between symphysis pubis and coccyx.

General modalities :

Aggravation – EARLY MORNING
SEDENTRY LIFE
HOT DRY WEATHER
EATING, DRINKING
STANDING, WALKING

Amelioration – COLD WATER
COLD WEATHER
DISCHARGE OF FLATUS AND STOOL

Relations :

Complementry – Sulphur in chronic cases with abdominal plethora, congestion of portal circulation.
Develops suppressed eruption.

Remedies that follow well – Kali bich, Sepia, Sulphur

Inimicals – Allium sativum

Antidotes – Camphor, Lycopodium, Nux vomica, Sulphur.

Important Questions ?

Q. 1. Give Indication of Aloes in :

Dysentry [1973, 75, 77 S, 78 S, 91]
Diarrhoea [1973, 74, 75, 77, 81]
Piles [1977, 79, 82, 93]

7. AMMONIUM CARBONICUM

Hahnemann

Common Name – Smelling salt

Miasm – Psora is in the backround

Constitution – Stout fleshy women with various troubles in consequence of leading a sedentry life.

- Delicate women who must have a *'smelling bottle'* always in hand.
- They readily catch cold in winter.

Relation with heat and cold – Chilly patient

Diathesis – Heamorrhagic diathesis [Fluid blood + degeneration of red blood corpuscles]

Amm carb is a deep acting constitutional medicine.

KEYNOTES

1) Patient is easily affected by *cold, wet weather* and *motion.*
2) It is a *right sided remedy.*
3) *Heamorrhagic diathesis* with easy bleeding of black, non coagulable blood.
4) Ulcerations tend to *gangrene.*
5) Children *dislike washing* (Ant crud/Sulphur)
6) *Nosebleed* – When washing the face (Arnica/Mag. C) and hands in the morning, after eating : Epistaxis from left nostril.
7) ***Stopping of nose at night.*** Must breathe through the mouth.
8) All fluids are *acrid* – saliva, tears, leucorrhoea.
9) Cough : Dry from tickling in the throat as from dust. Cough every morning at 3-4 A.M. (Kali carb)
10) Body red – as if from scarlatina.
11) ***Cholera like symptoms at the commencement of menses.*** (Bovista, Veratrum album). Profuse menses causing *fatigue* especially of *thighs* with gripping colic.

Particulars :

1) HEAMORRHAGIC DIATHESIS
2) SCARLATINA/SCARLET FEVER
3) MENTAL SYMPTOMS
4) HEAD
5) EYES
6) RESPIRATORY SYMPTOMS

7) HEART
8) FEMALE SYMPTOMS
9) SKIN

HEAMORRHAGIC DIATHESIS

Ammonium carbonicum Causes DISSOLUTION OF R.B.C.S due to poor oxygenation ⟶ GANGRENOUS ulcerations + Flabbiness of muscles + Spongy consistancy of gums and tissues ⟶ DARK CLOTTED Heamorrhages
↓
ANEAMIA
↓
Chilly patient [Aversion to washing, wet application cold wet weather.]

SCARLET FEVER (Virus)

- Malignant type of fever
- Drowsiness or somnolence is always present
- Body is **bluish red**. Bluish red lips (Due to lack of oxygen in blood)
- Miliary rashes – Faintly developed eruptions due to weakness of patients vitality.
- Throat is swollen internally and externally.
  Externally – enlarged cervical lymphatics, cellular tissues.
  Internally – Bluish/dark red swelling of tonsils
- Nose is obstructed at night that causes the child to start from sleep as if smothering.
- *Child has to lie with his mouth wide open to breathe*
- Enlarged *right parotid* gland

Scarlet fever :

AMMONIUM CARB	BELLADONNA
Similarities : 1) Right side of the throat affected. 2) Bright red rashes 3) Drowsiness.	

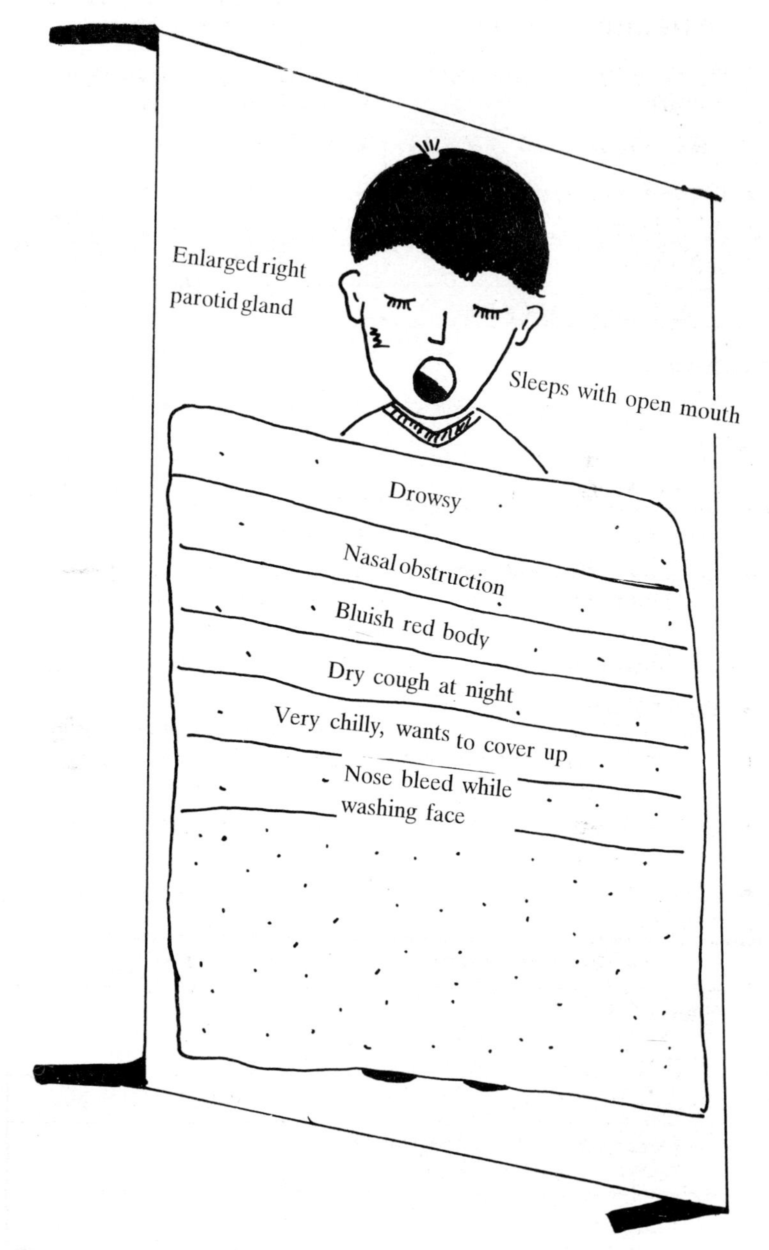

AMMONIUM CARBONICUM

AMMONIUM CARB	BELLADONNA
• Miliary eruptions on skin present • Dark red throat • Drowsiness is marked • Crying out in sleep due to suffocation	• Miliary eruptions on skin usually not present • Bright red throat • Less drowsy but more wild • Crying out in sleep due to *turmoil in brain*

AMMONIUM CARB	APIS
Similarities Miliary rashes, low type scarlatina, somnolence both affect the right side of throat. **Differences :**	
• Chilly patient • No dropsy. Inflamed and swollen throat	• Hot patient • Dropsical symptoms. Puffiness of throat and oedema of uvula.
Meningitis : • Stupid and non reactive state	**Meningitis :** • Inflammation or irritation of the meninges of the brain indicated by "*sudden shrill crying of the child*".
• Cold body with *cynoses and weak pulse*	• Child rolls the head on pillow
• Aggravation – Cold, wet weather.	• Aggravation – Warmth and heat.

AMMONIUM CARB	LACHESIS
Similarities 1) Complaints aggravate after sleep. 2) Blueness of the body surface. 3) Somnolence. 4) Engorgement of the neck 5) Dark red bluish swelling of the throat	

Differences :

• 1) Right sided remedy • 2) Chilly patient • 3) Not as extremely sensitive	• 1) Left sided remedy • 2) Hot patient • 3) Extremely sensitive – Patient cannot bear to have anything touched on neck.

MIND

- Hysterical females who always carry a bottle of ammonia hanging to their chain.
- Depressed patients with fainting fits, anxiety and uneasiness
- Mental and physical complaints aggravate in *cold, raw wet weather.*

HEADACHE

Cause – Wet, Cold weather

Sensation – Brain would ooze out through the forehead and eyes. *Pulsating, beating* in the forehead as if it would burst. *Aggravation* – Stepping, cold wet weather.

Amelioration – Warmth, pressure on the painful side.

EYES

- Eyelids fester and become dry and cracked from ***excoriating fluids*** from the eye.
- ***Sparks*** before the eyes with headaches, double vision and aversion to light.
- Large black spots float before the eyes after sewing.
- Remedy for cataract – Amm carb has helped clearing the crystalline lens.

RESPIRATORY SYMPTOMS

Nose :

- Nosebleed when washing the face in the morning.
- Bathing causes red mottled spots on the body as well as nosebleed.
- Ammon carb has cured acute or chronic *dry/stuffed coryza.*

Coryza :

- Patient is aggravated at night.
- Must breathe through mouth
- Discharge – Bluish coloured mucus
- Discharge from the nose is acrid and excoriates the upper lip
- Severe pain as if the brain is forcing itself out through the forehead.

Throat :

In Malignant scarlet fever/diptheria throat appears *purple, swollen, ulcerated, bleeding, gangrenous accompanied by great lassitude, enlarged tonsils*.

- Burning in the throat
- Glands outside the throat and neck are enlarged and felt as lumps.

Diptheria :

With the above symptoms :

- Nose is stopped
- Child starts from sleep gasping for breath
- Patient is aggravated from sleep and gets up suffocated

Cough :

Time – 3-4 O' clock in the morning

Character of cough – Catarrhal dyspnoea caused due to much rattling of mucus in the chest and air passages.

- Can hardly cough loud due to weakness
- Congestion of the lungs which fills up the chest and causes rattling

Concomitants –
- Coldness of body
- Prostration and weakness
- Weak heart with palpitation
- Pale and cold face

Aggravation – Cold, wet weather

Amelioration – Warmth lying on abdomen.

Amm. carb can be used in *bronchitis, last stage of consumption, pneumonia, emphysema*.

HEART

- Dilatation of heart
- Audible palpitation with great dyspnoea and retraction of epigastrium.
- Cough is accompanied with bloody sputum

Aggravation – Motion, ascending stairs, warm room.

Amelioration – Lying on the abdomen.

FEMALE SEXUAL SYMPTOMS

Menses :

Time – Too early

Quantity – Profuse

Duration – Long lasting

Character of blood – Blackish blood in clots. Blood is extremely acrid and makes the thighs sore.

Concomitants :

- Cholera like diarrhoea at the commencement of menses.
- Great fatigue of thighs during menses
- Gripping colic during menses accompanied with yawning and chilliness

Leucorrhoea :

Watery; acrid, profuse discharge from vagina with excoriation of vulva.

SKIN

- Body is red.
- A patient who has come down with severe internal troubles may develop unhealthy looking boils, erysipelas or ulcers on treatment – Amm carb can be used in such cases for cure.
- Panaratia/whitlow – Deep seated periosteal pain, red streaks run up the axilla from the inflamed area.
- Malignant scarlatina.

General Modalities :

Aggravation – COLD, WET WEATHER
WASHING
MENSES
WALKING

Amelioration – LYING ON ABDOMEN
LYING ON PAINFUL SIDE
DRY WEATHER
WARMTH

Relations :

Remedies that follow well – Belladonna, Bryonia
Lycopodium, Pulsatilla
Phos, Rhus tox , Sepia, Sulphur, Veratrum alb.

Inimicals – Lachesis

Antidotes – Arnica, Camphor, Hepar sulph

Important Questions ?

Q. 1. Give indications of Ammonium Carb in :

1) Female Symptoms [1977, 81, 95 S, 97]
2) Asthma [1995]
3) Bronchitis [1987]
4) Heamorrhage [1979]
5) Stoppage of nose [1982]

8. ANTIMONIUM CRUDUM

Caspari

Common Name – Sulphide of Antimony.

Miasm – Psora and Sycosis in background.

Constitution – *Greedy, fat, sentimental* with sore corners to mouth and crippled feet.

Relation with heat and cold – Antim crud patient is easily affected by extremes of heat and cold.

Diathesis – Rheumatic and Gouty diathesis.

KEYNOTES

1) Patient ***cannot bear heat of the sun*** and cannot bear cold bathing (child cries when washed or bathed in cold water).
2) Children and young people are inclined to grow *fat*.
3) Child ***cannot bear to be touched or looked*** at.
4) Great *sadness* with weeping.
5) Longing for *acids and pickles*.
6) Gastric affections are caused from bread, pastry, sour wine, *cold bathing, overheating.*
7) Gastric complaints are caused by *overeating* that causes weak digestion.

    Weak digestion is marked by :

    - Thickly white coated tongue. [Red line symptom]
    - Alternate diarrhoea and constipation.
    - Diarrhoea is watery with little hard lumps.
8) ***Disposition to abnormal growth of skin***.
    - Brittle and crushed finger nails.
    - Horny and sensitive corns on soles of feet.
    - Nostrils and labial commisures – Sore, cracked andcrusty
9) ***Symptoms change locality*** and go from one side of the body to another.
10) ***Mucous piles*** – Ichorous oozing staining cloth yellow.

Particulars :

1) MIND
2) HEADACHE
3) EYES

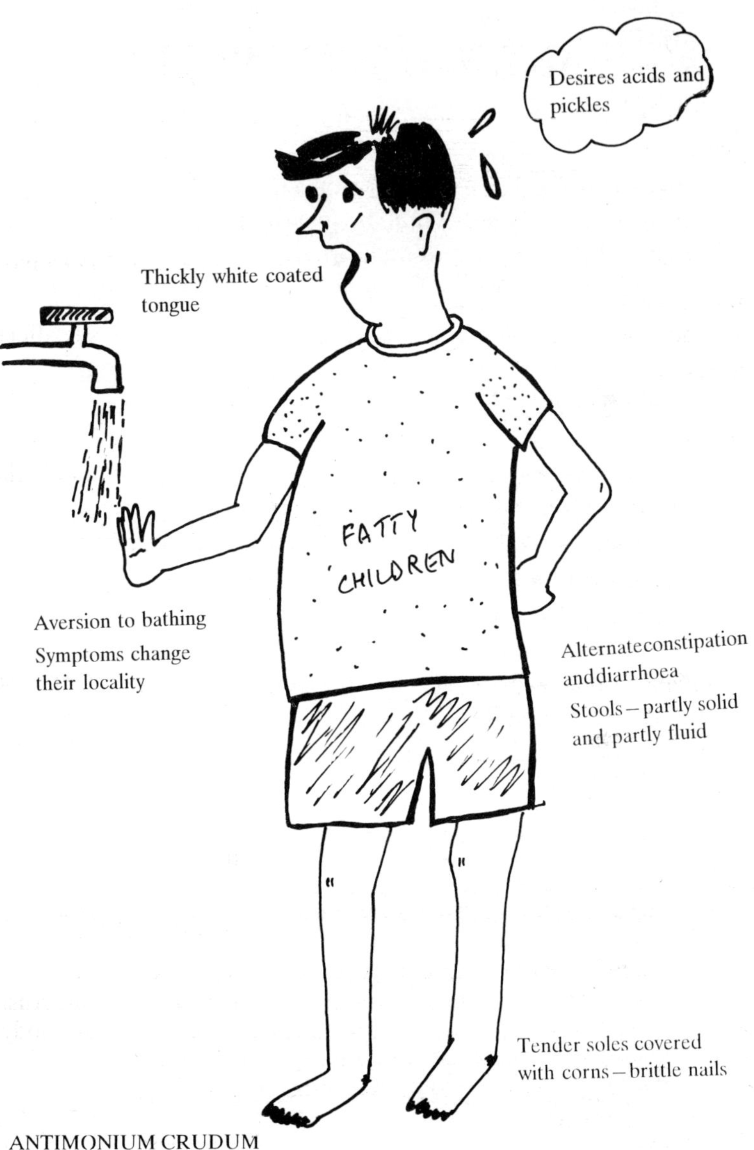

ANTIMONIUM CRUDUM

4) CATARRAH
5) GIT
6) FEMALE
7) SKIN
8) RHEUMATISM
9) CHILD

MIND

Child – Cross and peevish child cannot bear to be touched or looked at. Baby does not wish to speak or to be spoken to.

Adult patient – Morose, down hearted, gloomy . Patient is inclined towards commiting suicide. Loathing of life – total absence of desire to live. Irresistable desire to talk in rhymes and verses. Sentimental in moonlight;bad affects of disappointed love.

HEADACHE

Causes – Cold bathing, overheating, overeating – acids, fats, fruits; alcohol, chill, cold, suppressed eruptions

Sensation – Congestive and throbbing headache.

Location – Over the entire head especially the vertex.

Amelioration – Open air, lying down and keeping quiet, warm bath.

Headache alternates with catarrhal symptoms [Nose, stomach, rectum]

EYES

Inflammation of the eyes causing soreness of the canthi.

[*Graphites* – Inflammation involves the whole border of the lids]

Aggravation – Sunshine, bright light.

CATARRAH (Nose)

Cause – Taking cold, getting over heated, drinking sour wine.

Character :

- Increased flow of mucous membrane and nose gets stuffed up at night.
- Cough becomes chronic because of low and feeble circulation.
- In chronic cases coryza becomes associated with headache and as the catarrah lessens and becomes dry, the headache increases. Catarrah of nose alternates with crushing headache and catarrah of the stomach (causing increased vomiting)

Better – Open air.

GIT

Teeth Toothache is caused by eating, cold water.

Character – Pain in the hollow of the teeth.

Aggravation – Night, eating, cold water, touching with tongue.

Amelioration – Walking in open air.

Tongue – Thick milky white coated tongue.

Stomach :

Gastric catarrah is caused by – overeating, acids, sour wine, cold bathing, overheating

- *Thick white coated tongue* which may be interrupted with tinges of yellow.
- Constant nausea and a distended stomach with a feeling of being overloaded.
- Stomach feels distended and the person vomits the contents of the stomach. Prolonged vomiting leads to exhaustion.
- Violent thirst with dry lips.
- Belching with taste of what has been eaten

Diarrhoea :

Character – Watery with little hard lumps and undigested food. Diarrhoea may end in dysentery with inflammation of rectum and colon. Diarrhoea alternates with constipation.

Constipation :

Stools – White hard stools that are too large and look like undigested curd.

Piles :

Cause – Cold wet weather, cold bathing, sour wine.

Character – Mucous piles with constant burning, continuous mucous discharge that stains yellow. Discharge has a disgusting odour.

GASTRITIS :

AETHUSA CYNAPIUM	ANTIM CRUD
• **Cause** – Dentition, Summer	• **Cause** – Overeating, cold bathing
• Vomiting of curdled milk in infants during dentition or other times. • Vomited matter comes out with a rush. • After vomiting the patient is sleepy and prostrated. After a nap the patient is again hungry and it soon eats and vomits.	• Antim curd is generally not used for very severe cases of vomiting • Child is hungry as soon as it vomits milk.

IPECAC	ANTIM CRUD
Similarity – Vomiting after meal, acids, coughing.	
Difference :	
• More nausea.	• Vomiting and retching
• Clean tongue	• Thick white coated tongue

BRYONIA	ANTIM CRUD
Similarity – White tongue + Dry mouth + Constipation.	
Difference :	
• **Tongue** – White down the middle. Edges are not coated.	• **Tongue** – Whole tongue is white coated.
• **Diarrhoea** – Offensive (old cheese) and watery.	• **Diarrhoea** – Watery with hard lumps and undigested food.
• **Constipation** – Hard, dry and brown stools.	• **Constipation** – White hard stools that are too large.

PULSATILLA	ANTIM CRUD
Similarity – Gastric catarrah may be caused due to pork.	
Difference :	
• Thirstless	• Very thirsty
• No vomiting	• Intense vomiting
• **Stools** – Yellowish, green and slimy.	• **Stools** – Partly solid and partly fluid.
• Complaints may be caused due to – ice creams pastry and fatty food	• Complaints are caused due to – Overheating, cold bathing, acids, pickles.

FEMALE

- Prolapse of uterus with constant bearing down feeling as if something is pushing out of the vagina.
- Tenderness over the ovarian region when the menses have been suppressed by cold. Leucorrhoea is watery with lumps.

SKIN

Disposed to abnormal growth and horny excrecenses on skin.

Nostrils and labial commissures – Sore, cracked and crusty.

Nails – Finger nails grow in splints like horny warts.

Toe nails are brittle and grow out of shape.

Sole – Soles of feet are covered with corns and callosities which are very tender and the patient can hardly walk on them. Soles of feet are very painful.

Warts – may grow on the hands.

Eruptions – Thick and scabby eruptions. Pimples, furuncles which may arise primarily or secondrily with itching of skin. Rubbing causes tenderness and soreness.

RHEUMATISM

- Ant crud has cured long standing cases of chronic rheumatism that is guided by excessive tenderness of soles of feet.
- Rheumatism or gout alternate with stomach symptoms. There is persistent vomiting for days and all of a sudden vomiting stops and gouty symptoms come back to the extremities.
- Symptoms change *locality* and go from one side of the body to another.

Aggravation – Night, cold damp weather, overheating, open fire.

Amelioration – Applied heat, open air.

CHILD

- Tendency to grow *FAT*
- Mind – cross and peevish. Cannot bear to be looked at. Does not want to speak to anybody.
- Child cannot bear cold bathing.
- Great longing for acids and pickles.
- Gastric complaints with a thick milky white coated tongue.

General Modalities :

Aggravation – COLD BATHING
OVER HEATING

Overeating – ACIDS, FATS, PICKLES
SOUR WINE
SUPPRESSED ERUPTIONS

Amelioration – OPEN AIR
WARM BATH
LYING DOWN QUIETLY

Relations

Complements – Scilla.

Remedies that follow well – Calcarea carb
Lachesis, Merc sol
Pulsatilla, Sepia
Sulphur

Antidotes – Coffea.

Important Questions ?

Q. 1. Compare skin symptoms of Antim crud and Hydrocotyle.

ANTIM CRUD	HYDROCOTYLE
• Abnormal growth and horny excrecences of the skin.	• Dry eruptions.
• Sore cracked and crusty lips and nose.	• Thickening of epidermal layer with exfoliative scales.
• Nails grow in splints. Nails are brittle and grow out of shape.	• Hypertrophy and induction of connective tissue.
• Corns on soles of feet. Soles of feet are very tender.	• Intestinal inflammation and cellular proliferation.
• Thick and scabby eruptions with yellowish green discharges.	• Psoriasis gyrate
	• Pustules on chest
	• Copious perspiration
	• Intolerable itching on soles of feet
	• Used in syphilitic affection, acne, leprosy, ulceration of womb.

Q. 2. Give indication of Antim crud in following :

Skin [1987, 95]
GIT [1974, 75, 76, 77, 86, 88, 96]
Mentals [1973, 74, 75, 79]
Tongue [1977, 82]
Constipation [1979]
Cause of complaints [1977]
Modalities [1979]
Desires and Aversions [1991]

9. ANTIMONIUM TARTARICUM

Stapf

Common Name – Tartar Emetic (Induces Vomiting).
Miasm – Psora and sycosis are in the background.

Pathogenesis

- Depresses the heart and circulation.
- Increases sweat.
- Catarrhal inflammation of mucous membrane.
- Induces nausea, vomiting, purging, fainting, collapse.
- Skin – rashes, pustules.

Constitution – Adapted to sluggish and phlegmatic people. Person has a hydrogenoid constitution.

Diathesis – Scrofulous diathesis.

Relation with heat and cold – Complaints are caused by wet weather and over covering.

KEYNOTES

1) Complaints caused by ***exposure to damp basement cellars***, too much clothing or warming up, bad effects of *vaccination*.
2) ***Death rattle*** with large collection of mucous in the bronchi which is not expectorated due to feeble expulsive power of lungs.
3) *Expectoration* is *nil* or very scanty which is white in colour.
4) *Face* – Cold, blue, pale covered with cold sweat.
5) *Tongue* – Pasty thick white with reddened papillea and red edges. Tongue is red in streaks.
6) *Vomiting* in any position except when lying on the right side. *Nausea is relieved by vomiting.*
7) Intense ***drowsiness and prostration*** (Opium,Nux mosh.)
8) *Thirstlessness* is marked.
9) There is *craving* for apple, acids and cold drinks. Aversion – **Milk**, food, tobacco.
10) *Trembling* – Internal, head and hands.
11) *Asphyxia neonatorum* – Child at birth is breathless, pale and cynosed.
12) *Asphyxia* caused by drowning, mucus in bronchi, paralysis of lungs, foreign bodies in larynx and trachea attended with *drowsiness and coma*.
13) *Pustular eruptions* like small pox are cured by **Ant tart.**

Eye symptoms – Flickering before the eyes, dim vision etc. produced in eruptive diseases like small pox, measles, scarlatina are also cured.

14) *Cholera Morbus* (Ant tart is an excellent remedy)

- sharp cutting colic before stool
- burning at the anus after each stool
- tenesmus during and after stool
- drowsiness and coma
- profuse perspiration leading to prostration
- Pulse – rapid, weak and trembling

Particulars :

1) MIND
2) HEAD
3) FACE
4) RESPIRATORY SYSTEM
5) GIT
6) DROPSY
7) SKIN

MIND

Bad humor

- Irritable child who doesn't want to be looked at or touched.
- Child wants to be left alone.
- Child wants to be carried (Cham).
- Always in bad humor.

HEADACHE

Cause – Passive congestion of brain.

Location – Pain in right temple extending down to lower jaw bone.

Sensation – As if band is tied around the head.

- Head is confused with warmth of the forehead.
- Drowsiness and confusion in the forenoon.
- Vertigo alternates with drowsiness.

TONGUE

Tongue has a coating of white fur but the papillae are red prominent and edges are characterised by a band of red.

- Dry tongue with thirstlessness.
- Imprint of teeth on the borders.

FACE

Hippocratic countenance

- Face is pale and sickly.
- Nose is drawn and sunken.
- Eyes are sunken with dark rings.
- Pale lips with flapping and dilated nostrils.

- Face is covered with cold sweat and is blue and cyanosed.
- Cyanosis is caused by unoxydised or carbonised blood.

RESPIRATORY SYSTEM

Ant tart produces inflammation of respiratory mucous membranes.

Ant tart is indicated in :

- Atelectasis with symptoms of asphyxia
- Oedema of lungs
- Emphysema
- Paralysis of lungs
- Pneumonia
- Bronchitis

Cause – Damp basement cellars

Bad effects of vaccination.

Symptoms :

- Patient looks as if he is *sinking*.
- Great accumulation of *phlegm* in the chest and bronchial tubes.
- Steady filling up of the lungs with mucus which at first can be thrown out but later as *paralytic condition of the lungs* sets in the patient is unable to throw out mucus.
- Mucus in the chest causes breathlessness with orthopnoea. Person has to sit up and breathe. Lying down lessens suffocation.
- There is coarse rattling cough with catarrhal condition of the chest later leading to a death rattle.
- *Scanty expectoration* which is white.

Concomitants :

- Hippocratic countenance
- Blue pale, cynosed patient with cold sweat and cold body.
- Thirstlessness
- Drowsiness and sleepiness
- Tongue – thick white pasty coat with red streaks in the middle and raised papillae.
- Pulse – rapid, weak and trembling
- Internal trembling.

Asphyxia Neonatorum – Child is pale, blue and cyanosed at birth. Child is breathless and gasping though the cord still pulsates.

- Mucous rattles in the chest.
- Shortness of breath and child appears to be sinking.

G.I.T.

Dyspepsia :

- Constant nausea, vomiting and indigestion.
- Nausea is relieved by vomiting.

- Nausea causing great anxiety in stomach with loss of appetite and disgust for food.

    Desires – Apples, acids, cold drinks.

    Aversion – Food, milk, tobacco.

- Vomiting except when lying on right side.
- Vomiting with great retching. The person has to strain a lot for vomiting. Vomiting of large quantities of *thick white ropy mucus with bile*.
- Great yawning and drowsiness.
- Thirstless.
- Precordial anxiety with pressure and distension in the hypochondrium.
- Patient breaks into cold sweat while vomiting.

Cholera Morbus :

- Sharp cutting colic before stool.
- Burning in the anus after each stool.
- Drowsiness and coma.
- Profuse perspiration leading to collapse.
- Thready pulse with increasing prostration.
- Thirstlessness.
- Constant nausea with spasmodic vomiting.
- Patient has to gag and strain to vomit.

DROPSY

- In old broken down constitution at the end of pneumonia / fevers there may be dropsy with bloating of feet for 3-4 months after getting up from fever.
- 'Fever sores' may develop especially in the legs in place of dropsy following old fevers.

SKIN

Ant tart is used for :

- **Pustules** identical to small pox pustules may be found in conjunctiva, face, mouth, fauces, oesophagus, jejunum, genitals.
- **Variola** with backache, headache, cough and crushing weight on chest before or at the beginning of the eruptive stage.
- Pustules are bright red, hard with intense itching, pustules leave behind bluish red marks.
- Being a sycotic remedy – Ant tart produces *warts* behind the glans
- Due to checked gonorrhoea, secondary *orchitis* may be produced.

General Modalities :

Aggravation – DAMP COLD WEATHER
LYING DOWN AT NIGHT
WARMTH OF THE ROOM
COVERING UP
CHANGE OF WEATHER IN SPRING
(KALI S. NAT S)

Amelioration – COLD OPEN AIR
SITTING UPRIGHT
EXPECTORATING
LYING ON RIGHT SIDE

Relations :

Similar to :

Lycopodium – spasmodic motion of alae nasi

Veratrum alb – Diarrhoea, colic, vomiting, coldness and craving for acids.

Ipecac – Drowsiness from defective respiration, constantly nauseated.

Complementry to – Ipecac.

Remedies that follow well – Baryta carb, Cina, Cham, Ipec, Puls, Sep, Sulphur, Tereb. Carbo veg.

Antidotes – Asafoetida, China, Cocc., Ipecac, Opium, Puls, Rhus, Sepia.

Ipecac precedes Ant tart in catarrhal symptoms.

Baryta carb succeeds Ant tart when the latter only partially relieves orthopnoea or threatening paralysis.

Important Question ?

Q. 1. Give indications of Ant tart in : [1995, 76, 79, 82]
Respiratory symptoms [1986, 91]
Heart failure [1988]
GIT [1974, 92]
Desires and Aversions [1991]
Skin [1995]
Vomiting [1974, 77]

Q. 2. Compare Ant tart and Ipecac in Respiratory symptoms :

ANT TART	IPECAC.
• Great accumulation of *mucus* with weakness and *lack of reaction in the lungs.* Expectoration hence is very scanty.	• Great accumulation of *mucus* with coarse rattling but attended *with great expulsive power of the lungs.*

• Due to increasingly carbonised blood, the patient becomes more and more drowsy with cold sweat, cynosed face and lips.	• Violent dyspnoea with wheezing, great weight, anxiety about the precordia and threatened suffocation.
	• Whooping cough with nose bleed, heamoptysis (Bright red blood)
• Rattling cough with deep inspiration	• Patient turns pale, blue and rigid.
• Rattling that comes after *many days*	• Rattling in the first few days of sickness.
Tongue :	**Tongue :**
• Thick white pasty coat on tongue with red streaks. Clean tongue with thirstlessness.	• Very red and dry in the middle with thirstlessness
• **Nausea** is relieved by vomiting.	• **Persistent Nausea** – nothing relieves.

10. APIS MELLIFICA

Brauns

Common Name – Honey Bee (Apium Virus)
(Derived from poison of Honey Bee)

Miasm – Psora in the background. *Apis is slow in* its action; favourable action of the remedy is first shown by an increased flow of the urine.

Constitution – Strumous constitution (Goitrous)

- Enlarged and indurated glands.
- Scirrous or open cancer.
- Awkwardness runs through the remedy.
- Tendency to dropsy of external coverings.

Temperament – Irritable.

Relation with heat and cold – HOT patient.

Diathesis – Scrofulous.

KEYNOTES

1) Affects the *right hand side* (right ovary, right testes etc.)

2) *Aggravation* – heat / warmth.
Amelioration – cold water.

3) ***Oedema*** – bag like puffy swelling under the lower eyelids. [upper lids – Kali carb, around the eyes – Phos]. Swelling of the hands and feet. Dropsy of the external tissues – meninges, pleura, pericardium, serous membrane of joints, skin.

4) Dropsy and fever with *thirstlessness* [dropsy with thirst – Acetic acid, Apocynum]. Thirst only in chill stage of intermittent fever.

5)***Burning, stinging pain***, suddenly migrating from one part to another. [Kali bich, Lac can, Puls]

6) Extreme *sensitiveness* to touch.

7) ***Tongue—Fiery red, dry cracked, blistered.***

8) In *Fever* – Face is alternately dry and perspiring, wary and pale skin, scanty urine, thirstlessness; aggravation from heat.
Intermittent fever – Chill stage – 3 P.M. + Thirst; sweat stage; heat stage – thistlessness. *Aggravation* – Warm room.
Amelioration – Cold things.

9) ***Throat*** – Dropsical, swollen throat with a feeling of fullness – this causes laboured breathing.

10) ***Meningitis*** – Cri-encephalique. There is sudden shrill cry of the child in sleep caused due to cerebral irritation.

11) ***Diarrhoea*** – At every motion of the body the bowels move as though the sphincter ani had no power; as though the anus was wide open (Phos, Secale cor)

12) ***Constipation*** – Sensation of tightness in the abdomen as if something would break if much efforts were used.

13) ***Incontinence of urine*** – Frequent, painful, scanty and bloody urine.

14) Apis is an excellent remedy for *ovarian cysts and abortion caused in 3rd month*.

15) Patient is very awkward, fidgety.
   - Fear of impending death.
   - Jealousy and suspicion.
   - Muttering delirium, loquacity.
   - Cri-encephalique.

Particulars :

1) DROPSY
2) HEAD
3) EYES
4) DIPTHERIA
5) G.I.T.
6) URINARY SYSTEM
7) FEMALE SYMPTOMS
8) FEVER
9) SKIN

DROPSY

General features – Skin is transparent, with a waxen look, whitish yellow.

- Bag like puffy swelling under the eyes.
- Thirstlessness.
- Scanty urine.

Hydrocephalus – 'Dropsy of the brain'. Inflammation of membrane of the brain followed by accumulation of serum.

- Child bores its head backwards into the pillow and rolls it from side to side.
- Every little while the child arouses from sleep with a shrill piercing cry (shriek is due to pain).
- One side of the body twitches and the other lies as if paralysed.
- Strabismus is present.
- Pulse is rapid and weak.
- Urine is scanty.

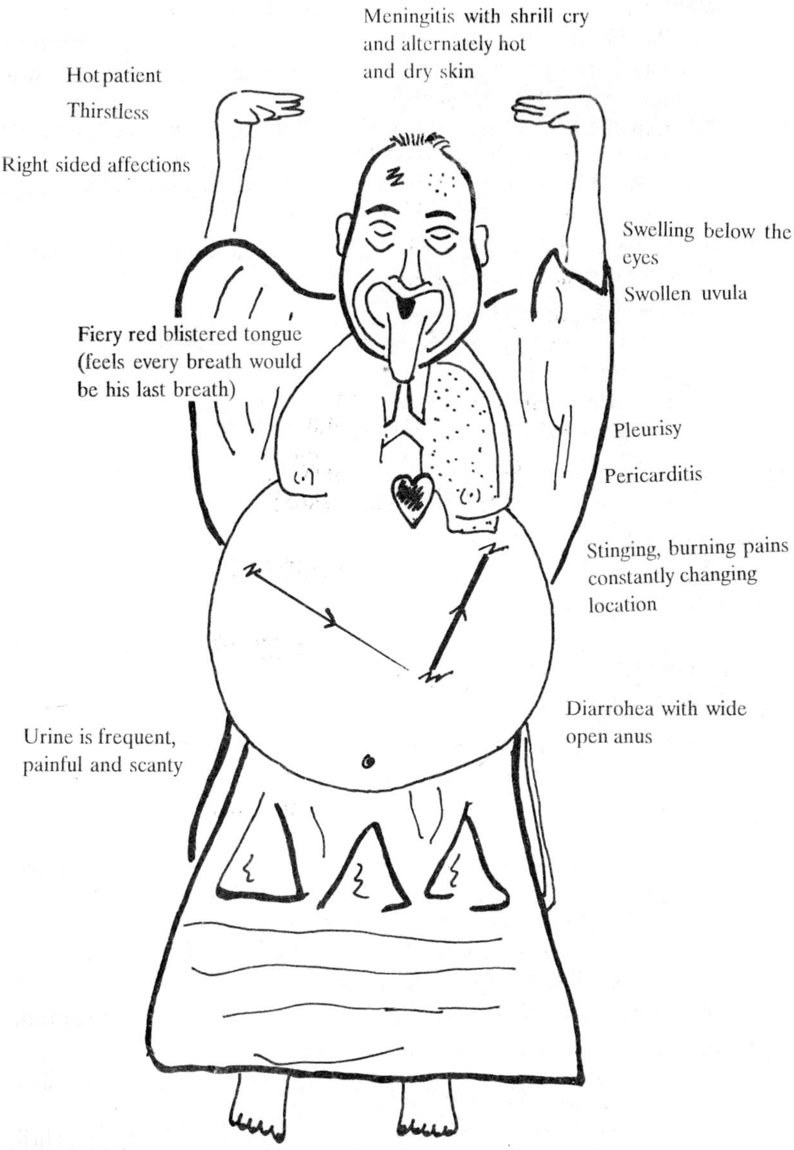

Meningitis with shrill cry and alternately hot and dry skin

Hot patient

Thirstless

Right sided affections

Swelling below the eyes

Swollen uvula

Fiery red blistered tongue (feels every breath would be his last breath)

Pleurisy

Pericarditis

Stinging, burning pains constantly changing location

Urine is frequent, painful and scanty

Diarrohea with wide open anus

APIS MELLIFICA

Hydrothorax – "Especially when the trouble is of cardiac origin."

- Oedematous feet.
- Intolerable burning and soreness.
- Constrictive feeling about the chest.

- Dry cough which seems to start from the trachea and does not cease until a small quantity of phlegm is loosened.
- A great suffocative feeling causing a laboured breathing.
- Patient has a feeling as if he is going to die.
- Fidgety anxiety is present.

Pleurisy – Apis is excellent for pleurisy.

Dropsy of renal origin –

- Urine is scanty, highly albuminous and contains casts of the uriniferous tubules.
- Bag like swelling under the lower eyelids.
- Surface of the body feels sore and bruised.

Synovitis – Apis acts particularly on synovial membranes of knee. It is indicated when there are *stinging pains* shooting through the joints with aggravation from slightest motion.

- Patient feels better from cold applications.

HEAD

Congestion from head to face in consequence of which a general aching through the brain is complained of.

Meningitis (Tuberculous) :

Cri Encephalique – Sharp stinging pains extort a shriek.

- Child goes into a state of unconciousness.
- Child lies in stupor – one side of the body twitching and the other side motionless.
- Head drawn back rigidly.
- Pupils are contracted or dilated with red eyes.
- Flushed face with semi conciousness.
- Child lies with eyes partly closed as if benumbed.
- Premonition of approaching death.
- Heat aggravates complaints.

EYES

Apis is indicated in asthenopia, staphyloma, keratitis of eyes.

- Inflammation of the eyes that leave thickening of mucous membranes and lids.
- Opacities or white spots are present over the eyes.
- Enlarged blood vessels.
- Oedema of the lids.
- Swelling of the mucous membranes may be so great that they roll out looking like pieces of raw beef.
- Tears may be burning and stinging.

Apis has a tendency to formation of pus in the eyes (Rhus tox)

APIS	RHUS. TOX
• Stinging pains. Lids – bluish red, watery, looking, semitransparent.	• Lids are dusky red in colour and together with cheeks are studded with small watery vesicles.
• Swelling of palpebral conjunctiva is more due to congestion. Worse – evening Relief – cold water	• True swelling of the lids due to chemosis with hot gushing lachrymation. Worse – night Relief – warmth

Apis is inimical to Rhus tox in eruptive diseases.

DIPTHERIA

- Child is prostrated with high fever and drowsiness.
- Throat has a varnished appearance – tonsils and fauces seem to be coated with a glossy red varnish.
- Membrane forms mostly on the right tonsil.
- Uvula hangs down like a bag of water causing a feeling of fullness.
- Rim of the glottis is swollen ,red and oedematous – causing laboured breathing owing to narrowing of the entrance of larynx.
- External throat appears swollen and erisipelatous. Red rash may be present over the skin.

G.I.T.

Tongue :

Dry + fiery red + Blistered tongue

Tongue feels scalded, red, cracked and trembling. Apis can cure "Cancer of Tongue".

Abdomen :

- Soreness and tightness throughout the abdomen and hypochondria.
- Abdomen is distended with gas causing great tension and fullness.
- In all inflammatory complaints [peritonitis, inflammation of liver, pelvis]. There is great tension and tightness that makes it impossible for the patient to cough. Cough makes him feel as if something will burst.

Constipation – Person cannot strain at stool because of the fear that something would burst. Feeling of tightness throughout the abdomen.

Diarrhoea :

Cause – Drunkards, eruptive diseases especially if eruption is suppressed.

Character of stool – Thin, watery, yellow in colour and worse in the morning. Stool may be offensive.

Sensation – Anus is wide open – as if the sphincter ani has no power. At every motion of the body the bowels move. Anus feels raw and sore before and after stool.

URINARY SYSTEM

- Frequent, painful, scanty, bloody urine.
- Urine is scanty and comes only in drops.
- Constant ineffectual urging – as soon as little drops collect in the bladder, urging to urinate comes on.
- Urine burns and causes the patient to shriek.
- Urinary troubles with swelling of genitals 'swelling is oedematous'.

In acute albuminuria – scanty foetid urine is present with albumen and blood corpuscles.

FEMALE

Ovaries – Apis is used in *right sided affection of the ovaries.*

It is indicated in ovaritis, ovarian cysts, tumors of ovaries.

Symptoms – Burning and stinging pain in ovarian region.

- Tumefaction (swelling) detectable over the pelvis.
- Numbness runs down the thighs.
- Tightness across the chest.

Abortion – Apis cures abortion before or at 3rd month.

(Apis should be given coutiously during pregnancy as it may cause miscarraige if given in frequent doses in low potency).

Menses – Amenorrhoea, at puberty.

Symptoms – Bearing down in uterine region Congestion of head due to suppression of flow, thirstlessness, intolerance of heat.

Concomitants – Awkwardness, Nervous women.

- For dysmenorrhoea with severe ovarian pain, Apis is a very good remedy.

FEVER

Intermittent :

Chill stage – At 3 P.M., thirst.

- Oppression of the chest as if too full.
- Aggravation – By heat.

Heat stage – Oppression of the chest, drowsiness, thirstlessness

Worse – Warm room

Sweat stage – No thirst.

Apyrexia – Patient complains of pains under the ribs on either sides.

Skin – Pale, waxy and oedematous; urticaria may break out.

Urine – Scanty.

Feet – Swollen and oedematous.

Nat mur chill – 10 o'clock

Apis chill – 3 o'clock

Remittent (Typhoid) Fever

- Muttering delirium.
- Pale, waxy, oedematous, flushed face.
- Dry skin which is burning hot at some places and cool in others.
- Increased prostration.
- Dry and cracked red tongue. Tongue may be blistered. Apis is also indicated in scarlet fever, cerebral fever.

SKIN

- Skin is waxy, oedematous and pale.
- Skin may be alternately dry and perspiring.
- During fever the patient is hot at some places and cool at others.
- *Erisipelas* – Inflammation commences about the right eye and spreads all over the face on the left side, parts quickly become oedematous and assume a pinkish rosy hue. Soreness soon becomes more severe with burning and stinging pains.

There is high fever + dryskin + thirstlessness.

BELLANDONNA	APIS
• Smooth bright red swelling with no tendency to oedema.	• Inflammation has a rosy hue with tendency to oedema.
• Acute throbbing pains.	• Stinging, burning pains.

Urticaria – Pinkish white blotches raised above the skin. Itching burning and stinging is intolerable. Worse in a warm room and better in cold air.

Boils / Carbuncles – Stinging pains and tendency to oedema.

Cancer – Oversensitive to touch.

Burning and stinging pains

Metastasis of cancerous affections takes place in cellular tissue with effusion.

General Modalities :

Aggravation – WARMTH /HEAT
MOTION / COUGHING
EVENING / NIGHT

SLEEPING
GETTING WET

Amelioration – OPEN AIR
COLD WATER
UNCOVERING

Relations :

Complements – Natrum mur.

Inimical to – Rhus tox.

Antidotes – Cantharis, China, Iodum, Digitalis.

Followed well by – Arsenic and Pulsatilla

Important Questions ?

Q. 1. Give difference between symptoms of **Apis and Arsenic album**

APIS	ARSENIC ALBUM
MIND **Similarities :** ● Changes place anxiously. ● Fear of impending death. ● Restlessness. ● Weakness. **Differences :**	
● Nervous restlessness	● Anxiety and fear
DROPSY **Differences :** ● Transparency of skin. ● Dropsy of renal, cardiac, hepatic origin.	
● Thirstlessness	● Intolerable thirst but drinks little at a time because water annoys stomach.
● Awkwardness	● Restlessness ● Eating and drinking causes vomiting

DIPTHERIA	
Differences :	
• Membrane forms on the right tonsil.	• Throat is swollen from inside and outside.
• Swollen tongue.	• Membrane has a dark hue with a foetid breath.
• Oedematous uvula.	• Nose has a thin and excoriating discharge.
• Glottis is swollen that causes a sense of fullness and laboured breathing.	• Restless (After midnight).
• Nervous anxiety and awkwardness.	–
• Prostrated, high fever and drowsiness.	–
• Scanty and frequent urine.	• Scanty urine.
• *Pulse* – Rapid but not strong.	• *Pulse* – Thread like, incompressible, weak.
EYES	
Similarities : Hot tears, violent pains, oedematous lids.	
Differences :	
• Lachrymation is less acrid.	• Lachrymation is more acrid.
• Lids are bluish red.	• Lids are pale.
• Nervous fidgetyness.	• Restlessness.
• *Relief* – Cold water.	• *Relief* – Warm application.

Q. 2. Give indication of Apis in the following :

Skin	[1985, 87]
Urinary Symptoms	[1975, 76, 77, 78, 81, 82, 94]
Diarrhoea	[1988]
Respiratory Symptoms	[1987]
Mind	[1981]
Tonsillitis	[1975, 76, 76 S]
Dropsy	[1976, 79]

Meningitis [1979, 81, 95]
Malarial Fever [1973, 81]
Keynotes [1977]
Modalities [1972, 74, 76, 79, 82]

Q. 3. Give difference between Cantharis and Apis in urinary symptoms.

APIS	CANTHARIS
• Frequent, scanty, scalding urine.	• Burning in the urethra causing intolerable pain while passing urine.
• Urine burns very much and causes the patient to shriek.	
• Constant urging to urinate – urine dribbles and the patient has to wait for a long time before he can pass urine.	• Intolerable urging to urinate before during and after urination.
• Urinary troubles with swelling of genitals where swelling is oedematous.	• Passage of few drops at a time which is mixed with blood.
	• Violent tenesmus and strangury.
• *Aggravation* – Warm / hot drinks	• *Aggravation* – Urination, touch, cold water, coffee
• *Amelioration* – Cold application.	• Amelioration – Warm, application.
CANTHARIS ANTIDOTES APIS	

Q. 4. Give difference between Apis and Phosphorus in diarrhoea.

APIS	PHOSPHORUS
Cause – Drunkards; eruptive diseases especially if eruption is suppressed.	**Cause** – Eating anything.
• Yellow watery stools worse in morning. Offensive odour. Stools may be intermingled with mucus, blood and food giving it an appearance of a tomato sauce.	• Profuse watery involuntary stools with offensive odour.

	• Burning in the rectum during stool.
• Anus protrudes with stools.	• Anus protrudes with stools.
• Sensation – anus is wide open.	• Sensation – anus is wide open.
• Movement of the stools with every motion.	• Before stool – Burning in anus.
• Anus feels raw and sore before and after stool.	• After stool – Painful cramps, burning in anus, tenesmus, sinking feeling in abdomen.
Concomitants	**Concomitants**
• Thirstless • No appetite • Dry and fiery red tongue	• Sharp sticking pains from coccyx up the spine to the base of the brain drawing the neck backward.
• Sore feeling in the abdomen with excess tenderness.	• Desire for ice cold things which disturb the stomach as soon as they warm up.
• Amelioration – Cold things Aggravation – Heat	• Restlessness is marked

11. ARGENTUM METALLICUM

Hahnemann

Common Name – Pure silver.

Miasm – Syphilis is in the background.

Argentum met is a deep acting remedy.

Constitution – Tall, thin and irritable persons. Constitutional affects of onanism and abuse of mercury.

Temperament – Irritable.

Relation with heat and cold – Chilly patient.

KEYNOTES

1) Argentum met is a *left sided remedy.*
2) Complaints are *aggravated by cold damp weather, becoming chilled.*
3) Memory and reasoning faculties are diminished.
4) Rending, *tearing pains* along the *nerves* especially in the lower extremities. Pains are aggravated during rest.
5) *'Inflamed cartilages'* infiltrate and form into hard knots. Ulcers form in the cartilagenous tissue with a copious discharge. Intense itching and the patient scratches until he bleeds.
6) *Articular rheumatism without swelling* (Hysterical rheumatism)
7) Argentum met is the principal remedy for *epileptic attacks.* Patient jumps about striking those near him.
8) Exhausting *fluent coryza with sneezing.*
9) *Hoarseness or loss of voice in professional singers, public speakers* (Alum, Arum T).
10) Laughing excites cough and produces *profuse grey mucus* in the larynx (Dros, Phos, Stannum met.)
11) *Raw spot* over the bifurcation of trachea.
12) *Males* – Bad affects of abuse of mercury, sexual excess etc.

- Crushed pains along the testicles.
- In gonorrhoea the discharge remains yellow instead of becoming white and gleety.
- Atrophy of penis.

14) *Prolaspe of Uterus* with pain and hea morrhage,ovarian cysts and tumors with pain extending forward.

Particulars :

1) MIND

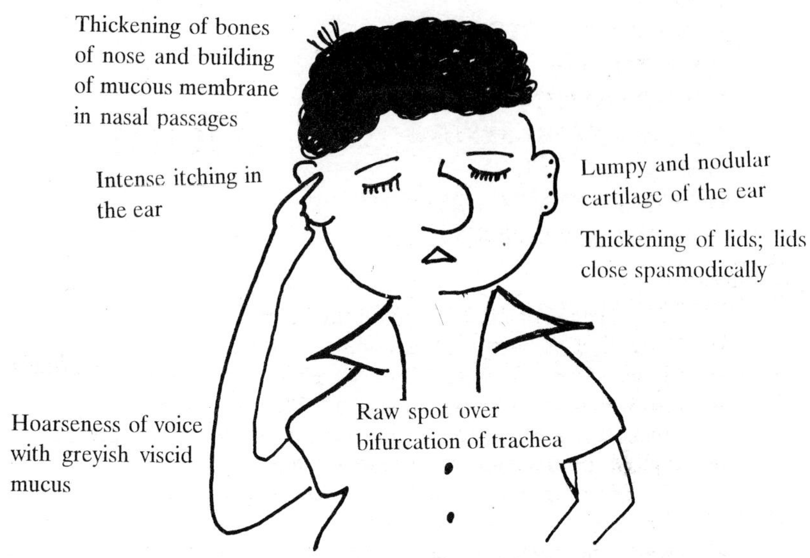
Thickening of bones
of nose and building
of mucous membrane
in nasal passages
Intense itching in
the ear
Lumpy and nodular
cartilage of the ear
Thickening of lids; lids
close spasmodically
Hoarseness of voice
with greyish viscid
mucus
Raw spot over
bifurcation of trachea

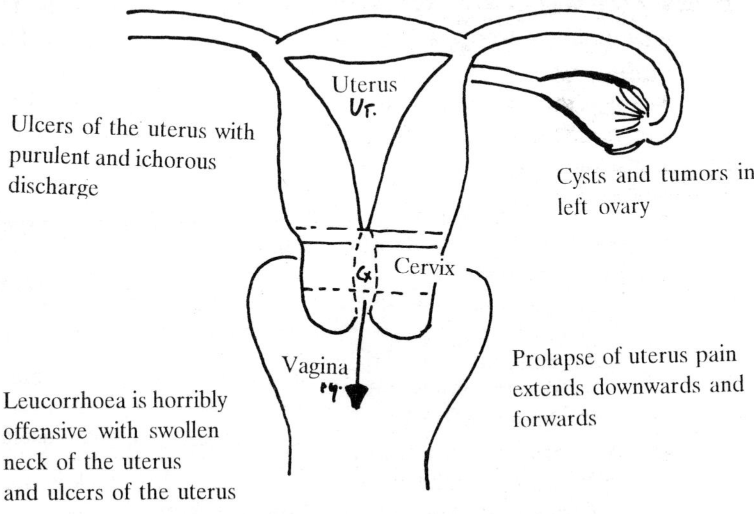
Uterus
Ut.
Ulcers of the uterus with
purulent and ichorous
discharge
Cysts and tumors in
left ovary
Cervix
Vagina
Prolapse of uterus pain
extends downwards and
forwards
Leucorrhoea is horribly
offensive with swollen
neck of the uterus
and ulcers of the uterus

ARGENTUM METALLICUM

2) HEAD
3) NERVOUS SYSTEM
4) CARTILAGE
5) RHEUMATISM
6) RESPIRATORY SYSTEM
7) MALE GENITILIA
8) FEMALE SYMPTOMS
9) CARDIAC DISTURBANCE

MIND

Arg. met has a profound action on the brain.

- Disturbed memory and reasoning faculties.
- Slightest mental effort brings on vertigo.
- All symptoms are aggravated by sleep and hence the patient wakes up in the morning with mental fatigue and weakness.
- Patient jumps from one subject to another.
- "In society indisposition to talk" because he is incompetent; he is mentally tired and looses thread of his discourse.
- Shocks on going to sleep – lower limbs jerk and twitch; he gets out of the bed and walks. Motion relieves symptoms.

HEADACHE

Location – frontal and occipital – one sided headache.

Sensation – violent neuralgia in the head on one side. Pain increases gradually reaching its acme and ceasing suddenly.

Aggravation – exposure to sun.

Scalp :

Tingling, itching and burning in the scalp that causes patient to constantly scratch but it gives no relief.

NERVOUS SYSTEM

- Tearing pains (*neuralgia*) along the nerves predominantly in the lower extremities. Tearing as if the nerves would be torn in pieces during rest.
- *Shocks* go over him when tired like an electric shock. Shocks appear on going to sleep; lower limbs twitch and jerk which make him move out of the bed.

  Worse – going to sleep.

  Amel – motion.
- Arg. met is a principal remedy for *epileptic attacks* which are followed by a delirious rage. As soon as the attack is over the patient jumps about striking those near him.

CARTILAGE

- Infiltrations of cartilages which form *hard knots*.

- Ulcerations begin in the cartilagenous tissue and break out in the cellular tissue with copious discharge.
- Broken down patient with necrosis of cartilage.

Ear – Cartilage of the ear is lumpy, nodular and infiltrated. Intense itching in the ear which involves the whole outside of the ear and the person scratches until it bleeds.

Nose – Thickening of the bones and building up of the mucous membrane and the cellular tissue in the nasal passages.

Eyes – Infiltrations of the lids, thickening of the lids until they are almost as hard as cartilage. Mucous membrane is infiltrated, hard and the eyelids cannot be opened up. Eyes spasmodically close and they cannot be pulled apart except by violence. Blepharitis with thickening and infiltrations.

RHEUMATISM

Cause – Cold damp stormy weather.

Symptoms – Rheumation without swelling. Tearing pains along the joints. Patient has to walk continuously to relieve complaints.

Aggravation – Cold damp weather.

Amelioration – Walking.

RESPIRATORY SYSTEM

Exhausting fluent coryza with sneezing.

Throat

- Throat feels raw and sore on swallowing or coughing.

Larynx

- Hoarseness caused due to overuse of voice in professional singers / speakers.
- Paralytic tendency with aggravation from exertion later leading to total loss of voice.
- When colds settle in the larynx there is a constant *tickling* in the larynx provoking cough.
- *Rawness and soreness* in the upper part of the larynx.
- *Laughing excites cough*, causes tickling in the larynx and the patient scrapes out quantities of grey mucus.
- *Raw spot* over the bifurcation of trachea when using the voice.
- When reading the person has to continuously *hem* and *hawk*.
- Cough is accompanied by *easy (greyish) expectoration*.

  Worse – Warm room.

  Better – Open air.
- *Paralytic weakness* in the chest causing difficult breathing, coughing (Stannum met).
- Arg met is indicated in *pthisis of larynx* which is *painless*.

Pthisis

- Rawness, soreness of larynx.
- Laughing excites cough with easy expectoration.
- Ulceration follows with loss of voice.
- Weakness in the chest.

MALE GENITILIA

Cause – Sexual excess, onanism, abuse of mercury.

Character – Hardness of testes with crushed pain in the right testicle.

- Gonorrhoea – When the discharge remains yellow.
- Pain ceases and urethra and mucous membrane loose their sensation to pain.

FEMALE SYMPTOMS

- **Ovaries** – Cystic tumors with hard and indurated ovaries (left ovary affected).
- **Prolapse of uterus** – Caused by weakness and relaxation of muscles through the whole body. Pain extends forward and downwards.
- *Concomitants* – Congested cervix with yellowish green bloody discharge.
- **Leucorrhoea** – With a horribly unbearable and offensive stench.

Concomitants – Neck of the uterus is swollen and corroded with ulcers in different directions (Kali s, Kali phos).

CARDIAC DISTURBANCE

A sense of trembling in the chest that is carried down to the whole body, hands and feet.

- Frequent palpitation and general weakness.
- Palpitation aggravated when lying on back and during rest.
- Limbs become stiff and numb.

Worse – Rest.

Amelioration – Motion.

General Modalities

Aggravation – REST
SINGING
READING
COLD WET WEATHER
REST IN RHEUMATISM
AND HEART COMPLAINTS

Relations :

Remedies that follow well – Calcarea, Puls, Sepia.

Antidotes – Merc, Puls.

Important Questions ?

Q. 1. Give respiratory symptoms of Argentum met.
[1973, 77, 87 S, 95]

Q. 2. Give difference between respiratory symptoms of Arg. met and Drosera. [1993]

ARGENTUM MET	DROSERA.
• Arg met is indicated in *laryngitis, laryngeal pthisis*.	• Drosera is indicated in *whooping cough, laryngitis, pthisis of larynx and lungs.*
• Throat and larynx feel ***raw and sore*** on swallowing and coughing.	• Sensation of ***feather*** in the larynx that excites cough. Cramping constriction in the larynx.
• *Hoarseness* caused due to overuse of voice in *professional singers*.	• Voice is *hoarse*, deep, toneless, cracked and requires *great exertion to speak.*
• *Paralytic* tendency of larynx with aggravation from exertion later leading to total loss of voice.	• *Clergymans sore throat* with rough scraping and dry sensation deep in the fauces.
• When cold settles in the larynx there is a constant *tickling* provoking cough.	• Deep hoarse barking *nocturnal cough*. With cough there is *vomiting of mucus* and *bleeding* from nose and mouth.
• Laughing excites cough.	• *Spasmodic difficulties* in the chest and larynx causing difficult breathing. **Pale, becomes purple** from *spasm* and *suffocation* later leading to copious sweat all over the body.
• *Raw spot* over bifurcation of trachea.	
• Cough is accompanied by easy *grey expectoration*	• No expectoration and even if there is, it is *greenish yellow*.
• **Aggravation** – Talking, singing, cold wet weather.	• **Aggravation** – Midnight, lying down, laughing, singing.

12. ARGENTUM NITRICUM

J.O. Muller

Common Name – Silver nitrate.

Miasm – Sycotic and syphilitic with psora in background.

Constitution – Adapted to impulsive, apprehensive people having a Carbonitrogenoid or Hydrogenoid constitution.

Look of the patient – Withered dried up old looking patients due to diseases caused by continued mental exertion.

Temperament – Bilious temperament. Very irritable and becomes angry easily.

Relation with heat and cold – Hot patient.

Diathesis – Neurosycotic.

KEYNOTES

1) ***Hot patient*** – Desires cold things, cold drinks which relieve all but gastric symptoms.
2) ***Withered dried up persons*** made so by disease. Complaints are caused due to mental exertion.
3) *Emaciation* is most marked in lower extremities (Abrot, Nat mur).
4) Great remedy for ***terrors of anticipation*** . When the patient is ready to go out for a public meeting or examination – ***diarrhoea*** *sets in* (Gels).
5) ***Time passes slowly*** – Patient is impulsive and wants to do everything in a hurry (Aurum, Lil. T).
6) *Hemicrania* – With a sensation as if head is *expanding.*

    Aggravation – Mental labour.

    Amelioration – Pressure of tight bandage (Apis/Puls).
7) Great ***longing for fresh air.***
8) Eyes – Granular conjunctivitis with *profuse mucopurulent discharge*. Opthalmia Neonatorum – with purulent discharge, cornea is opaque and ulcerated. Lids are sore and thick, swollen and agglutinated in the morning (Apis, Merc sol, Rhus tox).
9) Sensation of a *Splinter* in the throat when swallowing (Nit acid, Hepar sulph, Silicea).
10) *Chronic Laryngitis* of singers, higher notes cause cough.
11) *Craves sugar* – but diarrhoea results from eating sugar.

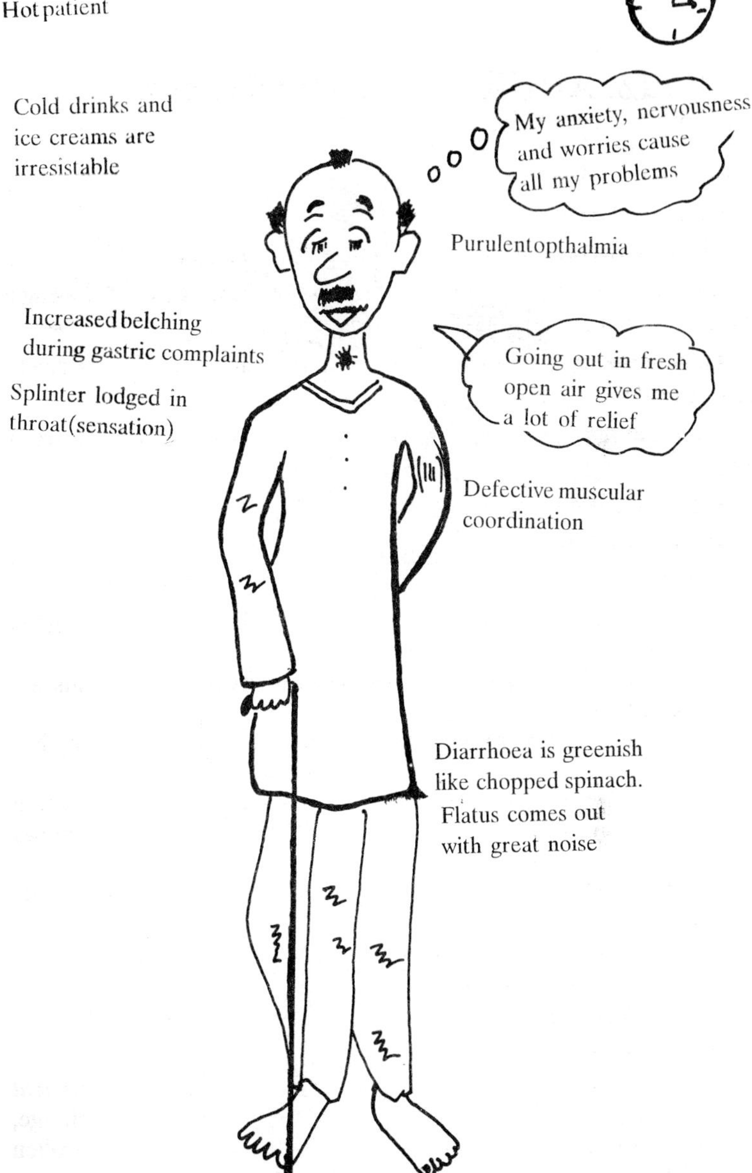

ARGENTUM NITRICUM

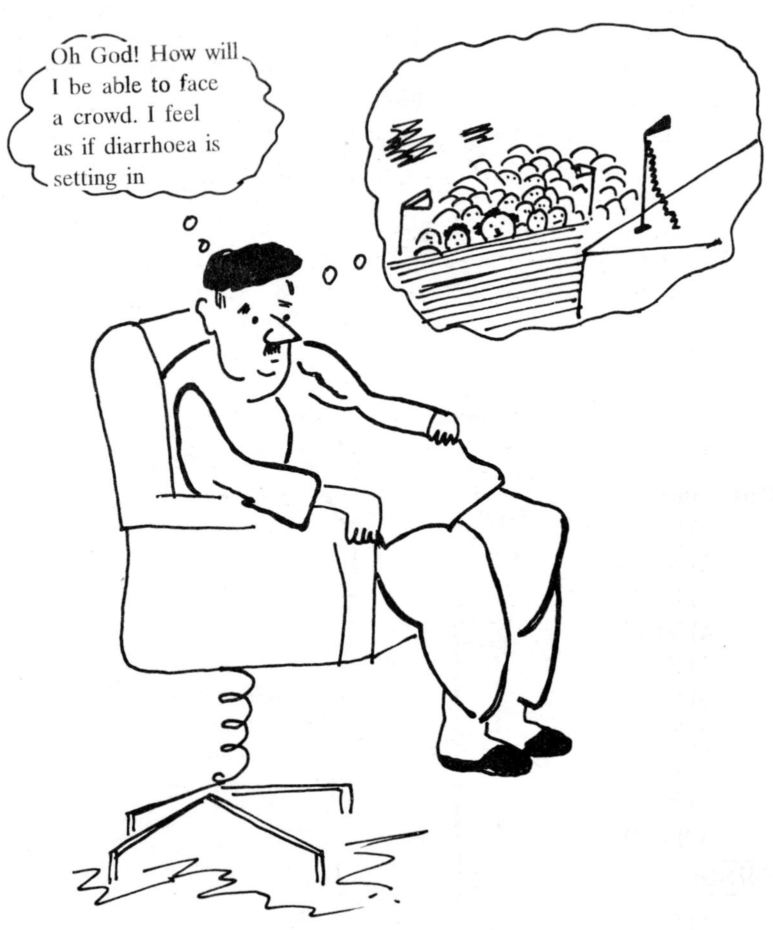
Oh God! How will I be able to face a crowd. I feel as if diarrhoea is setting in

ARGENTUM NITRICUM

12) *Belching* accompanies most gastric complaints.

13) *Diarrhoea caused due to sugar, mental exertion, apprehension, taking cold things*. Diarrhoea with *much noisy flatus*. Stools – chopped spinach flakes and turn green after remaining on diaper.

14) Urine passes unconciously day and night.

15) Coition painful in both sexes followed by bleeding from vagina.

16. *Metrorrhagia* – In young widows, in sterility with nervous erethism at the change of life.

17. *Defective coordination of muscles*. Great weakness of lower extremities with trembling. Cannot walk with eyes closed (Alumina).

18) *Epilepsy* caused by fright or during menses.
- Hours or days before the attack pupils dilate.
- Convulsions are preceded by great restlessness.

19) Chilly when uncovered, yet feels smothered if wrapped up.

Particulars :

1) MIND
2) NERVOUS SYSTEM
3) HEADACHE
4) VERTIGO
5) EYES
6) FACE
7) THROAT
8) G.I.T.
9) BACK
10) CHILD

MIND

1) Person has *terrors of anticipation* – His nervousness in anticipation may bring on diarrhoea (Gels).

2) Arg. nit is indicated in *examination funk*-anxiety caused due to fear of failure.

3) Patient is tormented by *troublesome thoughts*. He is always in a hurry and the faster he walks, the faster he thinks he must walk. He walks till fatigued.

4) *Inflowing of strange thoughts :*
- Patient *avoids going around the corner* of a street for the fear that he will do something strange.
- There is great *fear of projecting buildings* lest they would fall on him.

- While crossing a bridge or high place or while looking out of the window the patient thinks he might *jump off*.
- *Claustrophobia* – The patient wants to sit at the end of seat in a pew ; wants to be near the door so that he can have an easy escape.
- Sight of high houses makes him stagger and he becomes dizzy.

NERVOUS SYSTEM

Imperfect coordination of muscles

- Due to continued *mental exertion* or mental anxiety, nervous excitement, trembling, organic heart and liver diseases begin. This state of mind leads to weakness, trembling, paralysis, numbness, disturbed functions, palpitation and throbbing all over.

This nervous state continues until there is disorder of all the organs.

- Dyspepsia.
- Disturbed circulation with fullness of blood vessels and throbbing all over.
- Atheromatous degeneration and dilatation of veins.
- Ulceration on mucous membrane and skin.
- Heart becomes feeble – lips and extremities become cold and blue.

Aggravation – Mental exertion, stuffy and warm clothing suffocate.

Amelioration – Open air.

- *Paraplegia* after long continued diseases.
- *Post diptheritic paralysis*.
- *Numbness* in the forearms at night. There is numb sensitiveness of the skin of the arms i.e. increased sensitiveness to touch but diminished power of distinguishing sensations.
- *Epilepsy* – Arg nit is very useful where indications are :

  a) Dilatation of the pupils hours or days before the attack.

  b) Great restlessness following the attack with trembling of hands.
- *Locomotor Ataxia* :

  a) Defective coordination of muscles.

  b) Cannot walk with eyes closed.

  c) Legs are weak and calves feel bruised.

  d) Soreness and pain in back aggravated when rising from sitting. Amelioration-walking.

  e) Trembling of hands-patient drops things.

  f) Symptoms aggravate at 11 A.M.

HEADACHE

Hemicrania :

Cause – Mental excitation, emotions, loss of animal fluids.

Location – Left frontal eminance.

Sensation – Patient feels head is expanding. Boring pain in the head such that patient may loose consciousness.

Amelioration – Tight bandage, open air.

VERTIGO

Vertigo is accompanied with buzzing in the ears, general debility and trembling. Patient cannot walk without eyes open and the sight of high houses makes him dizzy.

EYES

Purulent Opthalmia – Inflammation with intense chemosis, strangulated vessels and most profuse purulent discharge. Cornea begins to get hazy and looks as if it would slough. With a *profuse purulent discharge*, lids are swollen from a collection of pus in the eyes or there is swelling of subconjunctival tissue.

Photophobia – With intolerance of light.

Blepharitis – Thick crusts on the lids with suppuration and induration of tissues.

In **Opthalmia neonatorum** Arg nit is a very useful remedy.

FACE

In *Prosopalgia* (Trigeminal Neuralgia) – Infra orbital branches of fifth pair and the nerves going to the teeth are affected. At the height of pain the face is sunken pale, bluish and looks prematurely old. This is accompanied with unpleasant sour taste.

THROAT

- Thick tenacious mucus in the throat causing hawking and cough.
- Sensation as if *splinter* is lodged in the throat (Hepar S. Nit acid).
- Wart like excrecenses which feel like pointed bodies when swallowing. This may involve the larynx in singers and clergymen.
- Uvula and fauces are dark red.

HEPAR	ARG. NITRICUM
• Desires warm room, warm clothing and the patient cannot put his hand out of bed or his head would begin paining.	• Desires cold room, cold air which relieves all his complaints, mental exertion, warm and stuffy rooms aggravate the patients complaints.

G.I.T.

Tongue – Red painful tip of tongue with erect papillae.

Dyspepsia – Pain caused due to over indulging in ice creams and other cooling dainties. Pain radiates from pit of stomach to all directions. When pain becomes excess there is vomiting of glairy stringy mucus.

Belching – After every meal belching is very violent. Eructation relieves the patient's uneasiness. Deathly and violent nausea.

Flatulence – Wind rumbles in the abdomen which the patient finds hard to expel. When the patient succeeds in expelling, it comes out with great noise. Stomach feels as if it would burst.

CHINA	CARBO VEG	ARG. NIT.
Distended stomach and every little while the patient gets up the gas with no relief.	Distended and full to bursting and he cannot get up any wind. Pain and distension are relieved finally by passage of wind.	Eructations relieve. *Frequent belching* and passage of noisy flatus.

Diarrhoea – a) Nervous Diarrhoea.

b) Due to gastric disorder.

Nervous Diarrhoea – It sets in when the patient is ready to go out in a public meeting or examination etc. Due to increasing anticipation and nervousness,diarrhoea sets in.

Character of stool – Watery stools with intolerable offensiveness. As the person starts performing his task,diarrhoea disappears and the patient feels fine.

Gastric Disorders :

Cause – Sugar (Irresistable desire to eat sugar but it causes gastric upset with diarrhoea.) cold drinks, ice creams, mental exertion.

Sensation :

As if abdomen would burst.

Stool – Green mucous like chopped spinach in flakes.

- Stools turn green after remaining in diaper.

- Stools expelled with much spluttering.
- Stools are shreddy, red, green, mucolymph epithelial substance.
- During stool there is emission of much noisy flatus.

Amelioration – After passing flatus, belching, open air and pressure.

BACK

- Pain in the back when the patient rises from the seat.
- Pain may be caused due to flatus.

Aggravation – Rising from a seat.

Amelioration – Walking, standing.

CHILD

- Child looks withered and dried up.
- Emaciation is more marked in the lower extremities.
- Great weakness and trembling of lower extremities.
- Patient cannot walk except with eyes open.
- Marasmus in children who crave sugar but have diarrhoea after that.
- Nervous children who have diarrhoea when taken to some gathering.
- Child is very hasty.
- Patient desires cold drinks, cold air and is averse to warmth.

General Modalities :

Aggravation – SWEETS
COLD FOOD, COLD AIR
ICE CREAMS
CONTINUED MENTAL EXERTION

Amelioration – OPEN AIR
BATHING IN COLD WATER
CRAVES – WIND BLOWING ON HIS FACE.
TIGHT BANDAGING.

Relations :

Antidoted by – Natrum mur for bad affects of cauterisation with silver nitrate.
Antidote to – Nitric acid, Sepia, Puls, Calc. carb.
Inimical to – Coffea.

Important Questions ?

Q. 1. Give indications of Argentum nitricum in the following :

1) Desires / aversions [1991]
2) Headache [1984]
3) Diarrhoea [1972 s, 73, 74, 75, 95]

4) Mind [1973, 74, 75, 79, 81, 87, 93]
5) Child / Marasmus [1973, 76, 82]
6) Eyes [1977, 79, 81]
7) Throat [1981]
8) Keynotes [1978, 82]

Q. 2. Give difference between mental symptoms of Arg nit and Cocculus. [1991]

Cocculus :

- Time passes too quickly.
- Thoughts are fixed on a single disagreeable subject – patient is absorbed in thoughts and notices nothing about her.
- Sits in deep revive.
- Sudden extreme anxiety.
- Ill effects of anger and grief.

Q. 3. Give difference between gastric symptoms of Merc cor / Arg nit.

ARG. NIT.	MERC. COR.
• Cause of Gastric disorder a) Mental anxiety b) Sugar c) Ice cold things	• Cause of Gastric disorder – Summer weather.
• Nausea after eating. • Painful swelling in pit of the stomach with great anxiety.	• Tenesmus persists before during or after stool.
• Vomiting and diarrhoea with violent colicky pains.	• Bloated abdomen which is very painful to least touch.
• Sensation as if abdomen would burst.	• Dysentry with violent urging to stool.
• Colic wakes the person from uneasy slumbers.	• Stools are hot, scanty, bloody, slimy and offensive. There may be passage of pure blood.
• Evacuation of greenish very foetid mucus with a great quantity of noisy flatus.	*Concomitants :* • Unquenchable thirst. • Swollen tongue • Scanty urine which is hot and bloody. • Cramps in calf muscles • Faintness, weakness and shuddering.
• Stools are greenish like chopped spinach flakes accompanied with noisy flatus.	

13. ARNICA MONTANA

Hahnemann

Common Name – Leopards bane (Compositae)

Miasam – Psora in the background.

Arnica is a *short acting remedy but prompt.*

Constitution – Nervous women, sanguine plethoric persons, lively expression with a very red face.

Relation with heat and cold – Chilly patient.

Temperament – Nervous temperament.

KEYNOTES

1) Arnica affects the ***walls of capillaries causing extravasation of blood*** and hence used in trauma.
2) ***Sore lame bruised*** feeling all through the body as if beaten; traumatic affections of muscles.
3) Whole body *oversensitive* – cannot bear pain.
4) Everything on which the patient lies seems *too hard* – patient is very *restless* due to pain and hence keeps moving from one place to another (Baptisia, Pyrogen, Rhus tox).
5) In concussions, contusions, results of shock or injury without laceration of soft parts. Arnica prevents *suppuration and septic* conditions and promotes absorption.
6) *Heat* of upper parts of the body and *coldness* of lower parts.
7) *Offensive* eructations or flatus, smelling like rotten eggs.
8) In *Delirium* – when spoken to, the patient answers correctly but unconciousness and delirium return at once (In Baptisia – patient falls asleep in midst of a sentence).
9) Stupor with ***involuntary discharge of feaces and urine.***
10) Conjunctival / *retinal heamorrhages* with extravasation from injuries or cough (Ledum, Nux vom).
11) *Child cries before a paroxysm of cough as if sore.*
12) Gout and rheumatism with great fear of being touched or struck by person coming near him.
13) *Soreness* of parts *after labor* – Prevents heamorrhage or pyemia.
14) Tendency to small painful *boils* one after another, extremely sore (small boils in crops-Sulph.).
15) Local application of Arnica produces extraordinary *growth of hair* and checks falling of hair.

Particulars :

1) INJURY
2) EYES
3) WHOOPING COUGH
4) G.I.T.
5) URINARY SYSTEM
6) FEMALE SYMPTOMS
7) JOINTS
8) FEVER
9) SKIN

INJURY

Acute Injury

Arnica is indicated from simple bruises to fracture of skull with compression of brain; headaches of long standing; meningitis; apoplexy; inflammation of eyes, retinal heamorrhages; expedites absorption of blood clots; deafness; epistaxis, affections from blows on stomach etc.

- Due to *relaxed blood vessels* there is easy exravasation of blood and blue spots come easily upon the skin and mucous membrane.
- ***Sore, lame, bruised*** feeling – oversensitive to pain.
- Everything on which the patient lies seems *too hard* so that patient keeps constantly moving.
- Arnica prevents sepsis.

Muscles (Myalgia)

Heamorrhages of mechanical origin; heavy lifting,when a person has been working labouriously and in consequence the whole body feels sore and bruised. This may later lead to hypertrophy of heart. [As a result of hypertrophy the patient complains of swelling of the hands on any exertion. Hands become red and arms swell when they are permitted to hang down. The heart feels as though tightly grasped by hands (Cactus)]

Fracture – Arnica relieves swelling and tumefaction of the limb and also relieves twitching of the muscles.

Meningitis – After mechanical injury, from falls, concussion of brain with involuntary evacuation from bowels and bladder.

Chronic effects of injury

Arnica is used in diseases which may be traced to a traumatic origin.

Injuries recieved years ago resulting in tremors, paralysis, rheumatism (Arnica is infallible). No matter what the disease may be of brain, eyes, lungs or nerves, if injury is the exciting cause administration of Arnica is proper.

Arnica : Suited to acute and chronic affects of injury. Injured parts turn blue and feel sore and bruised. Arnica prevents sepsis.

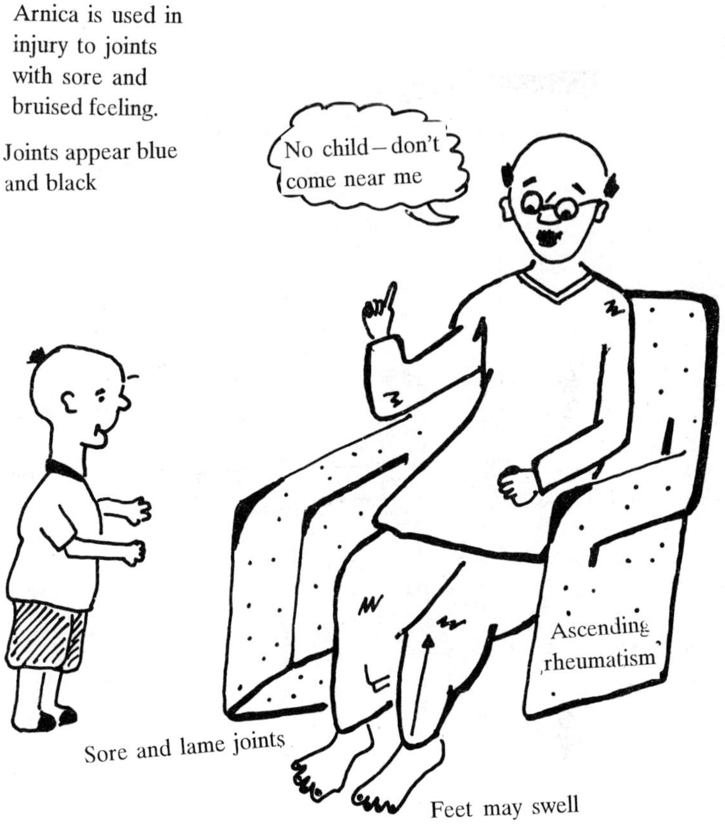

Arnica is used in injury to joints with sore and bruised feeling.

Joints appear blue and black

No child – don't come near me

Ascending rheumatism

Sore and lame joints

Feet may swell

ARNICA MONTANA

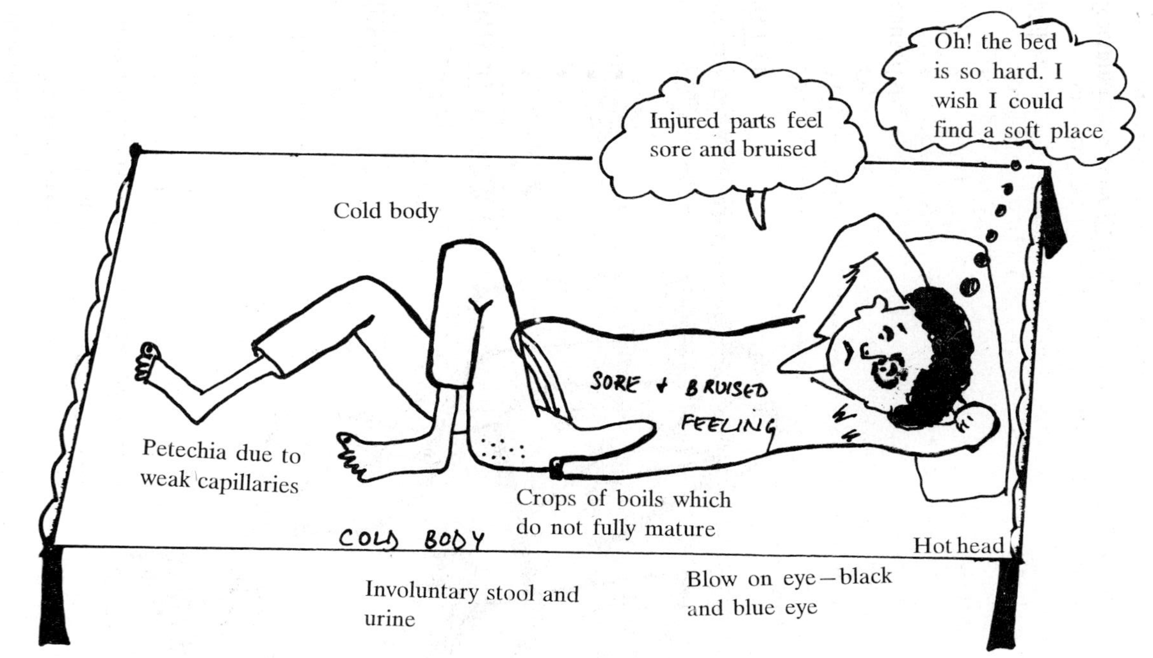

ARNICA MONTANA

Typhoid fever

Rhus tox : Ligaments of joints are involved in injury. Patient is very restless.

Calendula : Injury causes a ragged wound with loss of substance.

Hypericum : Nerves have been injured along with soft parts. Pain along the nerves.

Staphysagria : Smooth clean cuts made by surgeon's knife.

Ledum : Injuries inflicted by pointed instruments and hence used in punctured wounds. Punctured part feels cold to touch.

Symphytum : Mechanical injuries due to blow with blunt instruments. Used in bone injuries or irritable stump after amputation at point of fracture.

Conium : Induration of glands caused by contusions and bruises. Indicated especially when hardness becomes intense.

Anacardium : Tendons are affected.

EYES

Inflammation of eyes with suggilations after mechanical injuries, blows etc. In retinal haemorrhages Arnica expedites absorption of clots.

WHOOPING COUGH

Violent tickling cough excited whenever child becomes angry.

- Sore and bruised feeling all over.
- Child is cross and fretful.
- Child cries before paroxysms due to fear of soreness caused later.

Character of cough – Spasmodic cough with expectoration of blood or dark blood streaked mucus. Vomiting of food with black mucus.

G.I.T.

Aversion to meat, broth, milk.

Thirst – Patient is generally thirstless except in chill stage of fever.

Dyspepsia – Arnica is a great remedy for dyspepsia (dyspepsia caused due to injury).

- Discharges (stools and flatus) are offensive.
- Tympanites is excessive and the abdomen feels full to bursting.
- Loud and continuous belching.

Soreness in pelvis (Dr. Nash cured a case of dyspepsia caused by kick of a horse upon the region of stomach).

Constipation – *Cause* : Enlargement of prostate, retroverted uterus. Rectum is loaded with feaces which is not easily expelled.

Character of stool – Ribbon like stools. Stools and flatus are offensive.

Dysentry – With ischuria, fruitless urging and long intervals between stools.

URINARY SYSTEM

Used in bladder affections after mechanical injuries.

- Retention of urine from exertion.
- Tenesmus from spasms of neck of bladder.
- Constant urging while urine passes involuntarily in drops.
- Ischuria with dysentry.
- Heamaturia from mechanical causes.

In *nephritis* – violent chill followed by extreme nephritic pain with nausea and vomiting.

- Pain extends from right hypochondrium down to the groin.
- Retention with urging to urinate.
- Urine may be thick, with much pus and blood.

FEMALE

Arnica is used in *threatened abortion* due to falls and shocks. Sore and bruised feeling in the pelvis.

After Abortion / Confinement – Arnica promotes proper contraction of uterus and expulsion of any foreign substance such as portions of placenta or membrane that are left behind.

- Arnica cures constant dribbling of urine after labor.
- It has been known to check heamorrhage after parturition (Chin, Bell, Secale cor).

JOINTS

Gout / rheumatism

Cause – Winter weather, cold dampness as a result of chronic affects of injury.

Type – Ascending type of rheumatism (Ledum)

(Descending – Cactus, Kalmia)

Character of pain – joints are swollen, sore and lame.

- Rheumatic lameness with feeling as if bruised.
- Patient is oversensitive and does not want to be approached.
- Pain extends from legs and feet upwards.
- Feet often swell and feel sore and bruised.

Worse – Motion, touching.

Better – Lying down.

- *Injury* to joints with soreness, lameness, a black and blue appearance of it.

FEVER

Typhoid

- Passive congestion of brain causes drowsiness and indifference to those around him.

Delirium

- Patient falls asleep after answering a question and then delirium returns. Patient calls for a doctor and later refuses and says that there is no need for a doctor.
- Hot head and cold body.
- Sore and bruised feeling all over the body so that bed feels hard to him and he keeps searching for a soft spot on which to rest.
- Tongue shows a brown streak down the middle.
- When the lungs are affected there is cough with expectoration of mucus and blood.
- Pressure of blood on brain produces apoplectic symptoms and breathing becomes heavy and stertorous.
- Petechia appear on skin due to weakening of capillaries.
- Stool and urine are passed involuntarily.
- Tip of nose is cold to touch.
- Discharges (stool, flatus) are very offensive.

Arnica is also used in malarial fever with sore and bruised feeling, restlessness; thirst during chill stage and offensive discharges.

SKIN

Erisipelas – Parts look dark and blue.

- Numerous semitransparent vesicles with red basis merge together and the whole area becomes phlegmonous.
- Extreme tenderness with numerous bullae. Heat, swelling and shining hardness give it the appearance of septicemia.

Boils – Crops of boils all over the body. Arnica is indicated when boils and abscesses have partially matured but instead of discharging they shrivel up due to absorption of contaminated pus. (Arnica given internally and applied externally redevelops the abscess.)

Pyemia – Arnica promotes evacuation of pus and promotes the appearance of pus on surfare of a sore. It is thus used in operations to prevent pyemia.

General Modalities :

Aggravation – LEAST TOUCH
MOTION
DAMP COLD WEATHER

Amelioration – LYING DOWN.

Relations :

Complementry to – Aconite, Hyper, Rhus tox.

Follows well – Acon, Apis, Ham, Ipec, Vert alb.

Important Questions ?

Q. 1 Give indications of Arnica in the following:

1) Typhoid [1973, 74, 77, 81, 19]

2) Rheumatism [1975, 76, 77, 85, 95]
3) Injury [1973, 76, 78 S, 82, 89]
4) Mentals [1975, 77]
5) Cough [195]
6) Paralysis [1979]
7) Peurperal Sepsis [1979]
8) Threatened abortion [1978]

Q. 2. Give difference between Delirium of Arnica / Baptisia. [1991]

ARNICA	BAPTISIA
• Sore, lame, bruised feeling all over.	• Sore lame and bruised feeling all over.
• Low muttering delirium and stupor.	• Low muttering delirium.
• Patient answers correctly but again lapses into stupor.	• Patient falls asleep in the middle of the answer.
• Patient calls for a doctor but later says that he is fine.	• Delusion as if the body is scattered and tosses about to get the pieces together.

Q.3. Difference between injury of Bellis perennis / Arnica.

BELLIS PERENNIS :

- Princely remedy for old labourers especially gardeners.
- Acts upon muscular fibres of blood vessels.
- Venous congestion due to mechanical causes.
- Used in injuries to the deeper tissues after major surgical work.
- Indicated in injuries to nerves with intense soreness and intolerance of cold bathing.
- Sore and bruised feeling in pelvic region.
- Excellent for sprains and bruises.
- Complaints due to cold food or drink when the body is heated and in affections due to cold wind.
- Venous congestion due to mechanical causes.
- Boils are numerous and are sensitive to touch.

14. ARSENICUM ALBUM

Hahnemann

Common Name – Arsenious acid – Arsenic Trioxide (Deadly poison which produces cholera like symptoms).

Miasm – Psora, syphilis and sycosis.

Arsenic alb is generally not given in the beginning of diseases. Tendency of symptoms is deathward.

Constitution – Patient is anxious, fearful and restless. He has a pale, waxy, earth coloured skin with a tendency to emaciation and great debility.

Temperament – Fastidious patient.

Relations with heat and cold – Chilly patient (patient desires hot but wants to keep the head cool).

Diathesis – Scrofulous diathesis.

KEYNOTES

1) ***Mentally restless but physically too weak to move.***
2) Great ***prostration*** with rapid sinking of vital strength. While lying in the bed the patient is so restless that he keeps moving his limbs until he becomes so weak that he lies in perfect quietness. Restlessness goes towards cadaveric aspect i.e. towards death.
3) *Fear of death* – Patient thinks that it is useless to take medicines, that he is incurable and that he is surely going to die.
4) ***Burning pains*** – Sensation as if coals of fire were applied to the part. Burning pains are ameliorated by heat. (Burning pain in Ars. is due to progressing destruction of tissues and not merely from a nervous cause).
5) *Thirst* – Despite unquenchable thirst the patient drinks little water at a time. (This is so because as soon as the patient drinks water he vomits it out and hence drinks little at a time.)
6) *Cannot bear smell or sight of food* (eating and drinking cause vomiting and diarrhoea).
7) Discharges are *acrid, burning, corossive* and have a *cadaverous odour*.
8) Tendency to *bleeding* from mucous membranes.

9) *Periodicity* of complaints is marked. Patient has midnight aggravtion (1-2 A.M. and 1-2 P.M.).

10) Ars is excellent for *intermittent fever* because of its tendency to produce periodicity of complaints with intense restlessness, burning, prostration.

Chill Stage – Patient desires hot drinks. Sensation as if blood running through the vessels is ice-water.

Heat Stage – Desires cold drinks – drinks little and often.

Sweat Stage (sweat relieves) – Unquenchable thirst for cold drinks.

11) *Asthma* – Complaints are aggravated at midnight. Patient is unable to lie down for fear of suffocation.

12) Aggravation – Cold things, cold air, 1-2 A.M. motion.

Amelioration – Warm air or room, hot application, sweat.

Summary – ANXIETY
BURNING
CADAVEROUS ODOUR
RESTLESSNESS
PROSTRATION
MIDNIGHT Aggravation

Particulars :

1) MIND
2) INTERMITTENT FEVER
3) HEAD
4) EYES
5) HEART
6) RESPIRATORY SYMPTOMS
7) G.I.T.
8) MALE GENITALS
9) FEMALE SYMPTOMS
10) SKIN

MIND

- Patient is very *anxious* and *fearful.* He feels that there is no need to take a medicine as his disease is incurable. Patient does not predict the time of death unlike the Aconite patient.
- *Gold headed cane patient* – patient is very fastidious and wants everything in order, neat and clean. Even a picture hanging on the wall must be adjusted properly.
- Mental *restlessness* with physical weakness. Patient tries to move himself from place to place but because of the intense weakness he becomes exhausted.

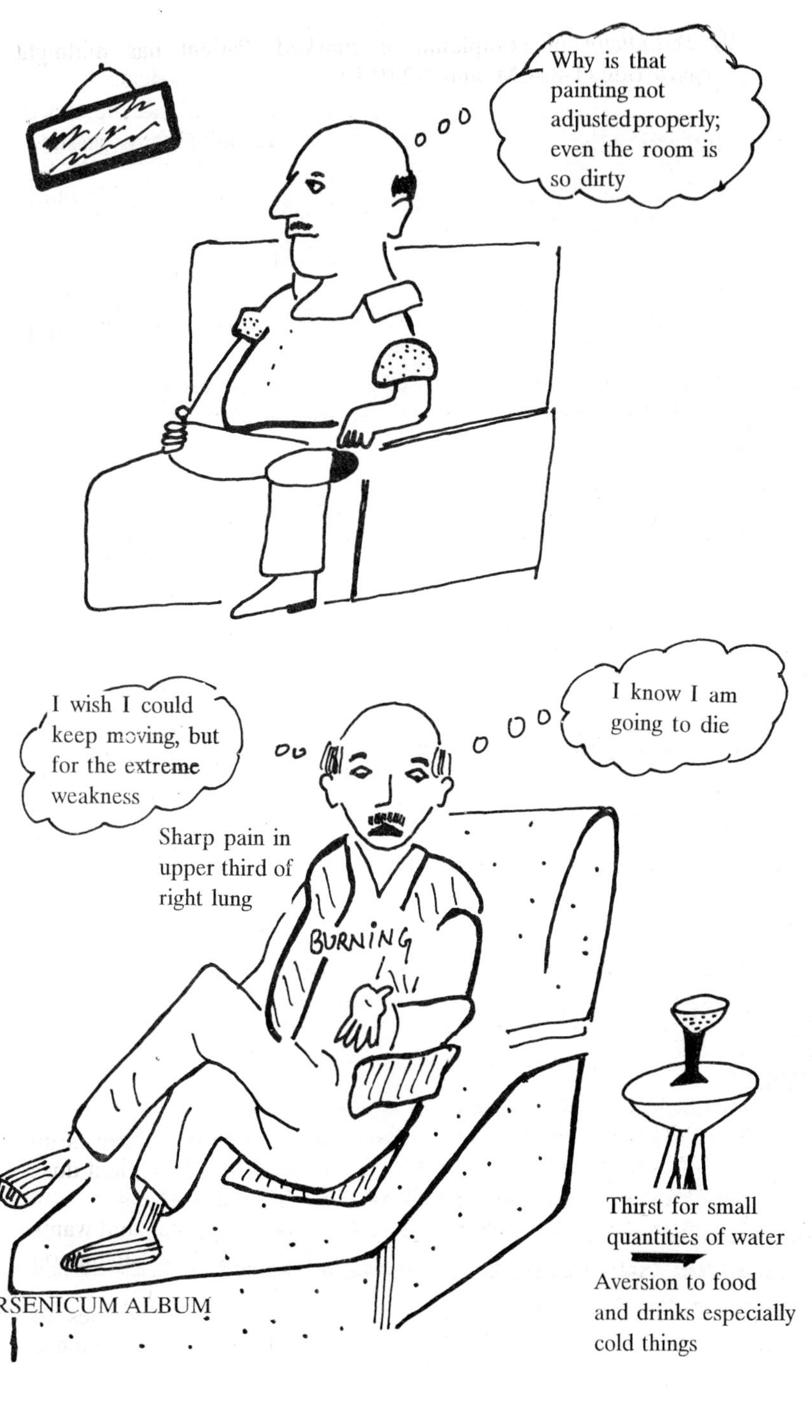
Why is that painting not adjusted properly; even the room is so dirty
I wish I could keep moving, but for the extreme weakness
I know I am going to die
Sharp pain in upper third of right lung
BURNING
Thirst for small quantities of water
Aversion to food and drinks especially cold things

ARSENICUM ALBUM

- Patient *loathes life* and has a tendency to commit suicide.

ARSENIC ALB	ACONITE
• Patient does not want to call a doctor as he feels that his disease is incurable.	• Patient feels that unless proper medicine is taken he will not survive and hence calls for a doctor.
• Does not predict the time of death.	• Predicts the time of death.
• Restlessness comes in later stages when the patient looses strength.	• Restlessness in early stages of the disease with high grade fever.
• Due to great weakness the patient becomes terribly exhausted on least exertion.	• Patient is strong and robust and hence constantly keeps moving.

INTERMITTENT FEVER

Arsenic produces marked periodicity. It thus is used in malarial fever and relapsing typhoid fever. Paroxysms generally occur between 1-2 P.M. and 12-2 A.M. Paroxysms come every 14 days or there may be yearly return of symptoms.

Chill Stage – desire for warm drinks and the patient wants to cover up warmly. There is intense restlessness with anxiety, fear and prostration. Sensation as if blood flowing through the vessels is ice water.

Heat Stage – patient desires cold drinks but drinks little and often. Sensation as if boiling water is flowing through the vessels.

Sweat Stage – Relieves complaints. Patient has unquenchable thirst for cold drinks.

Apyrexia – Patient craves for fresh drinks, wine, coffee, lemonade.

Concomitants – restlessness, prostration, anxiety, fear of death. Midnight aggravation of complaints.

HEAD

Headaches also show *periodicity* like malarial fever.

- There is *alteration of states* i.e. head symptoms alternate with physical symptoms.

Rheumatism that the patient is suffering from may disappear and sick headaches may come on. "There may be increased pressure on top of the head relieved by hard pressure. This may disappear leading to constant urging to urinate."

Character of pain – Congestive headaches with throbbing pain relieved by keeping the head cool. Intense anxiety and restlessness. Scalp is very sensitive to touch.

Aggravation – heat, motion.

Amelioration – cold application.

EYES

Ars is indicated in opthalmia, chronic trachoma, keratitis, iritis, retinitis etc.

- Eyelids are swollen and oedematous.
- Intense photophobia.
- Lachrymation is scalding making eyelids and cheeks sore.
- Everything the patient looks at seems green to him.
- Nocturnal aggravation.

Also indicated in half sights where the patient can see the lower half of the objects.

HEART

Ars. is indicated in angina, rheumatism of heart, hydropericardium.

- There is great weakness and palpitation.
- Any motion increases palpitation.
- Dyspnoea is aggravated on ascending.
- Pulse is frequent,small and thread like.
- Patient is pale and cold covered with cold sweat.
- In angina the patient is relieved by bending forward.
- Great restlessness and anxiety.

RESPIRATORY SYMPTOMS

Nose

Coryza – used in 'winter colds' with sneezing.

- Patient has a fluent discharge which corrodes the wings of the nose and the lips.
- Sneezing starts from irritation in one spot in the nose as from tickling with a feather.
- Repeated catarrah leads to thick yellowish mucopurulent discharge later forming ulcers and scabs in the nose.

Diptheria – Ars. is a valuable drug. Patient has a foetid breath with fever and a great deal of somnolence which is broken by starts, crying out and jerking limbs. Membrane looks dark and gangrenous.

Laryngitis

- Burning pain in the larynx.
- Hoarse voice.
- Constant tittilating cough induced by a sensation of sulphur vapour.

Asthma *caused due to suppressed eruptions (eczema, measles).*

Symptoms :

- Dyspnoea is aggravated at midnight and by lying down.
- At night the patient suffocates and becomes bathed in profuse perspiration.
- His limbs become cold and stiff.
- Wheezing respiration with frothy expectoration.
- Patient is unable to move without being greatly put out of breath.
- Air passages seem constricted.

Amelioration – Coughing and throwing off mucus with a tenacious viscid character.

Pneumonia – In last stage of pneumonia with gangrenous expectoration.

Important indications – ***Acute sharp darting pain in the apex and through upper third of right lung.***

G.I.T.

Mouth – dry and cracked lips

- Bleeding gums with foetid breath.
- Mouth is dry apthous, ulcerated or gangrenous.

Tongue – Dry and red tongue with raised papillae. Red with indented edge. Dry brown black as in typhoids.

Thirst – Unquenchable thirst but drinks little at time for fear of vomiting.

Stomach (Gastritis) :

Cause : Least food and drink especially cold, ice cream, cold drinks, alcohol, sausage, food poisoning.

Character – Least food and drink excite vomiting or stool or both together.

- Distressing heart burn with burning in the stomach like coals of fire.
- Vomiting of bile, blood and coffee ground substances.
- Extreme sensitiveness of the stomach and the patient does not want to be touched.

Amelioration – Drinking little hot water comforts the patient for sometime. Heat applied externally relieves the patient.

Diarrhoea – *Cause* – eating and drinking.

Character – Stools are watery. Black bloody and horribly offensive. Intense abdominal pain causes the patient to twist and turn in every direction.

Concomitants – Anxiety, pallor, fear of death and restlessness.

Dysentry

- Involuntary passage of urine and feaces.
- Stools – bloody, watery, black and horribly offensive.
- Burning in the anus as if there were coals of fire in the rectum.

Relief—Pain in the abdomen and rectum is relieved by hot application.

Gastroenteritis—Which takes on a gangrenous character (Ars. is an excellent medicine).

Cholera :

Cause—eating and drinking cold things, old and decayed food.

Symptoms—intense vomiting and purging.

- Dark black watery stool with horribly offensive odour.
- Burning in the anus during and after stools.

Look of the patient—Patient is prostrated with cold sweat, cold extremities and intense restlessness. Foul and pungent odour in the room.

Aggravation—Midnight.

MALE GENITALS

- Dropsy of penis or scrotum with oedematous appearance.
- Syphilitic bubo with ulcer on the genitilia which may be gangrenous.
- Granulations are florid and bleed from slightest touch.
- From the ulcer oozes a watery corossive and offensive secretion.
- Coffee coloured eruption on the skin may be present.

FEMALE SYMPTOMS

Menses—Profuse, acrid and excoriating.

Leucorrhoea—Excoriating the parts causing itching and burning.

After labor—Atonacity of bladder after parturition. Patient feels no desire to pass urine even if the bladder is full.

SKIN

Troubles caused by suppressed eczema or exanthemata. Skin is pale dry and waxy.

Urticaria—Wheals are attended with burning, itching and restlessness.

Gangrene—'Dry Gangrene'. Buccal cavity, scrotum, sexual parts, lower limbs are more prone to develop gangrene. Gangrene in internal organs, malignant inflammation, erisipelatous inflammations. Inflammation may take on a malignant character.

In bowels—inflammation will be attended with horribly offensive discharge, vomiting of clots of blood with burning in the bowels and tympanic condition.

Concomitants—anxiety, prostration, fear of death and chilliness (patient wants to be covered warmly).

(Secale cor—Similar condition but patient desires cold air and cold drinks.)

Ulcers – Ulcers of cancerous character with elevated edges having great burning. Discharge is thin, watery, bloody with fetid pus. Ulcers may become gangrenous.

Carbuncles and boils – Pepper box like openings and dipping deeply into cellular tissue. Burning pains like coals of fire with irritability of mind and body.

Aggravation – midnight.

General Modalities :

Aggravation – MIDNIGHT (1-2 A.M., 1-2 P.M.)
COLD – COLD DRINKS AND FOOD, LYING ON AFFECTED SIDE WITH HEAD LOW.

Amelioration – HEAT (OPP. SECALE) HEADACHE IS RELIEVED BY COLD BATHING OR KEEPING HEAD COOL.

Relations :

Complementry to – Sulphur, Thuja, Rhus, Carbo veg., Phos, Secale cor.

Antidotes – Camphor, Carbo veg, Graphites, China, Hepar, Ipecac, Nux vom.

Important Questions ?

Q. 1. Give indication of Arsenic album in the following :

1) Keynotes [1987, 88, 90, 93]
2) Intermittent Fever [1975, 79, 86, 89, 90, 93, 95]
3) Mind [1973, 74, 76, 81, 91, 93]
4) Diarrhoea [1986]
5) Respiratory Symptoms [1977, 79, 86, 93]
6) Skin [1979, 87, 93]
7) Dropsy [1976]
8) Peptic Ulcer [1981, 82]
9) Dysentry [1991]
10) Typhoid [1973, 77]
11) Puerperal Sepsis [1979]
12) Modalities [1972, 73, 74, 76, 82]

Q. 2. Give a complete drug picture of Arsenic album. [1977 – S, 78 – S]

Q. 3. Compare :

Heart affections – Ars alb / Ant. tart [1988]
Skin symptoms – Ars alb / Anthracinum [1988]
Restlessness – Ars alb/Aconite/Rhus tox [1973, 75, 78, 81, 93, 97]
Neuralgia – Ars alb/Mag phos [1988]
Cholera – Ars alb/Veratrum alb – [1991, 94 – S]

CHOLERA :

ARS. ALB	VERATRUM ALB
• *Cause* – cold food and drinks decayed food sausages, alcohol. *Symptoms :* • Profuse vomiting and purging. • Intense abdominal pains causing the patient to twist and turn. • *Stools* – dark black offensive stools with burning in the anus. • *Thirst* – Intense thirst but drinks little at a time.	• *Cause* – Fright, impure, drinks, tobacco. *Symptoms :* • Profuse vomiting, sweat and diarrhoea. • Cramps with cholera, cold and clammy sweat all over the body. • *Stools* – Profuse rice watery stool which gushes out. • *Thirst* – Intense and drinks large quantities of cold water.
Look of the patient	**Look of the patient**
Patient is prostrated with cold sweat and cold extremities. Intense restlessness and fear of death. Aggravation – Eating, drinking, midnight. Amelioration – Warm application	Hippocratic face – blue and pale face with sunken cheeks and eyes. Patient is cold as if dead – excessive weakness. Aggravation – Eating, drinking and least motion. (Before and during menses there is cholera like symptoms).

15. ARUM TRIPHYLLUM

Common Name – Indian Turnip.

Miasm – Psora is in the background.

In most of the complaints urine becomes scanty and hence starting up of *copious flow of urine is a good-sign* of the remedy.

Constitution – Arum triphyllum is an acute remedy and hence consideration of constitution is not very important.

KEYNOTES

1) *Left sided affections* – left nose, left side of throat etc affected.
2) ***Acrid, ichorous discharge*** excoriating the inside of nose, alae nasi and upper lip (Arsenic A, Allium cepa).
3) Constant ***picking at the nose until it bleeds.***
4) Nose feels ***stuffed*** up inspite of ***watery discharge***.
5) *Picks lips until they bleed.*
6) ***Corners of the mouth—sore, cracked and crusty.***
7) *Bites nails* until they bleed.
8) *Hoarseness* with *changing voice* when exciting it from high to low pitch and vice versa.
9) Children *refuse food and drink* on account of soreness of mouth and throat.
10) Scarlatina, typhoid guided by sore mouth, nose and suppressed scanty urine.

Particulars :

1) HEAD
2) NOSE
3) MOUTH
4) THROAT
5) DIARRHOEA
6) SCARLET FEVER

HEADACHE

Cause – Too warm clothing, hot coffee.

Symptoms – Child bores the head in pillow.

NOSE

- Acrid, excoriating discharge with rawness and smarting in the nose (esp. left side).

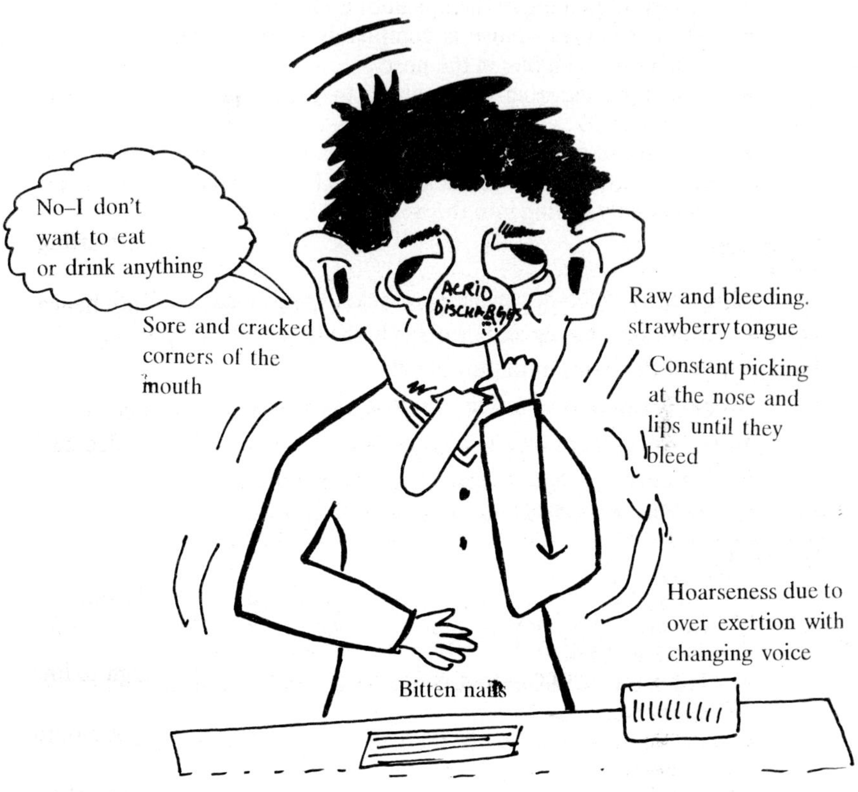
No–I don't
want to eat
or drink anything
Sore and cracked
corners of the
mouth
ACRID
DISCHARGES
Raw and bleeding.
strawberry tongue
Constant picking
at the nose and
lips until they
bleed
Hoarseness due to
over exertion with
changing voice
Bitten nails

ARUM TRIPHYLLUM

- Acrid discharge which excoriates inside of the nose, alae and the upper lip.
- Constant picking in the lips until it bleeds.
- During coryza – Nose is completely stopped with fluent acrid discharge. Tingling in the nose.
- Constant sneezing with aching in the bones as if the bones would break.
- In affection of the nasal duct there is constant tickling in the nose with acrid tears and nasal discharge. Child keeps constantly boring into the nose until it bleeds.

MOUTH

Lips – Lips become swollen, cracked and look as if they are chapped. Constant tingling and pricking in the lips. Constant picking of the lips (inspite of the pain) until they bleed.

Tongue – raw and bleeding : strawberry tongue.

Saliva – acrid saliva with excessive flow.

Buccal cavity – tingling, raw and sore condition which extends far back into the throat. Foul odour in the mouth with soreness.

THROAT

- Inflamed root of tongue, throat and soft palate leading to rawness and soreness due to which the child refuses to take food or drink.
- Hoarse voice from overexertion especially in singers and public speakers.
- Patchy inflammation of the vocal cords causing a continuously changing voice – now deep, now hoarse etc.

  Aggravation – talking, singing.
- Constant hawking with expectoration of much mucus.
- Lungs and chest feel sore especially left side.

HOARSENESS :

ARUM. T	RHUS. TOX	PHOS.	RUMEX	CAUSTICUM
Hoarseness caused due to overexertion of voice. Continuously changing voice.	Relief from hoarseness by constant motion i.e. use of voice.	Hoarseness is ameliorated by constant clearing the vocal cords of little mucus.	Hoarseness from exposure to cold or slightest inhalation of cold air.	Hoarseness due to weakness of vocal cords.

DIARRHOEA

Character of stool – Yellow like cornmeal, frequent feacal and thin mushy stools. Acrid stools that keeps the anus raw and burning.

SCARLET FEVER

- Acrid and excoriating discharges.
- Constant picking at the nose and lips until they bleed.
- Swollen tonsils and tongue.
- Restless and irritable child.
- Scanty urine.
- Well developed eruptions with double desquamation or dark and imperfectly developed rashes. Appearance of profuse urine is a sign that the remedy is acting well.

General Modality :

Aggravation – COLD DRY
OR
CLEAR FINE WEATHER (CAUSTICUM).

Amelioration – WASHING FACE OR WASHING THE AFFECTED PARTS WITH COLD WATER
DAMP WET WEATHER (CAUSTICUM).

Relations :

- **Similar to** – Causticum (in modalities).

Aloes, Arg. n, Merc, Pod, Puls, Sulph acid (Stringy, Shreddy stools).

- **Followed well by** – Bis, Caust, Puls, Sulph.

Important Questions ?

Q. 1. Give indications of Arum triph in.

Coryza [1986, 87, 89, 90, 95]

16. AURUM METALLICUM

Common Name – Gold.

Miasm – Syphilitic Miasm.

Constitution – Suited to sanguine, ruddy people with black hair and eyes. Old people who are tired of life. Pining boys – low spirited, lifeless, weak memory, undeveloped testes lacking boyish go. Constitution broken down by bad affects of mercury and syphilis.

Temperament – Melancholic and irritable.

Relation with heat and cold – Chilly patient.

Diathesis – Scrofulous diathesis.

KEYNOTES

1) Aggravation from *surise to sunset.*
2) Constantly ***dwelling on suicide.***
3) ***Profound Melancholy*** – feels quarrelsome, desire to commit suicide. Life is a constant burden and he feels hateful.
4) *Nodes and bone pains* – caries and necrosis of bones with great depression of spirits.
5) *Oversensitive* to smell, taste, hearing, touch and least contradiction.
6) *Hemiopia* – Sees only the lower half of the object.
7) Repeated attacks of *congestion* leading to *hypertrophy and induration of glands.*
8) *Induration* and *Prolapse of uterus* caused due to congestion and hypertrophy of uterus (weight of the organ rather than the weakness in ligaments is responsible for the prolapse).
9) Sensation as if the heart stood still, as though it ceased to beat and suddenly gave one hard thump.
10) Complaints are aggravated at night and by cold air..

Particulars :

1) MIND
2) HEAD
3) EYE
4) NOSE
5) EAR
6) HEART
7) LIVER
8) BONE AFFECTIONS

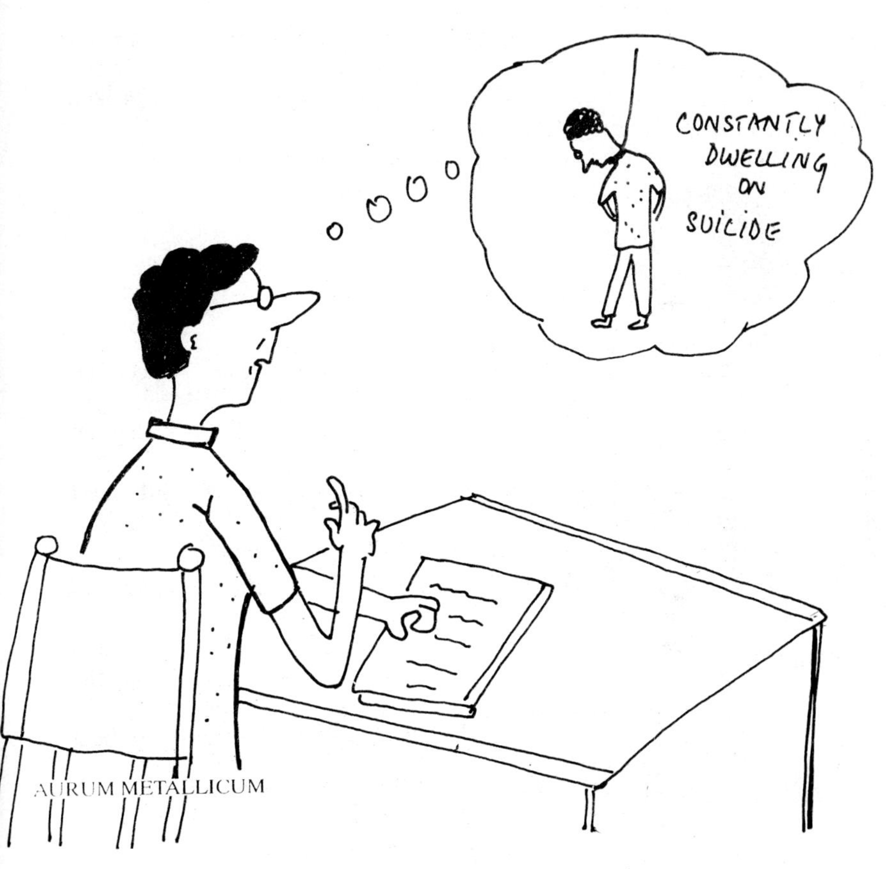

AURUM METALLICUM

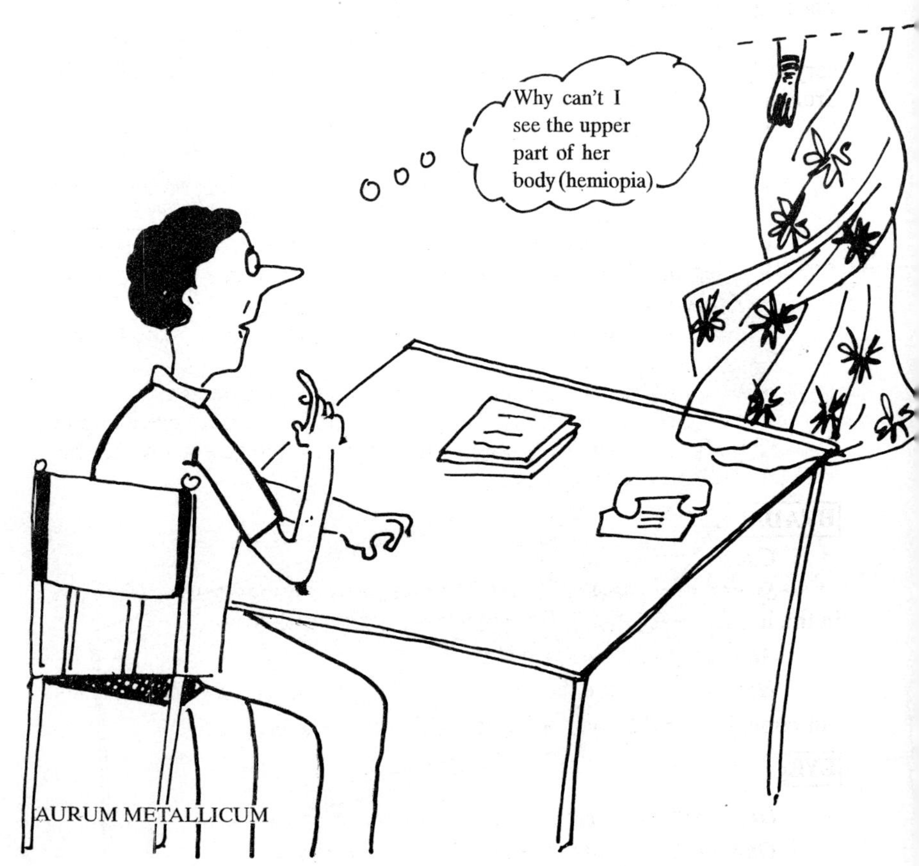
Why can't I see the upper part of her body (hemiopia)
AURUM METALLICUM

9) MALE GENITAL ORGANS
10) FEMALE SYMPTOMS.

MIND

Dr. Burnett made a short proving of gold upon himself–

its first effects were–"Exciting and Exhilarating" i.e. all day long he was in good humor and talkative.

In a few days–Dr. Burnett felt himself not upto the mark. He was very depressed and low spirited and nothing seemed worth while. He dreamt of death and corpses.

- All mental affections are due to bad affects of mercury and syphilis.
- Profound melancholy–person is very pessimistic, hopeless and despondent.
- Person is weary of life and seeks methods to commit suicide.
- Self condemnation, self reproach, self criticism are his constant companions.
- Person feels that he has neglected his duty and has commited a sin by doing so.
- Every little thing rouses him into anger and turmoil.
- To get rid of these troubles the person constantly dwells upon suicide. Patient wants to destroy himself. He has no love for his life and he thinks he is worthless.

HEADACHE

Cause–mental labour.

Symptoms–Rush of the blood to the head causing a sense of fullness in the head. Intense pain and the head feels sore and bruised.

Amelioration–Wrapping up.

Hair–In old mercurised cases with necrosis of skull, the hair falls out copiously and the head becomes bald for lifetime.

EYE

Hemiopia / half sight–can see only the lower half of the object.

Opthalmia–great vascularity is a characteristic.

Syphilitic Iritis–sore and bruised sensation around the eyes. Skull bones are sensitive to pressure.

NOSE

Used in catarrah and ozeana before the trouble has progressed to actual caries. Nostrils are agglutinated and ulcerated. Nose is filled with crusts and has an excessively foetid discharge.

In later stages of mercurial affections the bones of the nose may necrose and be discharged–the nose flattens down.

EAR

Aur. met is indicated in caries of mastoid, obstinate otorrhoea.

- Ears are congested.
- Foetid otorrhoea.
- As the disease spreads there may be entire loss of the ear drum and the bones of the ear.
- Hearing is lost.

HEART

Cause – Syphitic and Mercurial affections cause fatty degeneration, cardiac hypertrophy without dilatation.

Sensation – As if the heart stood still as though it ceased to beat. It actually stops for 2-3 seconds and then gives a sudden thump.

Characteristic of heart disease –

"Violent palpitation with anxiety and congestion of the chest and visible beating of the carotids and temporal arteries." Dyspnoea of cardiac origin.

LIVER

Hepatic congestion consecutive to cardiac disease.

- Swollen liver with cutting pain in the right hypochondrium.
- As hyperemia continues the liver later becomes cirrhosed or else undergoes fatty degeneration.
- Ascites appears.
- Stools are of greyish or white colour from defective secretion of bile.

BONE AFFECTIONS

Cause – Syphilitic and Mercurial affections.

Symptoms

- Thickening of periosteum with induration.
- Inflammation of the bones with caries and bone pains.
- The patient is driven out of the bed at night and continuously keeps waking.
- Caries of bones especially nose, palate and mastoid process.

(Caries of long bones – Flouric acid, Angustura).

MALE GENITAL ORGANS

Due to bad affect of syphilis or mercury there develops a strong tendency to erections and lasciviousness. There is epididimitis, orchitis, balanitis, induration of testes. Suicidal tendency with melancholy.

FEMALE GENITAL ORGANS

Hypertrophy and congestion of uterus causing prolapse from its great weight (prolapse is not due to relaxation of ligaments but due to weight of the organ caused by hypertrophy). Bruised pain worse after lifting a heavy weight with profuse and corroding leucorrhoea and backache.

General Modilities :

Aggravation – SUNSET >SUNRISE
COLD AIR, LYING DOWN
MENTAL EXERTION
WINTERS

Amelioration – WARM AIR
MORNING
SUMMERS

Relations

Remedies that follow well – Nitric acid, Aco, Bell, Calc, Chin, Lyc, Merc, Puls, Rhus, Sep, S, Syphilinum.

Antidotes – Bell, Chin, Cocc, Coffea, Cupr, Merc, Puls, Spig.

Important Questions ?

Q. 1. Give indication of Aurum met in the following.

1) Mental Symptoms [1973, 74, 76, 79, 81, 82, 87, 93]
2) Cardiac [1975, 82, 93, 96]
3) Female [1997]
4) Keynotes [1991]
5) Orchitis [1977]

17. BAPTISIA TINCTORIA

W.H. Burt

Common Name – Wild Indigo (Leguminosae).

Miasm – Psora is in the background.

Baptisia is a *deep* but *short acting* remedy suitable for complaints that are not lasting.

Dr. Nash says – Baptisia is generally indicated *after Gelsimium* stage is over in typhoid fevers.

Constitution – Face is flushed, dusky, dark red with a stupid besotted drunken expression (Gels.) Great prostration and disposition to decomposition of fluids with foetid discharges and ulceration of mucous membrane.

Temperament – Lymphatic temperament.

Relation with heat and cold – Chilly patient.

KEYNOTES

1) All exhalations and discharges are ***offensive and foetid*** – *breath, stool, urine, perspiration, ulcers.*

2) Parts rested upon feel *sore and bruised.*

3) Great ***prostration*** with disposition to decomposition of fluids and *ulceration* of mucous membranes.

4) *Tongue*

In the beginning – coated white with red papillae and dry brown in centre.

Later – dry, cracked and ulcerated.

5) *Face* – flushed, dusky, dark-red with a stupid besotted drunken expression (Gels).

6) *Stupor* – falls asleep while spoken to or in the midst of his answer.

[**Arnica** – answers correctly when spoken to but delirium returns at once.]

7) Cannot go to sleep because *head and body feel scattered* about the bed; tosses about to get the pieces together and feels that he cannot get them together and cover them up.

8) Can *swallow liquids* only (Baryta carb). Least solid food gags.

9) Painless sore throat – tonsils, soft palate and parotids are dark-red swollen; putrid with offensive discharge.

10) Abdomen sensitive in the right iliac region with rumbling.

11) *Aversion to mental exertion*, indisposed or want of power to think.

Particulars :

TYPHOD FEVER

Baptisia is suitable for typhoids that come on rapidly with remittent fever. All at once it turns continuous and takes on septic symptoms.

Look of the patient—Patient looks drunk. He has a besotted countenance. It is bloated, purple and mottled.

Delirium :

- The patient is in a confused state, falls asleep in the midst of his answer.
- Cannot collect himself—feels scattered and cannot get the pieces together and cover them up.
- Aversion to mental exertion and indisposed to think anything.
- Parts rested upon feel sore and bruised.

Temperature—High temperature ranging from 103-106 °F. Afternoon rise of temperature.

Pulse—Accelerated in proportion to the temperature. Pulse is full and strong.

Mouth :

- *Foetid* odour of mouth.
- Apthous patches which increase in size leaving a raw and denuded area oozing a thick saliva which is putrid.
- *Sordes on teeth and lips.*
- **Tongue**—Initially coated white with red papillae and dry yellow brown in the centre. Later—dry cracked and ulcerated. All discharges are ***offensive***.

Throat :

- Tonsils and soft palate is swollen and painless having a dusky red colour—the darker it is more likely is Baptisia indicated.
- Painless sore throat as if numb.
- Throat takes on ulceration and becomes raw and bleeding with offensive discharge.
- Throat is greatly swollen and hence the person can drink liquids only.

Oesophagus

- Oesophagus feels constricted from above down to the stomach.
- Smallest solid substance causes gagging associated with putridity and offensiveness;can swallow only liquids.
- Later there is paralysis of organs of deglutition.

Abdomen

Abdomen is very sensitive in right iliac region with rumbling.

Diarrhoea

Anus is ulcerated, raw and bleeding.

Stools – Foetid, involuntary stools and urine. Dark brown, mucoid and bloody stools.

Dr. Nash and Dr. Farrington have stated that *Baptisia is generally indicated after Gelsimium stage is over in typhoid fever.*

Similarities between Gelsimium and Baptisia

- Both have intense muscular soreness, prostration and drowsiness..
- Both have a feeling of expansion of some part of the body.
- Afternoon exacerbation of fever.

Gelsimium is indicated :

- On the first day.
- Malaise and muscular soreness.
- Patient suffers from chills and creeps which go down the back.
- Afternoon rise of temperature with accelerated pulse.
- Face is red and suffused.
- Gelsimium causes paralysis of motor nerves hence causing weakness of muscles.

Baptisia is indicated from the next day onwards when the fever rises.

Lachesis shares quite a few similarities with Baptisia in typhoid.

Similarities between Lachesis and Baptisia

- Dark red appearance of mucous membrane.
- Offensive discharges.
- Excessive prostration.

Distinguishing features in Lachesis :

- Trembling of tongue when attempting to protrude it.
- Blood escapes from every orifice.
- Intolerance of tight pressure.
- Worse after sleeping.

Relations :

Similar to – Arnica, Arsenic, Gels, Hyosc, Lach, Mur acid, Nitric acid.

Follows well – Arsenic alb.

Is followed well by – Nitric acid.

Important Questions ?

Q. 1. Give indication of Baptisia in.

1) Typhoid – [1973, 76, 77, 78, 79, 81]
1983, 86, 87, 93, 94, 95]

2) Delirium [1974, 77]

3) Tongue [1982]

18. BARYTA CARBONICA

Hahnemann

Common Name – Carbonate of Barium.

Miasm – Psora is in the background.

Baryta carb is a *deep seated, long acting* remedy.

Constitution :

Child – Appears like a Cretin. Scrofulous dwarfish children who do not grow and are imbecile.

- Mind and body are weak.
- Inclined to glandular swelling with swollen abdomen and general emaciation

Old Age – (especially when fat) Mental and physical weakness; childishness and thoughtless behaviour.

Temperament – Melancholic temperament.

Relation with heat and cold – Chilly patient

Diathesis – Tubercular and Scrofulous diathesis

KEYNOTES

1) Child is both ***mentally and physically weak.***

2) Scrofulous, ***dwarfish*** children who do not grow.

- Swollen abdomen with frequent attacks of colic.
- Bloated face
- General emaciation

3) *Deficient memory* – Forgetful child with threatened idiocy.

4) ***Swelling and induration of glands*** – especially cervical and inguinal.

5) Great *sensitiveness to take cold.* Cold settles in the throat resulting in sore throat, quinsy and tonsillitis.

6) *Inability to swallow anything but liquid.*

7) Dwarfish, hysterical women with scanty menses, deficient heat and always chilly and cold.

8) *Diseasesof old men* (especilly when fat) mentally and physically weak; hypertrophy of prostate and testes.

9) *Offensive foot sweat* – making the feet (especially toes and sole) sore. *Throat affections* are caused by checked foot sweat (Graphites, Psor, Silicea, Sanic).

10) *Aggravation* of complaints when *thinking* about them

Particulars :

1) MIND

2) GLANDULAR SWELLING

3) HEAD
4) EYE
5) MOUTH
6) TEETH
7) THROAT
8) RESPIRATORY SYSTEM
9) G.I.T
10) MALE SEXUAL ORGANS
11) FEMALE SYMPTOMS
12) PARALYSIS
13) CHILD

MIND

- Dwarfishness of mind and body
- Children are late coming into activity - late learning to talk, late learning to walk, to read etc.
- Child is easily frightened and is afraid of strangers.
- Child hides behind the furniture when the strangers come.
- Child cannot memorise or he cannot maintain a thought.
- Child refuses to play and he sits in one corner.
- He is full of imaginary cares and worries.
- There is inability to percieve anything. Child laughs at serious matters and becomes serious at laughable matters.

Girls in the age of 18-25 have a childish manner of doing things. They can be seen playing with dolls and saying foolish things. They lack the prudence of a woman.

Old and *fatty people* with mental and physical weakness. They have a childish behaviour.

All complaints are aggravated by thinking about them.

GLANDULAR SWELLING

- Lymphatic glands all over the body indurate especially glands of neck, groin, lymphatics in the abdomen.
- When a child suffers from any disease measles, mumps etc there is arrest of development with emaciation of the whole body except the abdomen.
- Patient is very sensitive to cold.
- Encysted tumors, growths of tuberculous character, sarcoma fatty tumors - Baryta carb has cured the above conditions and has mitigated the pains.

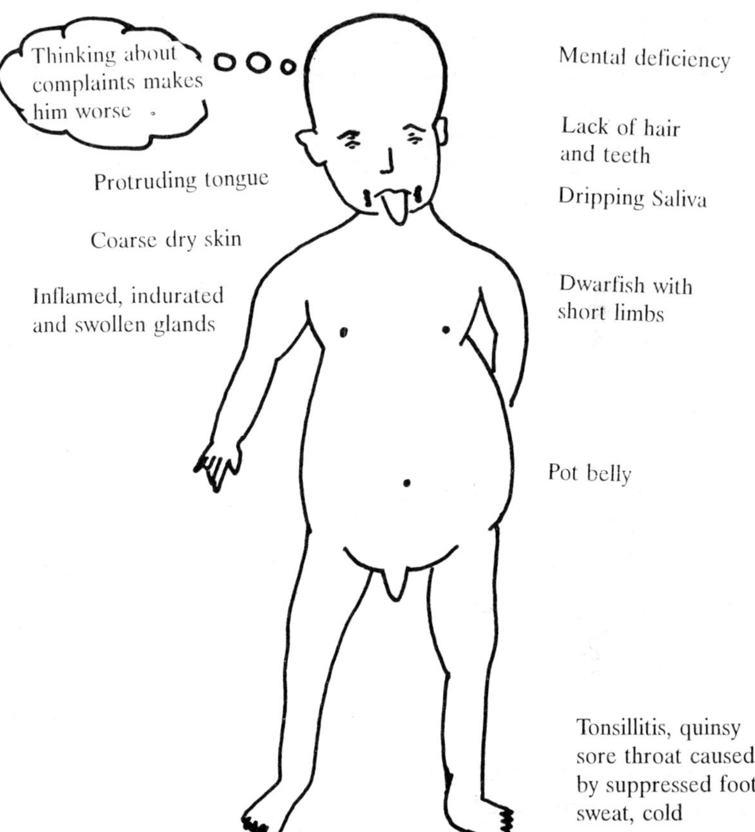

BARYTA CARBONICA

HEADACHE

Cause – Patient is sensitive to extremes of heat and cold

Character of pain

- Congestive headache
- Looseness of the brain with a sensation of motion of the brain when moving the head from side to side.
- Heat causes the blood to mount to the head thus favouring apoplectic conditions.

Amelioration – open air.

Scalp – Dry eruptions on the scalp. Falling of hair causing baldness.

EYES

- Granular lids
- Sensation of weight on the upper lids.
- Opacity of the cornea causing haziness
- Baryta carb has cured cataract.

MOUTH

- Dry mouth in the morning.
- Mouth is filled with inflamed vesicles and has foul taste.
- Paralysis of the tongue in old people.

TEETH

- Toothache in decayed teeth before menses or from thinking about them. Worse- thinking about complaints.

THROAT

Tonsillitis, sore throat, quinsy

Cause – taking cold
suppressed foot sweat

Symptoms :

- Pharynx looks shiny, studded with coarse granules which become inflamed with every cold spell.
- Tonsils are inflamed with swollen veins and may suppurate later
- Smarting pain when swallowing. Patient feels worse from empty swallowing
- Can only swallow liquids
- Right side is more prone to affections
- Chronic hypertrophy later.

Aggravation – Thinking about complaints, empty swallowing.

TONSILLITIS :

CALC. PHOS.	IGN.	HEPAR. S	LYC.	CALC. IOD	BELL	CHAM.	CONIUM
Chronic Cases; Bone diseases	Tonsils with small flat ulcers on them. Pain between the acts of swallo-wing	Large Tonsils; poor hearing. Sensation of fish bone in the throat	Large tonsils studded with indurated ulcers	Tonsils filled with little crypts and pockets	Tonsilliti s comes on with rapidity, Bright red tonsils.	Ear is involved and person is amelio-rated by applica-tion of heat	Enlarged tonsils without tendency to suppurate

Inflammation of parotid and submaxillary glands with induration and pain.

RESPIRATORY SYSTEM

Cause – Exposure to cold.

Catarrah – Accumulation of mucus in nose, throat, larynx, trachea with rattling respiration. Scabs form in posterior nares and base of the nose.

Larynx – Cause – exposure to cold, damp weather

Symptoms – hoarseness and huskiness of voice.

- Feeling in the larynx as if inhaling smoke.
- Coarse dry hoarse barking cough with impending paralysis of lungs.
- Chest is full of mucus and the patient is unable to expectorate. Relief – lying on the abdomen.

GIT

Oesophagus – spasm of the oesophagus with gagging and choking with little food (Kali, Graph, Merc cor).

Stomach – Weakness of digestion, stomach aches after eating.

Abdomen – Swollen and enlarged with emaciation of the limbs, enlarged glands with dwarfed intellect.

Constipation – hard and insufficient stools, heamorrhoidal protrusion during stool and urination (Mur. acid)

MALE SEXUAL ORGANS

- Enlarged and indurated prostate in old people
- Due to atrophy of cranial matters in old age the patient goes into his second child hood. There is sexual weakness amounting to impotence.
- Penis becomes relaxed and coition becomes impossible due to premature emission.

FEMALE SYMPTOMS

- Dwindling of ovary, mammary gland and yet lymphatics become enlarged and infiltrated.
- Menses - scanty.
- Leucorrhoea whitish thick copious discharge a week before the menstrual period.

PARALYSIS

- In old people there is paralysis following apoplexy, apoplexy of drunkards.
- Brain shrinks in old people and hence forming a vaccum or an effusion of serum takes place. This is followed by paralysis.
- Patient is childish with loss of memory
- Paralysis of tongue
- Trembling of limbs

CHILD

Look of the child – Dwarfishness of both mind and body. Mouth is kept partly open and saliva runs out freely. Child has a silly vacant look.

Mind –

- Idiocy and Imbecility is marked
- Late learning to do things.
- Afraid of strangers.
- Inability to percieve anything
- Becomes serious at laughable matters and vice versa.

Physical – Symptoms :

- All glands of the body are enlarged especially tonsils. Inflammation and induration of glands with a tendency to foot sweat.

Aggravation – cold, suppressed foot sweat.

- Enlarged abdomen, colic from eating anything.
- Inveterate constipation.

BARYTA CARB	SILICEA
Similarities :	
1) Offensive foot sweat. 2) Head is disproportionately large for body. 3) Both suffer from damp changes in the weather. 4) Sensitive to cold about the head.	
Differences :	
1) Not so.	1) Profuse sweat on the head.
2) Weakness of mind.	2) Not so.
3) Tonsillitis caused by suppressed foot sweat.	3) Complaints arising from suppressed foot sweat but Silicea has not the same affinity for throat.

General Modalities :

Aggravation – THINKING OF COMPLAINTS
LYING ON PAINFUL SIDE, AFTER MEALS
WASHING THE AFFECTED PARTS

Amelioration – WALKING IN OPEN AIR.

Relations :

Frequently useful before or after Psor., Sulph, Tuberculinum.

After Baryta carb, **Psor** will often eradicate the constitutional tendency to quinsy.

Similar to – Alum, Calc iod, Dulc., Flouric acid, Iod, Silicea

Incompatible after *Calc* in Scrofular affections.

Improtant Questions

Q1 Give indication of Baryta carb in

1) Tonsillitis [1973,95, 84]
2) Keynotes [1977]
3) Mind [1993]
4) Child [1972, 73, 75, 76, 79, 81, 83, 87, 89, 90,959]

Q2 Compare Glandular affections of Baryta carb and Conium. [1996]

Q3 Compare babies of Baryta carb / Calc carb. [1997]

BARYTA CARB	CALC. CARB
• ***Dwarfishness*** of both mind and body.	• Mental exertion causes ***profuse sweat*** and hence the child is unable to think.
• ***Late learning*** to walk and talk due to mental deficiency.	• ***Late learning to*** walk due to deficiency of bone tissue
• ***Fearful*** and shy child. Dull perception.	• ***Obstinate*** and self willed child.
• Perspiration is ***normal.***	• ***Profuse perspiration*** espically on single parts of the body. ***Sour smelling*** sweat.

19. BELLADONNA

Hahnemann

Common Name – Deadly Nightshade (Solanaceae) [Belladonna in its raw form is poisonous to man]

The name Belladonna is derived from 2 latin words

Bella – Beautiful, Dona - Lady. Venetian ladies used it as a cosmetic to brighten the eyes and flush their cheeks due to the property of two alkaloids *Atropin* and *Belladonna*]

Miasm – Psora is in the background.

[***Belladonna is the Acute of Calcarea*** which is often required to complete the cure. According to Kent – Bell is not suitable for those numerous recurrent complaints even though a single attack may be mitigated with Bell. After first 2-3 attacks for the same problem (eg-headaches, Bell is not suitable and its followers like Calc etc. are suitable for periodic complaints).

Constitution :

- Fleshy, phelgmatic and plethoric persons who are subject to congestions everywhere especially in the head. Women and children with light hair, blue eyes, fine complexion, delicate skin, sensitive, nervous threatened with convulsions.

Temperament – Bilious, lymphatic and nervous people.

Relation with heat and cold – Chilly patient.

Diathesis – Tuberculous diathesis.

KEYNOTES

1) Belladonna is a *right sided remedy.*
2) Belladonna is used in the ***first stage of inflammations*** which *localise.*
3) All complaints come on ***suddenly and violently*** and even subside suddenly
4) Inflammation is attended with *violent heat* . Heat is so intense that if we put our hand upon the patient we will suddenly withdraw it.
5) Inflamed parts are *very red*. Skin is bright red and shiny
6) *Intense burning* of inflamed parts
7) Swelling – inflamed parts swell rapidly and are extremely sensitive to touch
8) *Throbbing* with all congestions and inflammations

9) Patient is *oversensitive* to touch, light, noise. *Least jar* of the bed worsens all his complaints. Patient asks the doctor not to touch the bed, even before he has crossed the room.

10) Great *dryness* of mucous membranes - nose, mouth, tongue, throat

11) Bell causes *constriction* of circular fibres of blood vessels, spincters etc. A sensation of clutching is felt in the uterus, throat etc.

12) Bell-causes *congestion* everywhere is the body.

13) There is *turmoil in brain* (resulting from congestion /inflammation) leading to collateral symptoms of cerebral irritation.

a) **Congestion in the head** – from mild congestion to very severe headache with –

throbbing carotids
flushed face
hard and bounding pulse
hot and burning head
dilated pupils
jerking of limbs (extreme cases)

b) **Delirium** – (Trio of Delirium – Belladonna
Stramonium
Hyoscyamus

The patient is violent, tears clothes, strikes those near him, breaks, into fits of laughter and gnashes the teeth.

14) *Eyes* – red blood shot eyes. Pupils first contract then dilate.

15) *Heamorrhagic remedy* – Parts bleed easily. There is flow of bright red, hot blood. In uterine heamorrhages , there is copious flow of bright red blood mixed with clots (Sabina).

16) *Abdomen* – distended, tender with pain in the right ileoceacal region which is aggravated by least jar.

17) Patient is *sleepy but he cannot sleep.*

18) In acute and chronic *rheumatism* – Bell is one of the best medicines where joints are red, swollen and inflamed.

19) *Chilly patient* – Complaints are caused by exposure to cold.

Bell is an excellent remedy for headaches that come on suddenly due to exposure to cold air hence causing signs of congestion.

- *Stiff neck* caused by cutting the hair, getting head wet or exposure to cold air.

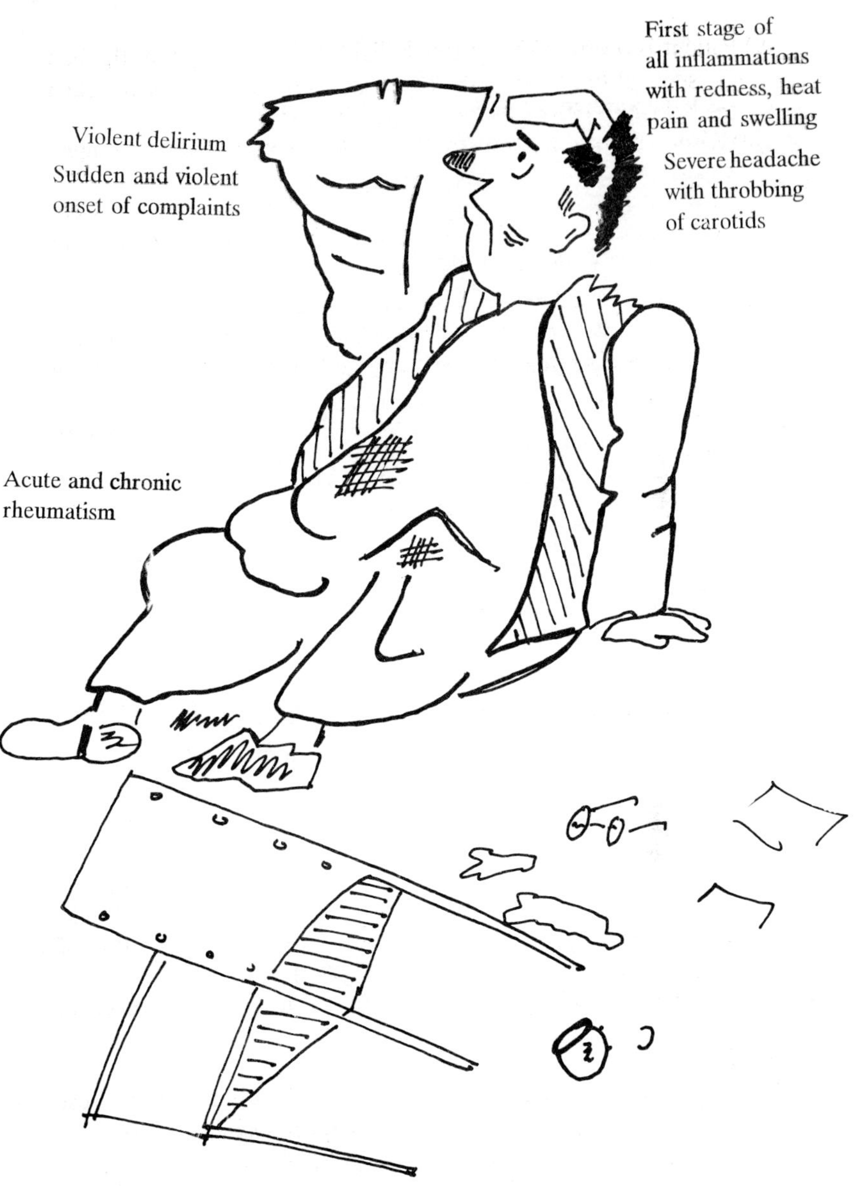
First stage of
all inflammations
with redness, heat
pain and swelling
Violent delirium
Sudden and violent
onset of complaints
Severe headache
with throbbing
of carotids
Acute and chronic
rheumatism

BELLADONNA

20) *Skin* – Uniform smooth shining, scarlet redness with intense heat which burns the touching hand. Sweat only on covered parts.

21) All complaints are :

Worse – Least jar, cold air, motion, light , noise, 3 p.m., lying down

Better – Warmth, being wrapped up, head high.

Summary – **C** – Congestion
Chilly patient
Clutching
B – Burning
I – Inflammation
R – Right Sided affections, Redness
D – Dryness, Delirium
S – Suddeness, Swelling, Sensitiveness

Particulars :

1) MIND
2) HEAD
3) VERTIGO
4) FEVER
5) NEURALGIA
6) EYES
7) G.I.T
8) RESPIRATORY SYMPTOMS
9) RHEUMATISM
10) URINARY SYSTEM
11) FEMALE SYMPTOMS
12) SKIN
13) EPILEPSY

MIND

Generally the patient is jolly and well behaved but sometimes rush of blood to the brain causes cerebral irritation and hence delirium. The patient becomes violent and there is great anxiety

- Heat, burning and redness.
- Pupils become dilated.
- Carotids throb violently.
- Sleepy but cannot sleep.

- Patient imagines that he sees ghosts, hideous faces, animals and insects. He fears these imaginary things and wants to run away.
- Patient breaks into fits of laughter or screams; he gnashes his teeth with inclination to bite others; strikes those around him.
- Patient loses his memory of all things and becomes wild
- He wants to run away from all his attendants.
- Aversion to noise, company and light.
- Hot head, cold hands and feet, hydrophobia. Finally the person becomes pale as the stupor increases.

In *meningitis* when the base of the brain and the skin become involved the muscles of the neck contract drawing the head backward; he moves the head from side to side. Burning redness of skin with dilated pupils

Trio of Delirium – Belladonna, Hyoscyamus, Stramonium.

BELLADONNA	STRAMONIUM	HYOSCYAMUS
• Violent mania.	• Religeous mania	• Lascivious mania
• Violent and furious with inclination to bite and tear things	• Wants to pray.	• Has lost all senses of decency and wants to uncover.
• Redness with intense burning of face and dilated pupils.	• Red face. No burning.	• Pale and sunken.
• Cannot bear light.	• Cannot bear dark. Wants light and company.	

HEADACHE

Cause – Standing in cold air with head uncovered, getting hair cut, sunstroke.

Congestive and nervous headaches caused suddenly and violently.

Location – Forehead, right sided headaches.

Sensation – Rush of blood to the head causing a hot head, flushed face with cold hands and feet Throbbing headache aggravated by inclining the head towards the part of the brain most congested. Expansive sensation as if head is enlarged.

Concomitant – Red face, red eyes, dilated pupils, throbbing of carotid arteries, patient becomes wild and excited.

Worse – least jar, bending forward .

- Any position that throws head out of perpendicular makes him worse.
- Cold air, 3 P.M.

Relief—Warmth, wrapping up drawing the head back. Both Belladonna and Glonoine are excellent remedies for headache caused by sunstroke.

Headache :

BELLADONNA	GLONOINE
Similarities :	
Cause—Sunstroke. throbbing, bursting headaches with intense pains.	*Cause*—Sunstroke. Hot flushed face with intolerance of least jar.
Difference :	
Aggravation—Cold Air, uncovering the head getting hair cut *Amel*—Wrapped up.	*Aggravation*—Heat, cannot bear head being wrapped up. *Amel*—Cold applications.

VERTIGO

Cause—Turning in bed,moving head.

Symptoms—Vertigo with pulsations Moving the head increases the pulsations and the vertigo. Patient lies in the bed and cannot hold the head up.

Sensitive Scalp—Women cannot have the head combed due to the over sensitive scalp and hence lets her hair hang down the back.

FEVER

Bell is indicated in remittent fever which comes on suddenly and violently commencing in night at 3 P.M

Symptoms— • Temperature —very high.
• Pulse—hard and bounding

- Much chilliness followed by much heat with intense burning within and without.
- Congestion of the brain promotes red face with dilated pupils
- Hot head, cold hands and feet.
- Throbbing carotids.
- Patient is sensitive to least jar.
- Sweat on covered parts.
- Thirstless.
- Scanty urine.
- Jerking of muscles.

- Furious delirium – Even in stupor there is never a complete profound sleep.

Aggravation – cold air, uncovering or getting hair cut, sun stroke

NEURALGIA

Neuralgia that comes on suddenly and violently and disappears suddenly.

Worse – motion, noise, least jar, lying down .

Better – sitting down.

Facial Neuralgia – Right side is involved and the face is red and hot

Sciatica – Pains worse in the hip joint at night.

Amel – Constantly changing position or constant motion.

EYES

Bell – As a poison dilates the pupils so much that the iris is hardly visible.

Physostigma – Contract the pupils by stimulating the 3rd cranial nerve.

Gelsimium – Dilates the pupils by paralysing the 3rd cranial nerve.

Conjunctivitis/Scleritis :

- Right eye is mostly involved.
- Sudden attack of congestion with severe and violent pains.
- Red hot and burning eyes.
- Intense photophobia and dimness of vision .
- Half open protruding eyes.
- Pulsation, tumefaction, lachrymation and intense pains.

G.I.T

Tongue :

- Dry, swollen tongue which feels dry hard like leather causing loss of taste and sensation. In congestion of brain tongue is bright red with erect papillae.

Parotid Gland – Right side is involved. Pain extends to the ear, gland is swollen, red and hot. Saliva is thick, yellow and gluey. Mucous coats the mouth and throat with a thick tenacious layer. Tongue is white and fissured.

Oesophagitis :

Sense of constriction " clutching" with painful swallowing and breathing.

Gastritis :

- Inflammation of stomach from becoming chilled.
- Intense heat, burning in the stomach with a red face.
- Pain in the the stomach extending through to the spine.

- Pressure in the stomach worse after eating with nausea and vomiting.

Worse – Pain is worse by least jar, slightest pressure.

Relief – Bending backward.

Liver – Sensitive especially when lying on the right side. Colic from gall stones.

Abdomen :

- Tympanic abdomen which is sensitive to least jar. Patient cannot tolerate the touch of bed clothes.
- Great pain in the ileo- ceacal region.
- Pressure downwards as if the contents of the abdomen would issue through the vulva.
- During pain (especially in children) transverse colon protrudes like a pad all the way across the abdomen.
- Pain is relieved by bending backward.

Stools :

Bell-causes spasmodic constriction of sphincter ani.

Diarrhoea with scanty fluid stool, marked straining and flushed face.

Dysentry – Stools are thin, greenish, bloody and mucoid.

RESPIRATORY SYMPTOMS

Throat (Inflammation of throat).

- Fauces are inflamed and bright red.
- Right tonsil is mostly swollen and enlarged.
- Sense of constriction of fauces and glottis causing a sensation of clutching.
- Burning and redness in the throat.
- Due to constriction both water and food are ejected out through the nose and mouth.
- Great dryness of mouth with constant desire to swallow.
- Swallowing of fluids is very painful.

Larynx – Dryness of larynx with a sense of clutching.

Dry spasmodic cough aggravated at night.

Whooping cough – Cough has a peculiar character.

- Cough comes with great violence.
- Patient gets relief after raising a little mucus.
- During the restful period air passages become drier and drier and ultimately tickling starts again bringing up a violent paroxysm of cough relieved by raising a little mucous.
- There may be expectoration of little blood after a violent paroxysm.

Pneumonia / Pleurisy

Bell affects the right side of the chest. Concomitants – congestion of the head, red face, burning.

Pleurisy – Right pleura is involved. Extreme pain and soreness aggravated by least jar.

Pleurisy :

BELLADONNA	BRYONIA
• Affects right lung.	• Affects right lung.
• Intense dryness.	• Intense dryness.
• Cannot bear least jar.	• Not so sensitive to jar.
• Intense heat throbbing and burning.	• Not present.
• Cannot lie on inflamed part.	• Relief by lying on inflamed part.

RHEUMATISM

Belladonna is excellent for acute and chronic rheumatism.

- Joints are swollen, red, shining and often have red streaks radiating from these along the limbs.
- Patient is sensitive to least jar and motion.
- Cannot bear least uncovering; draft of air.
- Inflammation of joints may be caused due to cold.
- *Stiff neck* – may be caused by cutting the hair, getting head wet, sitting with head and neck exposed to draft of air.

URINARY SYSTEM

Nephritis – Quantity of urine becomes greatly diminished and it looks turbid.

Cystitis – Urine becomes extremely hot It looks as if mixed with brick dusk and is strongly acidic.

- Sensation as if ball rolling inside the bladder.
- Constriction of the neck of bladder causing a clutching sensation.
- *Strangury* – Frequent desire to urinate with a scanty discharge of urine.
- Vesicular region is extremely sensitive to touch.
- When becoming chilled / cold – women loose their urine.

FEMALE SYMPTOMS.

Dysmenorrhoea – Violent dysmenorrhoea which comes suddenly with labor like pains and uterus feels clutched with strings.

Congested uterus :

- Uterus remains congested after parturition, menses and abortion.

- Uterine heamorrhages may be caused due to congestion with spasms and great sensitiveness.
- Great soreness with *copious flow of bright red blood mixed with clots;* blood feels hot.
- Cannot bear least jar.
- Bell relieves the hour glass contraction of uterus after confinement.
- Sensation as if inner parts were coming out which is worse from least jar.
- The patient must sit and cannot lean down.

Labor – Bell is used in labor when the os does not dilate due to spasmodic constriction of cervix.

Mastitis – Inflammation of breasts when the breasts are extremely sensitive to touch . Inflamed parts appear bright red and are hot to touch with tendency towards suppuration. Breasts become indurated and hard as stone.

SKIN

Erythema – Uniform smooth shining scarlet redness of the skin. Skin is hot and imparts a burning sensation to the hand.

Erisipelas :

- Smooth shining and tense surface.
- Bright red streaks start from a central point and radiate in all the directions.
- Rapid swelling and early involvement of cellular tissue beneath the skin.
- Violent and sharp pains.
- There may be metastasis of erisipelas to the brain causing cerebral iritation.

Bell is also indicated is cellulitis, boils, bubo etc with its violent congestive and inflammatory symptoms before pus formation takes place.

EPILEPSY

Cause – Taking cold, repelled eruption peurperal eclampsia.

- The child suddenly becomes rigid and stiffens out with fixed and staring eyes.
- Tonic and clonic convulsion. There may be opisthotonos.
- Symptoms of cerebral irritation - hot flushed face, throbbing carotids etc.
- Clutching sensation in the throat which makes it difficult for him to swallow.

Aversion – slightest motion, noise, touch light, cold air.

Amelioration – keeping still.

General Modalities :

Aggravation – LEAST JAR
TOUCH
MOTION
NOISE
COLD AIR
LYING DOWN
3 P.M.
UNCOVERING THE HEAD
SUMMER SUN
LOOKING AT BRIGHT SHINING OBJECTS

(Dr. Nash has qouted a case where he has cured a case of swelling and pain in the breast of long standing where the pains were aggravated by lying down.)

Amelioration – REST
STANDING/SITTING ERECT
WARM ROOM

Relations :

Complementry to – Calcarea (Bell is acute of Calcarea which is often required to complete the cure.)

Similar to – Acon, Bry, Cic, Gels, Glon, Hyosc, Opium, Stram.

Improtant Questions ?

Q.1. Give indications of Belladona in the following :

1) Fever [1972s, 73, 77s, 94, 95, 96]
2) Respiratory Symptoms [1973, 76s, 77, 95]
3) Headache [1973, 74, 75, 87s]
4) Sunstroke [1994]
5) Apoplexy [1985]
6) Desires and Aversions [1991]
7) Mind [1974, 75, 77]
8) Inflammatory Symptoms [1973s]
9) Uterine Troubles [1976, 77, 79 ,82]
10) Convulsions [1975, 76, 77, 81, 82]
11) Eye [1977]
12) Parotitis [1979, 81]
13) Skin [1981]
14) Modalities [1977]
15) Constipation [1977S]

Q2 Explain the 'Trio of delirium' with their keynote symptoms. [1987, 95, 97]

Q3 Compare Bell/Glonoine in Headache. [1993]

Q4 Compare/Bryonia in Headache. [1983]

Q5 Compare Bell/Mephitis - whooping cough.

Q6 Compare Bell/Aconite in fever.

ACONITE	BELLADONNA
1) Turmoil in circulation.	1) Turmoil in brain.
2) Distress in heart and chest.	2) Everything centres in the head.
3) Aconite acts on the sympathetic nervous system [in children the sympathetic nervous system becomes involved early]	3) Acts on cerebro-spinal nervous system.
4) Cerebral symptoms caused due to high temperature	4) Cerebral symptoms caused due to direct inflammation of brain.
5) Dry hot skin, no sweat.	5) Greater surface heat, redness. Sour sweat on covered parts which gives no relief and the more the patient sweats less is the sign of improvement.
6) Tosses about in agony with great fear of death.	6) Semistupor-Jerks and twitches in sleep. There may be a violent delirium.

20. BERBERIS VULGARIS

Common Name – Barberry (Barberidaceae).

Constitution – Face looks pale, earthy complexion, sunken cheeks and hollow eyes with blue circles around them.

KEYNOTES :

1) *Left sided affection* – left kidney, left ureter etc.
2) *Bruised pain* with numbness, stiffness and lameness in the region of the kidney and back.
3) *Soreness and bubbling* sensation in the region of kidneys aggravated by stepping or jarring motion.
4) *Rheumatic and gouty* complaints with diseases of the kidney.
5) *Wandering pains* – pains radiate in every direction from the centre.
6) *Urine* is greenish, blood red with thick slimy mucus. Urine may become, dark, turbid with copious sediments in chronic cases.
7) *Pale and earthy complexion* with sunken cheeks and hollow blue encircled eyes.
8) *Pain in the small of the back* aggravated when sitting or lying especially when lying in the bed in the morning.
9) ***Colic from gall stones.***
10) *Fistula in ano* with bilious symptoms and itching of parts. Lungs and chest complaints may follow operation for fistula.
11) *Aggravation* of complaints from motion, jar and fatigue.

Particulars :

1) LIVER
2) URINARY SYSTEM
3) RHEUMATISM
4) LUMBAGO
5) FEMALES

LIVER

Berb. is indicated in **gall stonic colic** when jaundice follows colic.

Character of pain – Violent stitching pains in the right hypochondriac region that causes him to hold his breath. Pains radiate from liver region to all directions.

Stools – Become clay coloured and bileless. Person appears pale with an earthy complexion and blue ring around the eyes.

Aggravation – motion, jar.

URINARY SYSTEM

Berb. is used in **renal colic**. Left kidney, ureter are generally involved.

Character of Pains :

- Radiating pains – Stitching, cutting pains in the left renal region which follows the course of the ureter into the bladder, urethra and thence into the hips.
- Bubbling sensation in the region of kidneys.
- Soreness, numbness, stiffness, lameness and burning with painful pressure in lumbar and renal regions.

Character of urine :

Acute cases – Urine is greenish, turbid flocculent having a copious mucous sediment.

In Chronic cases – Urine appears reddish, bloody, turbid with copious sediment. Urine flows slowly with constant urging.

RHEUMATISM

Rheumatic and gouty complaints with diseases of urinary organs.

Gout – Uric acid and urate deposits in the joints.

Rheumatism – Soreness and lameness in the joints with radiating pains.

LUMBAGO

- Prostration with a sense of weakness across the back.
- Numbness, stiffness and lameness in the lumbar regions.
- Backache worse when sitting or lying especially when lying in the bed in the morning – Patient rises from a seat with difficulty.
- Pains radiate in every direction.

Worse – Fatigue, sitting or lying down, jarring motion.

FEMALE SYMPTOMS

Berb. is indicated in menstural troubles associated with urinary difficulties.

Character of pains – Sticking, radiating pains. There is great sensitiveness and soreness of vagina.

GENERAL MODALITIES

Aggravation – MOTION
WALKING
ANY SUDDEN JARRING MOVEMENT.

RELATIONS

Similar to – Canth, Lyc, Sars, Tab in Renal Colic

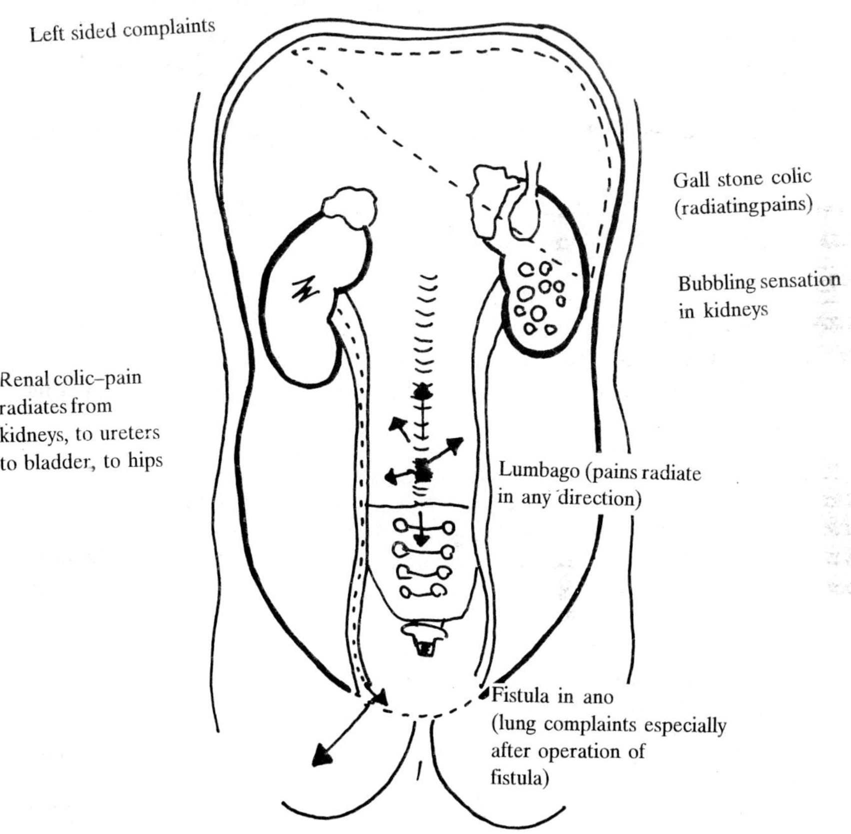
Left sided complaints
Gall stone colic (radiatingpains)
Bubbling sensation in kidneys
Renal colic–pain radiates from kidneys, to ureters to bladder, to hips
Lumbago (pains radiate in any direction)
Fistula in ano (lung complaints especially after operation of fistula)

BERBERIS VULGARIS

Acts well after—Arn, Bry, Kali bich, Rhus, Sulph in Rheumatic affections.

Important Questions ?

Q.1. Give indications of Berberis vulgaris in :

1) Keynotes [1974]
2) Liver disorders [1986]
3) Urinary disorders (Colic)
[1976, 77, 78 S, 79, 81, 84, 88, 94, 96]

21. BORAX VENETA

Hahnemann

Common Name – Borate of sodium.

Miasm – Psora is in the background.

Constitution – Borax is suited to a dirty and unclear patient whose hair is constantly tangled and knotted; eyelids are loaded with a gummy exudate; nostrils are crusty and inflamed with constant flowing of excoriating coryza; mouth is full of apthous sores that prevent eating; tongue is dry and cracked.

Patient is excessively nervous. Borax helps in red nose of women.

Relation with heat and cold – Hot patients.

KEYNOTES

1) ***Apthous sore mouth*** is the keynote for the use of Borax.

2) *Mouth is very hot* and is worse eating salty or sour food.

3) *Apthae* in mouth, tongue, inside cheeks, bleed easily on touch and prevents child from nursing.

4) ***Dread of downward motion*** – In all complaints child clings to the nurse on laying him down or going downstairs.

[Reason – Child suffers from *cerebral aneamia* and this downward motion causes a feeling as though it were going to fall.]

5) Child is excessively *nervous*, *anxious* and *restless* – easily frightened by slightest noise.

6) Anxiety increases until *11 P.M.*

7) *Inflamed and crusty nostrils.*

8) *Pain in right pectoral region* – cough with expectoration of an offensive herby taste.

9) Child has frequent urination and *screams before he passes urine*. Urine when passed is ***HOT*** and has a peculiar pungent foetid odour.

10) *Leucorrhoea* – albuminous, strachy and hot.

11) *Skin* is unhealthy and slight injuries suppurate.

12) *Hair splits* and becomes tangled.

13) *Eyelashes* become loaded with gummy exudation especially in the morning. Tendency to "wild hairs" which turn inward and inflame the eyes.

Particulars :

1) MIND
2) HAIR
3) FACE
4) EYES
5) EAR
6) NOSE
7) G.I.T
8) RESPIRATORY SYSTEM
9) URINARY SYSTEM
10) FEMALE SEXUAL SYMPTOMS

MIND

- Anxiety, fidgetiness and sensitiveness are prominent.
- Anxious about trifles – patient starts at every noise – hearing an unexpected noise, hearing something drop from a chair to the floor or if the door opens unexpectedly.
- Aggravation from downward motion when the mother is in the act of laying down the child, it rouses up in sleep and cries out in fright.

Downward motion causes an anxious feeling of exaggerated intensity with confusion and vertigo.

(Dr. Kent has said that this keynote is used to cure all problems like diarrhora, apthae, rheumatism and menstural troubles etc.)

- Patient is restless – He changes from one work to another and roams about indefinitely.
- Anxiety, nervous troubles and mental state keep up until 11 p.m. Insane people may start behaving normally (lucid interval) as if nothing happened – thus a great change at 11 P.M.

HAIR

- Hair becomes frowsy and tangled; splits stick together at the tips .
- Hair form bunches (Plica polonica) which if cut off form again. (Flour. acid, Lyc, Psor, Tub)

FACE

- Face is pale and clay coloured.
- Children have small vesicles around the mouth and on the forehead.

EYES

- Eyelashes are loaded with gummy exudation; agglutinated in the morning.

Restless, anxious, nervous child

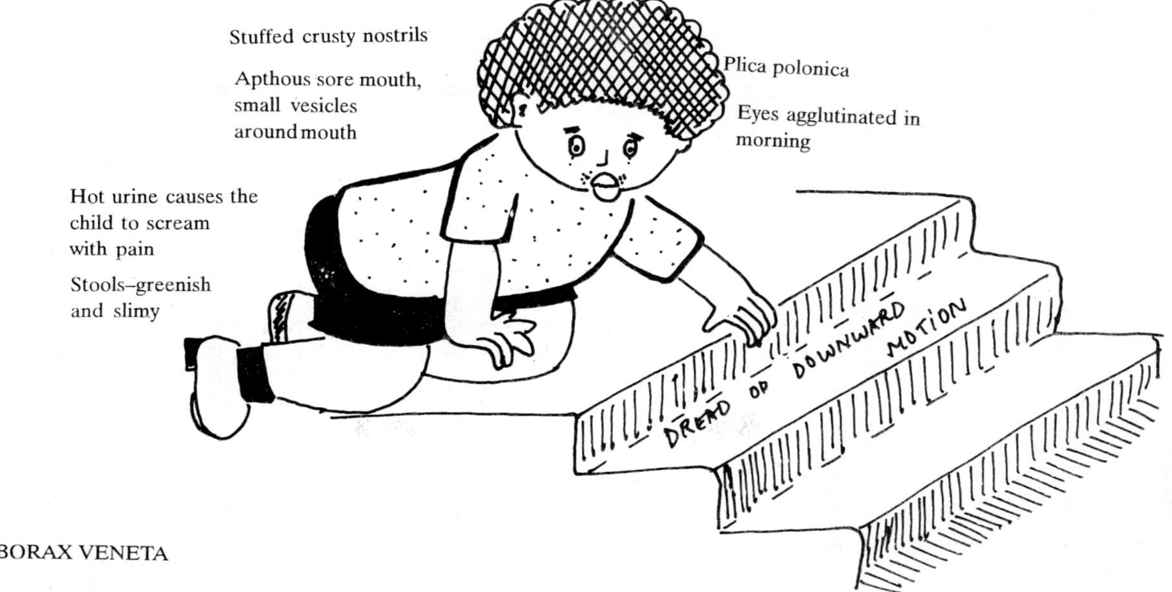

BORAX VENETA

- They turn inward and inflame the eye especially at the outer canthus.
- Tendency to wild hair.

EAR

- Earache accmpanied with soreness swelling and heat of the ear.
- Each paroxysm of pain causes the child to start nervously.
- There is muco purulent otorrhoea.
-

NOSE

- Borax has cured red nose in women.
- Chronic inflammation of mucous membrane-dry crusts form in the nose and reform if removed.
- Stoppage of right nostril and then left with constant blowing of nose (Amm. carb, Lac. can, Mag mur).

G.I.T

Mouth – apthous sore mouth – apthae form in the pouches on the inside of the cheeks, tongue and the fauces. Mouth is *HOT* which the mother notices when the child takes hold of the nipple. Mucous membranes around the apthae bleed easily.

The child lets go off the nipple and cries with pain and vexation or else refuses the breast altogether.

Apthous condition extends throughout the gastro intestinal tract. Borax patient with 'Stomach apthae' gags retches and coughs which is called stomach cough.

Stools

- Greenish slimy stools are passed day and night and the child keeps up a petiful crying with apthous sore mouth.

RESPIRATORY SYSTEM

- Pain in the right pectoral region.
- Cough with expectoration of an offensive herby taste.
- *Pleurisy* – Borax has cured pleuritis of the chest in the right pectoral region. These pains are very sharp and they make the patient wince and catch his breath.

URINARY SYSTEM

Urethritis – Child has frequent urging to urinate and screams before passing urine.

Urine passed is hot and has a peculiar pungent foetid odour.

(Lyc, Sars, Berb, Benz acid – Child cries before urinating but there is deposit of **sand** in the diaper or vessel.)

FEMALE SYMPTOMS

Menses

Dysmenorrhoea – Membranous dysmenorrhoea with violent labor like pains before and during the flow and it seems uterus would expel itself through the vagina. Violent pains keep on until expulsion of membrane.

Bleeding :

Time – Too early

Quantity – Too profuse

Character of blood – Very hot accompanied with stitching and pressing pains in the groins.

Concomitants – Throbbing in the head and rushing in the ears. Dread of downward motion.

Leucorrhoea

- Clear copious and albuminous.
- Leucorrhoea feels like hot fluid flowing down the legs.
- Due to acrid, profuse and scanty leucorrhoea, false membrane is formed causing sterility in women.

General Modalities :

Aggravation – DOWNWARD MOTION, SUDDEN SLIGHT NOISES, SMOKING – WHICH MAY BRING ON DIARRHOEA, DAMP COLD WEATHER, BEFORE URINATING.

Amelioration – PRESSURE
HOLDING PAINFUL SIDE WITH HAND.

Relations

Borax follows – Calc, Psor, Sanic, Sulphur.

Is followed by – Ars, Bry, Lyc, Phos, Sil.

Incompatible – Should not be used before or after Acetic acid vinegar, wine.

Improtant Questions ?

- Q.1. Give indication of Borax in.

1) Leucorrhoea [1972s, 77s, 78, 78s, 79, 82, 86]
2) Action of Borax on female genitilia [1978, 86, 93]
3) Apthae [1987]
4) Compare *dysmenorrhoea* of Borax and Vibernum opulus [1993]

BORAX	VIBERNUM OP.
Membranous dysmenorrhoea – Violent labor like pains before and during menses and it seems that uterus would expel itself from the vagina. Flow starts slightly but violent pains keeps on until explusion of the membrane.	Pain begins in the back and goes around to the loin and to uterus ending in cramps there.

22. BRYONIA ALBA

Hahnemann

Common Name – White Bryony (Cucurbitaceae)
(Wild Hop)

Constitution – Suitable to dry spare nervous, slender persons of irritable disposition and rheumatic tendency.

Temperament – Irritable temperament.

Relation with heat and cold – Hot patient.

Maism – Psora is in background.

Diathesis – Rheumatic and Gouty diathesis and prone to Bilious Attacks.

KEYNOTES

1) All complaints are ***aggravated by least motion and ameliorated*** **by** ***absolute rest, lying on painful side and pressure.***
2) Bryonia is a *right sided remedy.*
3) ***Dryness of mucous membranes*** especially of mouth and stomach (dryness is caused due to lack of secretion). Lips and tongue are dry and parched. Tongue is coated white down the middle; stool is dry as if burnt and expelled with difficulty; cough is dry hard and racking with scanty expectoration.
4) ***Great thirst*** for large quantities of cold water at long intervals
5) ***Constipation*** is a guiding feature of Bryonia. Stool is dry and hard as if burnt. It is expelled with difficulty as there is no moisture about the parts and no mucous to soften the hard stools.
6) *Pressure as from ston*e in the pit of the *stomach* relieved from eructation (secretion of gastric juice is insufficient and so the food lies undigested in the stomach).
7) *Sitting up causes nausea and faintness.*
8) Bryonia acts powerfully on the *serous membranes* (meninges, pleura, peritoneum). It causes *inflammation and effusion* with sharp stitching pains worse from any motion.
9) *Stitching pains* in serous membranes and joints worse on motion.

(Kali. carb – stitching pains irrespective of motion).

10) *Cough* is *dry, hard racking* with *scanty expectoration* and splitting headache. Worse – eating, drinking, warm room.
11) *Vicarious menstruation* – Nose bleeds when menses should appear (Phos); hemoptysis, blood spitting.
12) Breast are heavy of a *stony hardness*. They are hot and painful.

13) ***Rheumatism of joints,*** with pale swelling and great pain aggravated on touch and least motion.
14) Patient is *angry and irritable* – Sufferings are increased by physical and mental exertion.
15) *Delirium* – Talks constantly about his business. Desire to get out of the bed and go home.
16) *Desires things and refuses when offered.*
17) All complaints are *aggravated by eating* (vegetable foods).
18) *Aggravation* – motion, exertion, touch, sitting up *(causes nausea and vomiting), warmth, heat, ironing* (motion and heat), *chilling when overheated, suppressed discharges.*

Amelioration – *Lying on painful side.*

Particulars :

1) FEVER
2) HEADACHE
3) G.I.T
4) RESPIRATORY SYSTEM
5) RHEUMATISM
6) FEMALE SYMPTOMS
7) SKIN

FEVER

- Bryonia is indicated in fevers mostly of remitting type, rheumatic, gastric, bilious, traumatic and typhoid fevers in all of which gastric symptoms predominate.
- Fever develops slowly with gradually increasing severity (Gels sudden onset – Aco, Bell).
- Increased action of the heart giving rise to a frequent, tense pulse which is increased by least motion and hence the patient has to keep perfectly quiet.
- Dull and throbbing headache with sharp pain over the eyes.
- Least attempt to raise head from the pillow causes nausea and faintness.
- Dry mouth with a white coated tongue in the centre. As fever grows bilious symptoms predominate.
- Tongue becomes yellowish, dry, brown and cracked with a bitter taste in the mouth and splitting headache.
- Patient drinks large quantities of cold water at long intervals.
- Sensation of heavy pressure in the stomach as if a stone were lying there.
- Constipation – hard, dry and burnt stools expelled with difficulty due to atonacity of rectum.
- Sweat is provoked by least exertion.
- Dry and hard cough with stitching pains in the chest.

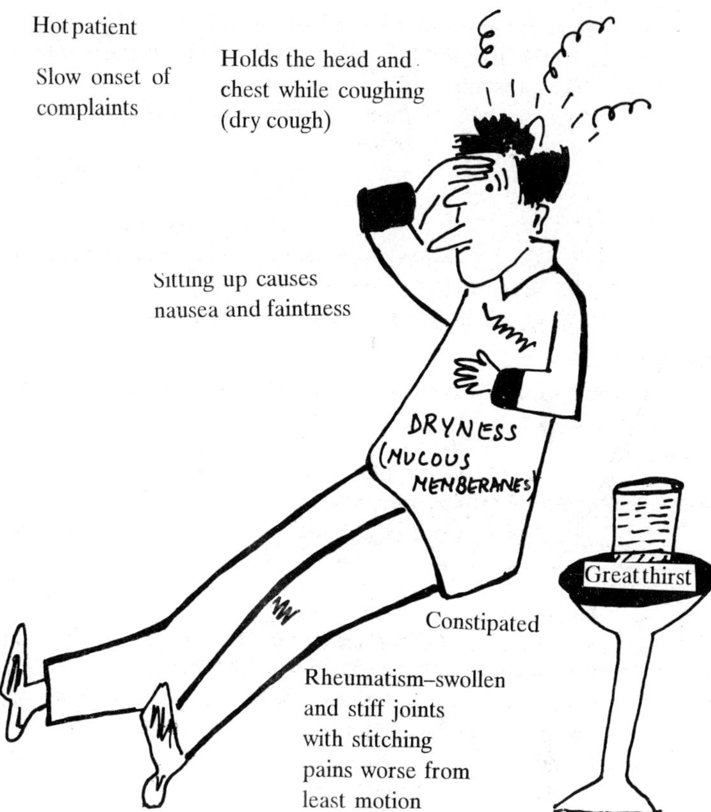
Hot patient
Slow onset of complaints
Holds the head and chest while coughing (dry cough)
Sitting up causes nausea and faintness
DRYNESS (MUCOUS MEMBERANES)
Great thirst
Constipated
Rheumatism–swollen and stiff joints with stitching pains worse from least motion

BRYONIA

DELIRIUM

- There is confusion of mind and sensorium is depressed.
- Extreme irritability—every word which compels him to speak aggravates him.
- Sluggish state of mind. Thinks he is away from home and wants to be taken home.
- Patient desires things and refuses them when offered.
- Talks constantly about his business.
- Full of fear and anxiety and wants to keep still.
- In brain affections—continual lateral motion of the lower jaw.

Constant motion of one arm and one leg.

Aggravation—Hot summer weather. Taking cold in hot summer, slightest motion.

Amelioration—Lying on painful side, complete rest, perspiration.

HEADACHE

Headaches are commonly the forerunner of other complaints like coryza, bronchitis, fever, constipation.

Causes—Overheating, overexertion, chilling up when overheated.

Symptoms:

- Headaches occur in the morning.
- Sensation as if the skull would split open and the contents of cranium would be pushed out.
- Pains are aggravated by heat, motion—winking the eyes, talking or any mental exertion.
- Congestion with a sluggish mind.
- Face is mottled and purple with congestion.
- Patient grasps the head while coughing as coughing causes a sharp stabbing pain.
- Obstinate headache with constipation.
- Headaches are often accompanied by nose bleed.

Worse—Slightest motion, eating, warm room, ironing (warm room and motion of hands)

Relief—Tight Pressure, Lying down, keeping quiet

G.I.T

Lips :

- Parched and dry lips with a tendency to bleed.

Toothache

Cause—Warm drinks, warm food, warm room, smoking, eating.

Stitching and tearing pains of nervous origin (teeth are not decayed).

Amelioration—Cold water, laying head on painful side.

Tongue

- **Thickly white coated tongue in the middle with clean edges.** Insipid and flat taste.

Thirst

- Dry mouth with great thirst for large quantities of cold water at long intervals.

Stomach

- Craves in mind the things he has an aversion to in the stomach (no secretion of gastric juice and hence food lies undigested).
- Patient craves acids.
- Thirst for large quantities of water at long intervals.
- Desire for cold drinks but stomach is better from warm drinks.

Gastritis / Gastroenteritis

Cause – Taking cold, becoming overheated,drinking ice water when overheated.

Symptoms :

- Soreness, tenderness and stitching pains in the stomach.
- Heavy pressure in the stomach as if a stone were lying there (due to deficient secretion of gastric juice the food lies undigested in the stomach).
- Sensation as if stomach would burst.
- Every inspiration, every motion of the chest, body or cough aggravates his complaints.
- Patient lies perfectly quiet with knees drawn up.
- Dreadful nausea and faintness when rising up, relieved by lying still.
- Vomiting of bile with bitter eructation.
- All except stomach complaints are better from pressure.
- Patient is relieved by warm drinks.

Liver

- Inflammation of liver when the right lobe is affected.
- Every motion, deep breath causes a stitching pain in the right hypochondrium.

Better – Lying on the right side.

Diarrhoea

Cause – Overeating, heat of summer.

Symptoms – Morning diarrhoea.

Before stools – Patient is siezed with sudden gripping pains doubling him up.If while lying he makes least motion he has to hurry for stools.

Character of stools – Yellow mushy or bilious stools with smell of old cheese.

After stools – Patient is completely exhausted and lies down almost dead covered with sweat.

Aggravation – Least motion.

Relief – Lying perfectly still.

Constipation

Due to difficult secretion of mucous membranes there is no moisture about the parts and no mucus to soften the hard stools.

Character of stools – Dry hard as if burnt, stools are expelled with difficulty. Obstinate headache with constipation.

Concomitants – Excess thirst with dry white coated tongue in the centre.

RESPIRATORY SYSTEM

Nose – Vicarious menstruation – Nose bleeds at the time of menses. If menstrual flow is checked suddenly from cold, nose bleed will appear.

- Dryness of nose with frequent sneezing and loss of smell.

Throat

- Constitutional tendency to apthous formation in the throat, sore with stitching pains, dryness and parched appearance of the throat. Thirst for large quantities of water at long intervals.

Bronchitis

Cause – Heat, coming from open air into warm room.

Character of cough – Hard and dry cough with no or little expectoration.

- There is soreness and stitching pains in the chest when the patient coughs.
- *"Cough hurts the head and chest and the person holds them with hands".*
- Pressure is felt over the sternum.

Pleurisy

Bryonia has marked affect on the serous membranes.

- Right lung is mostly affected.
- Bryonia is useful in the second stage of inflammation after the serous effusion has set in.
- *Stitching pains* are present in the chest.
- Rapid short breaths because breathing increases pain. There is constant disposition to sigh and expand the lungs.
- Pains are aggravated by least motion.

Amel – Lying still, pressure on painful side.

Pneumonia

Croupous pneumonia and pleuro pneumonia.

Symptoms :

- Right side mostly affected.
- Constriction in the chest with stitching pains and scanty expectoration.
- High fever with profuse perspiration and intense thirst.
- Expectoration has a reddish tinge with a rusty colour.

RHEUMATISM

- Local inflammation is violent.
- Joints are red swollen, stiff with stitching pains from slightest motion.

Aggravation – Least motion.

Amelioration – Lying still, pressure on painful side.

(Rhus tox: Joint pains are ameliorated by continued motion).

Synovitis of rheumatic or traumatic origin. Affected joint is pale, red and tense. There is effusion into the synovial sac with sharp stitching pains.
Worse – Motion.

Muscular System – Bryonia produces inflammation of muscular system. Muscles are sore to touch and at times they are swollen.

Worse – Least motion.

FEMALE SYMPTOMS

Menses

Bryonia is very useful when the normal flow of blood has been suppressed and there is vicarious menstruation. Remedy for heamoptysis, heamatemesis, epistaxis.

Amenorrhoea/Threatened abortion – caused by becoming overheated from exertion, ironing, washing etc.

Breast

Mastitis or mammary abscess.

- Breasts are stony hard and heavy.
- Hot and painful breasts and the patient must support them with hand.
- Stopping of milk in lying in period.

Worse – Least motion.
Better – Perfect rest, supporting the breast with hands.

SKIN

Bryonia is used in *eruptive fevers* – nettle rash, measles, scarlet fever etc when there is slow development of rash or sudden receding of rash with appearance of cerebral symptoms.

- Child becomes drowsy with a pale face and twitching of muscles of the face, eyes and mouth.
- Any motion causes the child to scream with pain.
- Dry mouth, increased thirst and tongue coated white.

In other cases instead of cerebral symptoms inflammation of chest may develop.

- Bronchitis/pneumonia.

Modalities

Aggravation – MOTION
EXERTION, TOUCH
CANNOT SIT UP – GETS FAINT OR SICK
WARMTH, WARM FOOD
EATING
SUPPRESSED DISCHARGES

Amelioration – LYING ESPECIALLY ON PAINFUL SIDE
PRESSURE ON AFFECTED PARTS (EXCEPT STOMACH IN ABDOMINAL COMPLAINTS)
REST
COLD THINGS, DRINKS

Relations

Complementry to – Alumina, Rhus tox
Similar to – Bell, Hepar for hasty speech and drinking.
Ranunculus – pleuritic/rheumatic pains of chest.
Followed well by – Alum, Ars., Kali carb, Nux vom, Puls, Rhus tox, Sulphur.
Antidotes – Alum, Merc, Rhus tox.

Important Questin ?

Q1 Give indications of Bryonia in the following

1) Keynotes	[1974, 78,89]
2)Delirium	[1974, 91]
3)Respiratory Symptoms	[1974, 82, 86, 94, 96]
4) Pleurisy	[1979, 95]
5) Toothache	[1985]
6) Fever (Typhoid)	[1973, 76, 77, 81, 86, 93, 95]
7) Headache	[1972, 73, 75, 86]
8) Rheumatism	[1976, 79, 82]
9) Breast	[1982]

10) G.I.T [1974, 75]
11) Modalities [1972, 75, 82]

Q2. Compare Conium mac / Bryonia in Mastitis – [1994 s]

CONIUM MAC	BRYONIA
• Sore hard and painful breast caused from taking cold, suppressed menses, bruises and injuries	• Breasts are heavy, stony hard
• An abscess of the breast becomes surrounded by lumps and nodules.	• Stopping of milk flow in lying in-period
• In malignant affections it takes hold of the gland from the beginning and infiltrates them causing stony hardness	• Milk fever – pain and swelling of the breast *Aggravation* – Least motion, heat *Amelioration* • supporting the breast with hand • Absolute rest and pressure

Q.2. Compare Opuim / Bryonia in Constipation. [1977, 79, 94]

OPIUM	BRYONIA
• Opium causes *inertia of rectum* and hence there is no inclination for bowels to move.	• Bryonia causes *dryness of mucous membranes* and hence there is no mucus or moisture about the anus to soften the hard stools. Atony of rectum later develops
• Bowels become impacted with feaces and flatus accumulates in upper part of the intestines and presses on upward against the chest	• **Ch. of stools** – Dry hard stools as if burnt and are expelled with difficulty
• Character of stools – Little hard dry like black balls. Opium in repeated doses restores peristaltic movements with colicky pains.	• Obstinate constipation with headache.

Q.3. Compare Belladonna/ Bryonia in Headache. [1987 s]

BELLADONNA	BRYONIA
• Headache develops suddenly with violence. First few hours of exposure to cold or sun	• Pain develops with gradually increasing severity. 'A day after exposure to cold or sunstroke.
• Throbbing headache with flushed face, red eyes and heat of the skin	• Bursting headache as if skull would split open. 'Dryness is marked'
• Congestion is marked	• Obliged to keep perfectly quiet
• Obliged to sit up (maintain perpendicular position)	
Amelioration – Warmth, wrapping up. Sensitive to least touch / pressure, cold air.	**Amelioration** – • Cool application. • Tight pressure lying on affected side.

Q.4. Compare Aconite / Bryonia in Fever. [1992]

ACONITE	BRYONIA
• Given in beginning of fever. There is congestion and chill before the inflammatory fever with full pulse and hot and dry skin.	• Bryonia is given in advanced. stages (second stage of the inflammatory fever or when effusion has set in).
• **Mind** – Full of fear Restlessness – Cannot keep still and constantly keeps moving.	• **Mind** – Irritable angry patient. Person is perfectly quiet as least motion aggravates his complaints

Q.6. Compare Sulphur / Bryonia in morning Diarrhoea. [1976]

SULPHUR	BRYONIA
• Early morning diarrhoea driving him out of the bed. Rectum feels too weak to retain the contents.	• Morning diarrhoea driving him out of bed. If while lying he makes least motion he has to hurry for stools.
• Burning about the anus.	• Patient is relieved by lying perfecty still.
• Anus feels red and excoriated.	

• *Concomitants* – craving for sweets.	• *Concomitants* – Dryness of all mucous membranes.
• Empty all gone feeling in epigastrium at 11 a.m.	• Empty all gone feeling in epigastrium at 9 a.m.
• Diarrhoea alternates with constipation.	• Thirst for large quantities of water at long intervals.

23. CALCAREA CARBONICA

Hahnemann

Common Name – Carbonate of Lime (Middle layer of Oyester shell).

Miasm – Deepest antipsoric and antisycotic remedy.

- *Calc. carb is the chronic of Belladonna* (congestion and constitution of both the remedies is the same but Calc. carb is needed to complete the cure).
- Calc. carb is a *deep acting remedy.* (In adults it should not be repeated again and again. It should be given in low potency in children) .

Constitution

Dr. Tyler has given the following description –

With the chalky complexion goes

Fatness without fitness

Sweating without heat

Bones without strength

Tissues of plus quantity and minus quality

Mere flabby bulk with weakness and weariness.

Child -- Teething picture

Rickety child

Teething picture – Fair, fat and flabby child; pale and waxy face, big head and open fontanelled; sour smelling; sweats profusely especially on back of the head. Difficult and delayed dentition.

Rickety child – Weak bones with flabby muscles. There is great weakness and weariness. Stomach is swollen like an inverted saucer. (Bell. does a temporary spadework in these constitutions but real constitutional work is done by Cal. carb.)

Aneamic Type – Aneamic/Chlorotic fat women with a pale complexion. There is great chilliness, weakness, breathlessness and palpitation. Menses are too early, profuse and long lasting.

Tuberculous Type – Enlarged and indurated lymphatic glands. Young men who grow very tall, are very susceptible to tuberculous infiltration especially in upper lobe of right lung.

Old Man – Old men with fatty degeneration of heart causing palpitation, dyspnoea and weariness on least exertion.

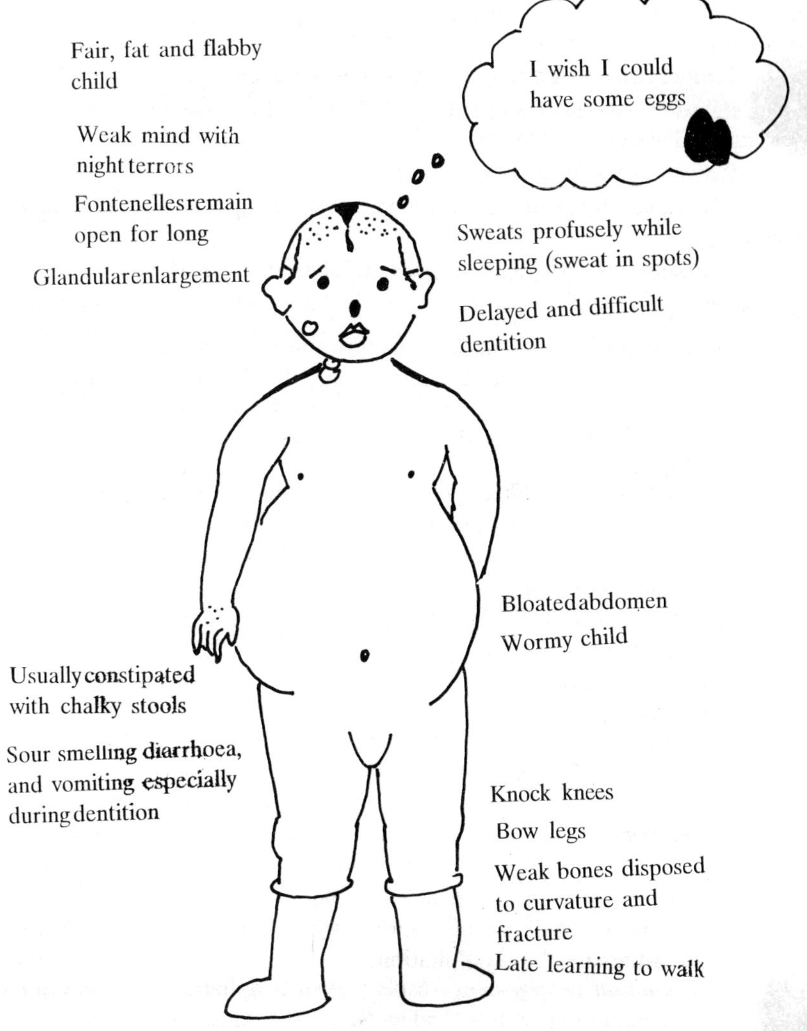

Very chilly patient.
sensation as if legs
had cold damp
stockings on (cold in spots)

CALCAREA CARBONICA

Mental Picture – Confusion of senses and dullness of the whole head. There is fear with restlessness. During epilepsy there is a sensation of a mouse running up and down the arm (Bell, Sil) .

Temperament – Leucophlegmatic temperament.

Relation with heat and cold – *Chilly* patient disposed to catch cold very easily. Patient sweats when cold.

Sweat and coldness come in spots

(Dr. Kent – Sulphur has heat in patches. Calc. has cold and sweat in patches.)

Diathesis – Scrofulous, rachitic and tuberculous diathesis.

KEYNOTES

1) ***Congestion*** – is a marked feature and more marked is the congestion of the internal parts, colder the surface becomes.

2) (i) *Chilly Patient* – Patient is very susceptible to cold. Least bit of cold air goes right through him and brings on all kinds of ailments.

(ii) ***Coldness in spots*** or single parts – head, stomach, feet etc. Patient finds it very difficult to keep these parts warm.

(iii) *Feet* and *legs* are habitually cold and damp as if they had ***cold damp stockings on.***

3) (i) ***Sweats profusely while sleeping*** – All over the body especially on back of the head and nape of the neck. While sleeping the pillows get wet far around.

(ii) ***Sour smelling sweat.***

(iii) *Sweat in spots* or single parts – head, arms, axillae, chest, knees, feet etc.

4) ***Sour smelling discharges*** – stools, vomiting, sweating etc. are all sour smelling.

5) Calc. produces *aneamic or chlorotic* states in plump, pale and waxy people and even in emaciated states. Chlorotic state is produced in young girls with weakness, weariness, breathlessness and palpitation.

6) *Glandular enlargement* – especially of lymphatic glands of neck and abdomen with a tendency to tuberculosis and induration. There is emaciation of neck and limbs while abdominal fat and glands increase.

7) ***Base of ulcers become indurated,burn and sting*** (Calc has a marked affect in cancerous ulcers having an indurated base. *It palliates and restrains the growth of these ulcers).*

8) Pyeamic states – absesses develop deep in the muscles, neck, thigh and abdomen. Calcarea favours resorption and encourages the part to become calcareous when the symptoms agree.

9) *Imperfect ossification* – Bones take long to develop and even after maturing they remain fragile. Weak bones with a tendency to curvature. *Late learning* to walk with open fontanelles and enlarged glands in children.

10) Calcarea babies are almost always more or less *wormy.*

11) Feels better when *constipated* – stool has to be mechanically removed (Aloes, Sepia,Sil, Thuja).

12) Calcarea grows and *cures polyps* anywhere on the body.

13) Children *long for eggs*. They are better by eating eggs.

- Eats, undigestible things – Lime, slate, pencil, earth, chalk. (Alum, Nit acid, Cina, China, Psor).

Desire to be magnetised.

Aversion to meat, milk, coffee.

(Aversion to meat – Alum, Graph, Mur acid, Puls).

14) *Mind* – Great weakness of mind. Person is full of fear and apprehension. Night terrors in children.

- *Least mental excitement causes profuse return of menstrual flow.*

Particulars :

1) CHILD
2) MIND
3) HEAD
4) EYE
5) EAR
6) FACE
7) RESPIRATORY SYSTEM
8) G.I.T.
9) FEMALE SYMPTOMS
10) SPINE
11) SLEEP.

CHILD

- *Fair, fat and flabby* child with a chalky complexion.
- *Defective assimilation and impaired ossification* – Tardy development of bony tissues with lymphatic enlargement. Bony tissues are irregularly nourished. Softening of bones leading to curvature of long bones. Extremities are crooked and deformed. Bones of leg give way under heavy weight of the body and so knock knees and bow legs develop with late learning to walk.
- *Delayed and difficult dentition.*
- Night terrors – children going through difficult dentition have a dreadful time in the night and screach out in the night.

- *Bones* are *unevenly nourished* leading to their irregular development while soft parts suffer from overnutrition thus the tendency to obesity.
- *Lymphatic enlargement* in neck and abdomen while the limbs are emaciated.
- Child is very sensitive to cold and takes cold easily. *Cold in patches.*
- *Profuse sweat on the head of large headed open fontanelled children.* Sweat in spots. Patient sweats profusely as a consequence he takes cold readily.
- *Sour smelling discharges.*
- Child is usually *constipated* but there may be offensive sour smelling diarrhoea during dentition.
- *Child longs for eggs and undigestible things.* Aversion to meat and milk.
- Swollen "*stomach like an inverted saucer.*"
- Babies are almost more or less *wormy.*
- *Hydrocephalus*—Slow formation of bones of skull and hence the fontanelles remain open. In hydrocephalus there is effusion in the membranes and the bones do not grow and keep pace with the bones of the head. Hence the head grows wider and larger with hydrocephalus.

MIND

Weakness—Great weakness of mind and the patient becomes very tired from least mental and physical work.

Fear—Fear that something is going to happen to herself or someone else. That people will notice her confusion of mind. Fear of death, consumption, misfortune dreadful dreams.

Night terrors—Child screams out at night due to dreadful dreams during dentition.

Restless patient—Patient sits and fidgets with small things.

Despondency—Despairs life and reason and broods over little things that have no importance.

Epilepsy—Sensation of mouse running up the arm or leg.

Confusion of mind and vertigo from least mental exertion.

- Desire to be *magnetised.*
- Slight mental effort produces heat.
- *Least mental excitement causes profuse return of menstrual flow.*

HEAD

Sweat— • Sweat on the head on slightest exertion. Patient sweats even in a cold room.

- Head sweats profusely while sleeping, wetting the pillow far around (Sil).

- Patient sweats profusely as a result he becomes chilly and catches cold easily.This brings on headache.
- Coldness of the whole scalp so he has to wrap the head.
- Congestive, periodical headache.

Cause – Stopping of catarrhal discharges, taking cold.

Location – Tearing headache above the eyes down to the nose.

Headaches in the temples, supraorbital region running down to the nose.

Sensation – Feeling of tightness and great tension in the forehead. Hammering headache with a sensation of strong pulsation in the forehead.

Burning in the vertex with coldness of the whole head. Sensation of coldness and numbness in the head and more the congestion, the colder the surface becomes.

Worse – During the day time, noise, talking, taking cold.

Relief – Lying down in the dark, evening.

EYES

- Calc is used in fat and flabby constitutions where cold settles in the eye and produces inflammation. Inflammation may lead to dim vision, photophobia and even ulceration of cornea.
- Calc is excellent for *eyestrains* caused by exertion of eyes like reading or looking steadily at one thing (Onosmodium). Eye complaints are aggravated by any exertion of the eyes, taking cold.

EAR

- Thickness of tympanum with defective hearing.
- Otorrhoea with mucopurulent discharge affecting the right ear. Catarrhal condition of the ear is brought on by taking cold or sudden change to cold damp weather.

FACE

- Sallow pale, sickly and dropsical face covered with cold sweat. Cold sweat on the face appears on slightest exertion.
- Cracked and bleeding lips.
- Hard, painful and swollen glands – submaxillary, sublingual and parotid.

RESPIRATORY SYSTEM

Nose

- Catarrah is caused due to exposure to cold.
- Calc is a great remedy for chronic nasal catarrah. Wings of the nose are thickened and there is offensive discharge which is both purulent and bloody.
- Stoppage of discharge may lead to headache.

- In nasal polyps with loss of smell Calc produces excellent results.

Throat

Sore throat

Cause – Exposure to cold/draft of air.

Symptoms – Red patches with little ulcers in the throat which extends to the roof of the mouth with a sore tongue and constant choking extending to the posterior nares filling with thick yellow mucus. Uvula is painful and swollen. Throat is painful on swallowing.

Painless hoarseness aggravated in morning (evening – Carbo veg, Hepar, Phos; Causticum – rawness and soreness).

Cough

Cause – Brought on by exposure to cold or damp weather.

Sensation – Plug going up and down the throat.

Character of cough – Tickling cough which occurs in a single paroxysm

2 Paroxysms – Merc sol, Puls.

3 Paroxysms – Cup met, Stannum.

Character of sputa – Yellowish, lumpy and sweetish sputa; when thrown into water it resembles a falling star which draws behind it a long trail of mucus. Sputa may contain blood. Tickling cough is troublesome at night. Dry and free expectoration in the morning.

Aggravation – Evening, playing piano, eating.

Concomitants – Chest is sore and sensitive to touch and feels tight, fills up with blood.

Tuberculosis

- Calc is used in the first stage of T.B. in persons with a leucophlegmatic constitution.

In tall slender rapidly growing young people with pthisis of upper lobe of the right lung (Ars, upper left lung – Sulph). Weak heart and weak chest, patient is too tired to make any efforts at breathing. There is great dyspnoea and weakness from going upstairs or walking against the wind.

Calc turns the tuberculous deposits from caseous into calcareous forms.

G.I.T.

Mouth

- Sour taste in mouth, sour vomiting and sour smelling diarrhoea in children during dentition. Toothache aggravated by cold air.

Stomach

- Longing for eggs, undigestible things.
- Aversion to meat and milk.

- Great indigestion of milk in children especially during dentition – vomiting in sour curds or ejected through the rectum in white curdled lumps.
- Food taken into the stomach remains and does not digest – it turns sour and there is sour vomiting and diarrhoea and hence there develops aversion to food.
- Feeling of fullness in the stomach after eating.
- Pit of the stomach is swollen like an inverted saucer and is sensitive to touch.
- Pain in the left hypochondrium and cannot tolerate tight clothes.

Abdomen

- Enlarged and flabby abdomen with general emaciation.
- Abdomen is distended with flatulence and is sensitive to pressure. Gurgling in the right side of the abdomen.
- Mesentric glands become enlarged and hard due to tuberculous deposits.
- Enlarged liver – with pain in the hepatic region aggravated by every movement.

Diarrhoea

Cause – Taking cold, during dentition.

Character of stool – Copious watery, whitish, sour, foetid stools with undigested food particles is a sure indication of Calc. carb.

Calc. babies are wormy. Worms lead to indigestion and may be passed out in stools or vomited out.

Constipation

Patient feels better when constipated. Stools are whitish and sour smelling.

FEMALE SYMPTOMS

Chlorotic – Women who are flabby and plethoric. They are weak and get easily tired, breathless with palpitation on least exertion. They get cramps and even sprain themselves very easily. They grow rapidly and their menses start early and profusely provoked by overexertion and emotions.

Menses

Calc. is indispensable in curing catamenia when the menses appear early with a profuse flow. A little physical exertion or least mental excitement causes return of menstrual flow.

Time – Too early.

Quantity – Too profuse.

Duration – Too long lasting.

Concomitants – Great tendency to catch cold, leading to ailments, headache, aching in back and hips, pain and swelling in breast, leucorrhoea, amorous dreams which are troublesome before menses and even linger on later.

Leucorrhoea

"Thick, yellow, profuse and acrid" leucorrhoea causing itching and rawness in the vagina. Leucorrhoea occurs between menses.

Labor

- Calc. is used when conception does not occur due to great weakness and relaxation of the organs.
- When menses continue even after pregnancy or threatened abortion.
- In false labor pains that move upward and reduce the strength of the mother, Calc is used.

Breast

- Calc. checks galactorrhoea, scantiness of secretion of milk and even improves quality of secretion of mother's milk.
- Sometimes when child does not take milk due to disagreeable taste – a few doses of Calcarea sweetens the milk and makes it digestible.

SPINE

- Weak and sensitive spine – the patient cannot sit upright. He always tries to lean back on the chair.
- Calc is indicated when the lime element is deficient which leads to curvature of spine.
- In caries of vertebra Calc. is a very good remedy.
- Rheumatic complaints of joints are caused by every cold, change in weather, stiffness in all joints on beginning to move.

SLEEP

- Sleepless for a good part of the night due to overactivity of mind.
- Patient is full of ideas and on closing the eyes he sees horrible visions.
- Cold feet at night in bed.

General modalities :

Aggravation – LEAST EXPOSURE TO COLD AIR OR WET WEATHER, MENTAL AND PHYSICAL EXERTION.

Amelioration – LYING ON PAINFUL SIDE.

Relations :

- Calcarea should not be given before *Nitric Acid* or *Sulphur* as it brings on complications.

- In children Calcarea may be repeated in low potency.
- In adults Calcarea should *not be repeated* often; especially if the first dose benefitted, it will usually do harm.

Complements – Bell, Rhus.

Inimicals – Nitric acid, Sulph.

Antidotes – Nitric acid, Bry, Camph, Chin, Ipec, Nux, Sep, S.

Remedies that follow well – Nitric acid, Bell, Borax, Bism, Dulc, Graph, Ipec, Kali Bi, Lyc, Nux, Phos, Puls, Plat, Pod, Rhus, Sil, Sep, Sars.

Important Quesions :

Q.1. Write drug picture of Calc. carb. [1974, 75, 76, 82, 87, 91]

Q.2. Give indications of Calc. carb in the following :

1) Nettle Rash [1987]
2) Child [1973, 76, 77, 775, 82, 86, 87, 91, 95, 96]
3) Female disorders [1972, 77, 79, 83, 85, 95, 94 S, 96]
4) Sinusitis [1987]

Q.3. When will you prescribe Calc. carb in case of intolerance of milk ? [1972]

Q.4. Compare Alumina/Calc. carb in Leucorrhoea. [1991]

Q.5. Compare child of .

Baryta carb/Cal. carb [1996]
Sanicula/Cal. carb [1993]
Silicea/Cal. carb [1997]
Cina/Chamomilla/Aeth/Cal. carb [1991]

24. CALCAREA PHOSPHORICA

C. Hering

Common Name – Phosphate of Lime (Calcium phosphate).

Miasm – Psora is in the background.

Constitution – Person is aneamic, dark, complexioned with dark hair and eyes. Thin and spare subject.

Child – Emaciated children with sunken flabby abdomen, weak bones with a tendency to curvature and late learning to walk.

Relation with heat and cold – Chilly patient.

Diathesis – Scrofulous and gouty diathesis.

KEYNOTES

1) ***Dark complexioned, thin and emaciated children*** with sunken and flabby abdomen and weak bones. Lack of animal heat with general *coldness* of the body.
2) ***Rachitis*** – Cranial bones are thin and brittle. Fontanelles and sutures remain open for too long or reopen after closing.
   Cal. phos – Anterior and Posterior fontanelle.
   Cal. carb – Anterior fontanelle.
3) Delayed and complicated *dentition*.
4) *Weak neck* which is unable to support the head; *weak spine which is disposed to curvature and is unable to support the body.*
5) Due to *defective nutrition* bones are weak and are disposed to curvature, child is slow in learning to walk.
6) ***Non union of bones;*** Calc. phos promotes the formation of callus in such cases.
7) Complaints *aggravate* by *thinking about them*.
8) ***Girls at puberty are aneamic***, tall, thin and rapidly growing. They usually suffer from **vertex headache** with flatulent dyspepsia aggravated by eating. There is a tendency of the bones to soften and the spine to curve.
9) Craving for *salted and smoked meats* (Calc. carb – eggs).
10) ***At every attempt to eat there are colicky pains in the abdomen.***
11) Diarrhoea where stools pass with flatulence and spluttering noise.
12) *Fistula in ano* alternating with *chest* complaints.
13) *Rheumatism* of cold weather.
14) Oozing of *blood* from the *navel of infants*.

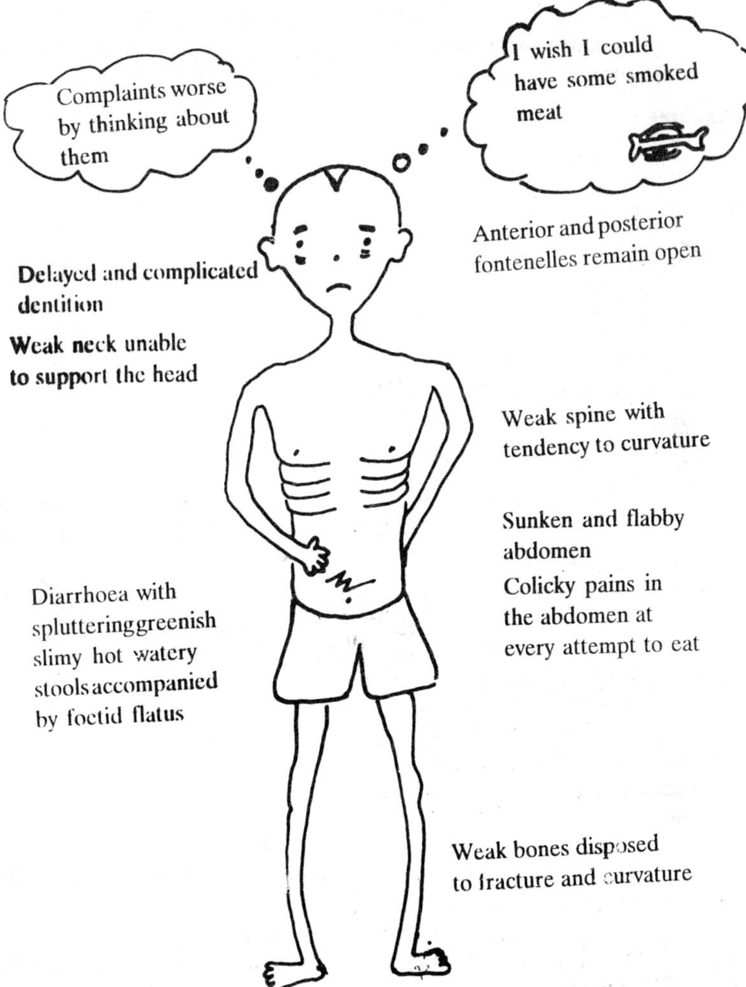

CALCAREA PHOSPHORICA

15) Dr. Grawvogl recommended Calc. phos highly in *chronic hydrocephalus*. Calc. phos is a prenatal remedy given during pregnancy to women who have given birth to hydrocephalic children.

Particulars :

1) CHILD
2) HEAD
3) FACE
4) EYES
5) EARS
6) NOSE
7) TEETH
8) RESPIRATORY SYSTEM
9) G.I.T.
10) URINARY SYSTEM
11) FEMALE SYMPTOMS
12) BACK and EXTREMITIES
13) NEURALGIAS

Calc. phos works with albumin as a cement and carries it to any part of the body i.e. bone, tissues etc. If for any reason phosphate of lime decreases – albumen not having sufficient phosphate of lime is thrown out of the body thus resulting in.

- Brights disease – Thrown off by the kidney.
- Nasal catarrah – Thrown off by nasal passage.
- Cough – Thrown off by the lungs.
- Eczema, pimples, freckles – thrown off by the skin.

CHILD

Look of the child – Thin and emaciated child with a sunken and flabby abdomen, weak bones and glandular enlargement.

Head – Large head with open fontanelles. Cranial bones are unnaturally thin and brittle. Mentally the children are dull and have a slow comprehension. In chronic hydrocephalus – Cal. phos is given to pregnant ladies who have repeatedly given birth to hydrocephalic children.

Dentition – Delayed and difficult dentition.

Rickets – Due to defective nutrition the child has weakbones – due to this there is late learning to walk. Weak neck which is unable to support the head. Weak spine with a tendency to curvature and is unable to support the body. Bones are disposed to curvature and fracture. Non union of fractured bones.

G.I.T. :

- Child vomits milk persistently whether it is breast milk or artificially prepared.

- Child desires salted bacons or smoked meat.
- Colic after every feeding.

Stools – Green, slimy, lientric stools accompanied by passage of a great deal of foetid flatus. Calc phos is also used in cholera infantum.

Complaints are aggravated by thinking about them, exposure to cold weather.

Fever – Chilliness and shivering in beginning of fever.

- Cold and clammy sweat on face and body.
- Lack of animal heat causes general coldness of the body.

HEAD

Aneamic school girls are disposed to constant headaches at puberty.

Location – Worse near sutures in vertex.

Sensation – Throbbing and burning in head with a tight feeling.

Aggravation – Jar, pressure, mental exertion.

Amelioration – Head being washed in cold water, being quiet.

FACE

- Aneamic and chlorotic,pale and waxy face.
- Rheumatic faceache in every cold spell of weather.
- Acne on the face of young girls especially at puberty.

EYES

- Inflammation of the eyeballs with pain in the eyes, spasm of the lids and photophobia.
- Calc. phos is markedly indicated in neuralgic pains of the eyes when Mag phos fails.

EARS

- Rheumatic pains in the ears with a characteristic albuminous and excoriating discharge. Enlarged and painful parotid glands.

NOSE

- Disposition to chronic catarrah of the nose with tough, thick and albuminous discharge.
- Calc phos has cured polyps of the nose.

TEETH

- Cal phos is the chief remedy in all teething disorders.
- Delayed and difficult dentition (Phosphate of lime is a constant material of teeth and when this material is deficient, dentition is slow and painful often causing convulsions).
- Teeth decay as soon as they appear.
- If gums are pale this remedy is especially indicated.

RESPIRATORY SYSTEM

Throat—Every cold settles in the throat. Calc phos produces excellent results in acute stage of chronic enlargement of tonsils. There is threatened suffocation with sticking pains in the throat on swallowing.

Larynx—Hoarseness with dry hacking cough. There is constant hemming and scraping of mucus while talking. Hence public speakers are greatly benefitted.

Lungs—Rheumatic pains in the lungs with involuntary sighing. Emaciation of the chest with great weakness and prostration. Rattling in the chest with difficult expectoration. Calc phos is very useful in pthisis and blood spitting.

G.I.T.

Tongue—White coated swollen tongue.

Stomach—The person desires salt bacon and salted meat. Cause of disorder of stomach—cold drinks, ice creams and fruits.

- Colicky pains in the stomach from least food.
- Burning and sinking sensation in the abdomen.
- Later there is nausea, vomiting and diarrhoea.

Diarrhoea :

Character of stools—Slimy, greenish, undigested spluttering stools due to copious offensive flatus.

- Also there is diarrhoea in young girls alternating with headache.

Piles—Heamorrhoids which ooze an albuminous substance resembling the white of an egg especially noticeable in aneamic persons. Painful piles; anus is cracked and fissured.

Worse—Standing, walking, night, sudden change of weather.

Better—Heat.

URINARY SYSTEM

As mentioned before due to deficiency of phosphate of lime, balance between albumen and phosphate of lime is disturbed and hence albumen becomes a disturbing element and is thrown out of the kidney leading to **brights disease, catarrah of bladder**—frequent urging to urinate, sharp shooting and cutting pains in the neck of the bladder. Albuminous urine calls for Calc. phos.

FEMALE

Nymphomania— intense sexual desire especially before menses. Sexual pains feel alive with blood and she feels pulsations in the parts with increased sexual desire. Even urination brings erection of clitoris.

Menses – Dysmenorrhoea from taking cold. Labor like pains in the beginning of menses. Amelioration when the flow begins. Throbbing pains in genitals going upwards to symphysis pubis and down to thighs.

Metrorrhagia in young girls with aneamia.

Time – Too early or too late.

Character of blood – Dark red blood with clots and membranes.

Concomitants – Pain in the back with flushed face and cold extremities.

Leucorrhoea – Albuminous and tenacious, acrid discharge like white of an egg. Worse after menses or with sexual excitement.

Uterus – Weakness in uterine region from prolapse of uterus and other uterine displacements. Uterine symptoms are aggravated by every change of weather.

Pregnancy – Aching in the limbs, during pregnancy aggravated by every change of weather. Child refuses to nurse and vomits sour and curdled milk due to poor watery and saltish taste of the milk.

BACK AND EXTREMITIES

Rheumatism :

Cause – Change of weather.

Rheumatism of joints and in the back between the shoulders.

Aggravation – Night, when air is full of melting snow, cold stormy weather, morning.

Lower limbs – Cold sensation in the lower limbs as if cold water has been poured on them. Intense pain in the lower limbs and the joints caused by abscesses and inflammation.

Aggravation – Night, cold damp weather.

NEURALGIAS

- Intense nerve pains with sensation of creeping numbness and coldness. Pains are worse at night..

(Cal. phos is used after Mag. phos fails to relieve the neuralgias.)

General Modalities :

Aggravation – CHANGE OF WEATHER
NIGHT
DAMP COLD WEATHER
MELTING EXERTION
MELTING SNOW

Amelioration – WARM WEATHER
WARM ROOM.

Relations :

Complementry – Ruta,.
Similar – Carbo animalis, Calc. flour, Calc. carb, Flour acid, Kali phos.

Psor. – **Debility after acute diseases.**

Silicea – Sweat of head is wanting.

Acts best before – Iod, Psor, Sanic, Sulph.

Acts best after – Ars, Iod, Tuberculinum.

Important Questions ?

Q. 1. Give indications of Calc phos in the following :

1) Guiding symptoms [1991]
2) Child [1975, 78, 79, 82, 87, 90]
3) Constipation [1973]
4) Mentals [1979]
5) Dentition [1973 S, 86]
6) Diarrhoea [1974, 79, 85]
7) Marasmus [1981]

Q. 2. Compare Symphytum and Calc. phos in **Bone** symptoms. [1993, 95, 96]

CALC. PHOS	SYMPHYTUM
• Rachitis – It occurs due to constant non deposition of lime in osteoid tissues due to **defective nutrition.** Calc phos helps in deposition of Calcium. • Bones are soft and friable.	• **Symphytum is used in case of injuries to soft tissues as well as periosteum and bony tissues.**
• Late learning to walk in children.	• **It helps curing injuries to orbital plates of the frontal bone in irritable stump after amputation, irritability of bones at the point of fracture or non union of fracture. Symphytum favours formation of callus.**
• Delayed and difficult dentition.	• It stimulates growth of epithelium or ulcerated surface especially gastric and duodenal ulcers.
• Bow legs. • Bones are disposed to curvature and fracture. • Weak neck and spine which is unable to support the head and body.	• Symphytom is effective in defective reunion of bone.

Q.3. Compare Cal carb and Cal phos child.

[1972. 73S, 76, 78]

CALC. CARB.	CALC. PHOS
• Enlarged abdomen.	• Sunken and flabby abdomen.
• Craving for eggs.	• Craving for salted or smoked meats.
• Stools – Greenish watery white mixed with curds.	• Stools – are green, slimy hot and watery accompanied by foetid flatus.
• Anterior fontanelle remains open.	• Anterior and posterior fontanelles are open.

25. CALCAREA SULPHURICA

C'arence Konant

Common Name – Sulphate of lime.
Miasm – Psora is in the background.
Calcarea Sulphate is a *deep acting remedy*.
Relation with heat and cold – Affected both by heat and cold.

KEYNOTES

1) Pathologically – Calc. **sulphate** has a ***tendency to form abscesses*** in the body.
2) Calc. **sulphate is used in the** ***IIIrd stage** of **all catarrahs***, **lung** troubles, **boils, carbuncles**, ulcers or abscesses. Calc. sulph **closes** the **process** of suppuration **at the proper time** (Silicea hastens the process of suppuration).
3) An *abscess that has ruptured* and is slow to heal having a continuous *yellow thick lumpy, mucoid discharge* is a strong indication of Calc. sulph.
4) Patient is distinctly *better in open air* (Hepar sulph cannot stand even a draught).
5) Inflammation anywhere in eyes; nose; throat; respiratory tract; cut, wounds; brights disease etc are led by discharge of thick yellow purulent secretions.
6) *Pimples on the face* of young people at the age of puberty with purulent and bloody secretions.
7) *Burning and itching of soles of feet*.

Particulars :

1) HEAD
2) EYES
3) EARS
4) NOSE
5) FACE
6) MOUTH AND TONGUE
7) RESPIRATORY SYSTEM
8) G.I.T
9) URINARY SYSTEM
10) FEMALE SEXUAL SYSTEM
11) SKIN

HEAD

- *Eruption* on the scalp leading to suppurations when the discharge is yellow and purulent.
- *Chronic headaches* with hyperemia of the brain, sense of constriction in the head > evening, warm room, stimulants, mental exertion, suppressed menses < open air.
- **Vertigo** is generally present in all complaints with a tendency to fall. Vertigo is better in open air.

EYES

- Inflammation of the eyes with yellowish purulent discharge.
- Itching and burning in the eyes in morning.
- Calc. sulphate has cured cataract, ulceration of cornea, photophobia etc,.

EARS

- Calc. sulphate is used in case of catarrah of eustacean tube, swollen parotid glands, eruption behind the ears when the symptoms agree.

There is thick yellowish purulent discharge from the ears occasionally accompanied with blood.

NOSE

- Catarrah of the nose with thick yellow and purulent discharge tinged with blood.
- Clinically Calc. sulphate is used in one sided discharge from the nose.
- In chronic catarrah of the head when the discharge is either from anterior or posterior nose—Calc sulph is a useful remedy.

FACE

Pimples and pustules on the faces of young people at the age of puberty with purulent and bloody secretions.

MOUTH and TONGUE

- Inflammation of the mouth with purulent secretions and offensive odour.
- Inflammation of tongue with swelling and difficult speech. Thick yellow coating on base of the tongue.
- Bitter sour and metallic taste in the mouth.

RESPIRATORY SYSTEM

Throat—Calc. sulph is used for ailments of throat (sore throat, quinsy, tonsillitis) in the IIIrd stage of the inflammation when suppurating or before pus is formed. Calc. sulph prevents the formation of pus.

Choking is the characteristic indication of this remedy (Hepar). In inflammation mucus drawn from the posterior nares is thick and yellow.

[Calc. sulph.—Better by open air. Patient throws off the covers and wants air—thus he seems to breathe better and croups less.

Hepar—Aggravation by uncovering the hand, throwing off covers. Patient is sensitive to least draft and cold air.]

Cough :

Character of cough—Short dry spasmodic cough coming in paroxysms.

Character of expectoration—Thick yellowish purulent discharge tinged with blood.

Calcarea sulph. is used in last stage consumption, croup, pneumonia or bronchitis.

G.I.T

Tongue—Inflamed tongue causing swelling and difficult speech. Thick yellow coating on base of tongue.

Liver—Abscess of the liver with soreness in the region of the liver causing a purulent discharge.

Diarrhoea—Painless and purulent diarrhora mixed with blood. Moisture about the anus causing smarting and itching,. Painful abscesses about the anus in case of fistula.

Constipation—Difficult and insufficient stools. Pain during and after stool.

Character of stools—Stools are bloody, dry, hard, knotty, yellow and purulent.

URINARY SYSTEM

Calc. sulph is valuable remedy when urethral discharges are yellow. bloody and gleety. There is burning in the urethra during urination.

FEMALE SEXUAL SYSTEM

Leucorrhoea—Thick, yellow and bloody leucorrhoea is present before and during menses.

Menses

Duration—Too frequent or too late.

Character of blood—Dark red.

Quantity of blood—Copious.

Concomitant—Dragging down pain in uterus during menses.

Impotency—Calc. sulph is excellent when other symptoms agree.

Pregnancy—Inflammation of breast when suppuration has taken and pus is discharging.

SKIN

Eruptions on the skin – boils, pustules, eczema, vesicles with a thick yellow purulent discharge.

- Neglected wounds that do not heal and continue to discharge pus. Calc sulph causes the wound to heal (Dr. Carey – Calc. sulph when given after Silicea gives good results).
- Ulcers discharge bloody pus that is offensive, thick and yellow.

Modalities :

Aggravation – GETTING WET
WALKING
GETTING OVERHEATED
(WALKING OVERHEATS THE PERSON)
WARM ROOM.

Amelioration – OPEN AIR.

Relations :

Similar to – Hepar, Silicea.

26. CALCAREA FLOURICA

J.B. Mill

Common Name – Flour spar.

Miasm – Psora.

C. Flour is a chronic remedy. It needs some time before manifesting its affections. It should not be repeated too frequently.

Relation with heat and cold – Chilly patient.

KEYNOTES

1) Calc. flour has marked action upon ***indurated infiltration*** in glands, cellular tissues, bony formations etc.
2) *Indurations* threatening *suppuration.*
3) *Discharges* in catarrah are usually *offensive thick and greenish yellow.*
4) Calc. flour is an integral part of *elastic fibers of blood vessels*, epidermis and hence is used to cure varicose veins, heamorrhoidal tumor, uterine heamorrhoids, relaxed abdominal viscera (caused due to lack of Calc. flour.)
5) In affections of *bone* and *osseous* growth, suppurations, affections of teeth where the *enamel* becomes rough and brittle, teeth become loose too early Calc. flour is indicated well.
6) Symptoms are *worse* in cold weather, during rest. Better – Warmth.
7) *Relaxation is the keynote* – relaxation of all parts – blood vessels, muscles, abdominal viscera, epidermis etc.

Particulars :

1) HEAD
2) EYES
3) EARS
4) FACE
5) G.I.T
6) RESPIRATORY SYSTEM
7) CIRCULATORY SYSTEM
8) MALE SEXUAL ORGANS
9) FEMALE SEXUAL ORGANS
10) BACK AND EXTREMITIES
11) SKIN

HEAD

Calc. flour is used in conditions of head involving defective and relaxed condition of elastic fibers.

Used in blood tumors of new born infants, bruises on scalp which become hard, ulceration of the bone of scalp.

EYES

- In cataract, ulceration of the cornea when the edges become hard Calc. flour has excellent result.
- Blurred vision caused by exertion of eyes and ameliorated by rest (this is caused due to relaxed state of blood vessels).

EARS

Diseases of ear where bone/periosteum are affected. Calcareous deposits causing hardening of tympanum.

Chronic suppuration of middle ear.

FACE

Hard swellings on the cheek with pain and toothache.

Osseous growth on the jaw bone which is painful.

G.I.T

Mouth – Gum boils with hard swelling of the jaw. Cracked hard and inflamed tongue.

Teeth – Enamel of the tooth is mainly composed of Calc. flour and hence Calc. flour is used when teeth become loose from their sockets. Teeth are sensitive to touch.

Gastritis – Acute indigestion caused by fatigue and brain fag. Vomiting of undigested food.

Piles – Due to relaxed blood vessel there is easy formation of heamorrhoids. Itching piles accompanied with pain in the back and constipation.

After confinement – There may be piles accompanied with accumulation of feaces in the bowels due to relaxed pelvic musculature.

RESPIRATORY SYSTEM

- **Nose :** Catarrah causing offensive thick stuffy discharges. In diseases affecting bones of nose especially when thick yellow crusts are formed.
- *Relaxed condition of the throat* – elongation of uvula causing a tickling cough by drooping into the throat. Relaxed blood vessels of the throat.
- Dryness and tickling in the larynx with desire to clear the vocal cords.
- **Cough** – *cause* – eating, cold air.
  Expectoration – difficult and consists of small yellow lumps.
- Large indurated *tonsils* are also cured by Calc. flour.

CIRCULATORY SYSTEM

- Calc. flour is excellent for vascular tumors with dilated blood vessels. Due to its tendency to relax the blood vessels it is of great use in varicose veins.
- Calc. flour removes fibroid deposits about the endocardium and restores normal endocardial structures.

MALE SEXUAL ORGANS

Hardening of testicles.

FEMALE SEXUAL ORGANS

- Calc. flour gives good results in *uterine fibroids* and varicose veins of the uvula.
- In displacements of the uterus Calc. flour helps to tone up the uterine muscles.
- *Uterus* may be *relaxed and flabby* or hard like stone due to irregular distribution of flouride of lime molecules.

BACK and EXTREMITIES

Calc. flour is used in recurrent fibroids in extremities. Dr. Kent has referred to a case of fibroid :

"A patient suffered from a recurrent fibroid in the hollow of the knee which was cut by a knife but grew to the size of a fist. The leg was drawn up to 45° and the knee became immobile. C.F. was thus prescribed on the symptoms of the case and the hardness of the tumor. The tumor gradually dwindled and the limb became normal.

C.F. is used for painful varicose veins in the legs which grow harder with time.

SKIN

- Chapped hands and cracked skin.
- When a fibrinous exudation is not dissolved by suppuration but has become hardened C.F. is given in indurations of stony hardness.
- Suppuration with callous and hard edges.

General Modalities :

Worse – REST, CHANGE OF WEATHER.

Better – HOT APPLICATIONS.

Relations :

Remedies that follow well – Phosphoric acid, Calc. phos., Nat mur, Silicea.

27. CALENDULA

Common Name – Marigold.
Calendula is used as an **antiseptic** and is intensly soothing.
It can be used both internally and externally in the form of *tinctures*.
Dilute Calendula used locally keeps the wounds odourless and reduces the amount of pus, favours granulation and thus it assists the surgeon in healing up of the surface wounds. It takes away local pain and suffering.

KEYNOTES

1) It ***helps cuts and lacerated wounds to be healed by first intention***.
2) In *external wounds* with or without loss of substance, post surgical wounds, it ***promotes healthy granulation*** and prevents excessive suppuration and disfiguring scars.
3) *Neuritis* – from lacerated wounds with loss of blood and excess pain.
4) In *rupture of muscles*, *tendons*, lacerations during labor, wounds, penetrating articulations with loss of synovial fluids – Calendula is very useful.
5) Tendency to develop *erisipelas.*
6) *Ulcers* that are inflamed, irritable,painful with excess secretion of pus – Calendula is specific.
7) Used as a *heamostatic in tooth extraction.*
8) Great *disposition to take cold* especially in damp weather.
9) Used in *cancer* as an intercurrent.
10) *Deafness* that is **worse** in damp surrounding with eczematous condition. Patient hears best in a train.

Modalities :

Aggravation – Damp heavy, cloudy weather.

Relations :

Complementry to : Hypericum in injuries to parts rich in santient nerves where pain is excess and out of all proportion to injury.

Similar to *Arnica* – traumatism without laceration of soft tissue.
Calcarea phos – Non union of bones.

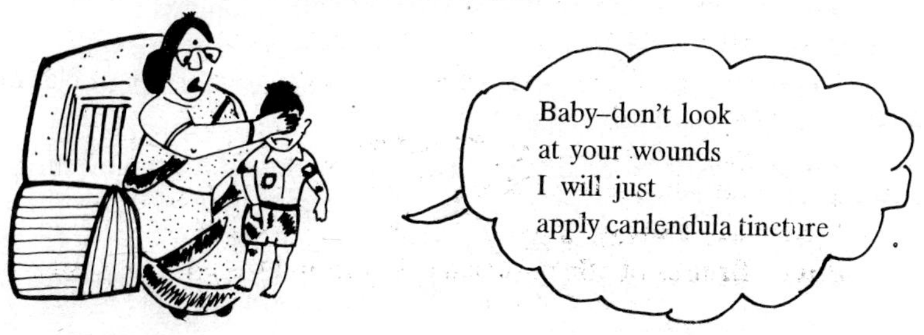
Baby–don't look
at your wounds
I will just
apply canlendula tincture

CALENDULA

Rhus, Ruta – Sprains or injuries of single muscles.

Salicylium acidum – prevents excess suppuration and gangrene.

Sulp. Acid – Painful, gangrenous wounds that destroy septic germs.

Remedies that follow well – Nitric acid, Arnica, Arsenic alb, Bryonia.

Inimicals – Camphor.

Antidotes – Arnica.

Important Questions ?

Q.1. Give indication of Calendula in Injuries.

[1976,78, 82, 87, 93, 94, 95]

Q.2. Compare injuries of

Calendula : Ledum pal [1996]
Calendula : Ruta : Staphysagria [1994]
Calendula : Hypericum : Arnica : – [195]
Symphytum : Ruta : Allium cepa

Ledum Pal –

1) Punctured wounds by sharp pointed instruments, insect stings.

2) Discolouration of injuries – black and blue parts become green.

3) Easy spraining of ankles.

4) Contusion of eye and lids especially with much extravasation of blood.

5) Used in complaints of people who are cold all the times due to lack of animal heat.

Rhus – Used when ligaments of joints, muscles, tendons are involved. Rheumatism that comes on during storms and wears of with continued motion.

Hypericum – When nerves have been injured along with other soft parts.

Staphysagria – Smooth, clean cuts made by surgeon's knife and hence it is called for in symptoms which are traceable to surgical operations.

Example – Colic after lithotomy or ovariotomy.

Symphytum – Bone injuries, irritable stump after amputation.

Arnica – Used in acute and chronic affects of injuries.

Acute – from simple bruises to concussion of brain and spine.

Chronic – any disorder or disease where injury is the exciting cause – Arnica has a marked affect.

Allium cepa – Neuralgic pains like a long thread. Chronic neuritis in a stump after amputation with burning and stinging pains.

Used when feet are rubbed and sore from friction.

Ruta – Bruises of bone, cartilage, insertion of tendons in joints.

28. CARBO VEGETABILIS

Hahnemann

'A VERITABLE CORPSE REVIVER'

Common Name – Vegetable Charcoal.

Carbo veg is *a broad acting, deep acting, long acting medicine.*

Constitution – Carbo veg is indicated in *advanced life* and consequently debilitated people. It is called for in weak, delicate *old dyspeptics* especially if they have abused their digestive organs by debauchery.

- General *sluggishness* is marked with *external coldness and internal heat.*
- Used in persons who have *never recovered from the exhausting affects* of some *previous illness.*
- *Hippocratic face* – Pale, greyish, yellow, greenish cold with cold sweat.

Temperament – Sanguine temperament.

Relation with heat and cold – Hot patient external coldness and internal heat. Due to *deficient oxygenation* of the system – Carbo veg patient desires to be *fanned* constantly and hard. The patient as if tries to inject oxygen into his body by fanning.

Miasm – Antipsoric remedy.

Diathesis – *Heamorrhagic diathesis*. Due to a general relaxed and sluggish condition there is heamorrhage of dark decomposed unclotted blood from every orifice. This causes an indescribale paleness and a hippocratic face.

KEYNOTES

1) Carbo veg is indicated in ***bad affects of any exhausting disease*** like injury, asthma, typhoid etc. Used in persons whose vitality has become exhausted or weakened due to previous illness.
2) ***Vital force exhausted*** with complete collapse. Blood stagnates in capillaries with venous turgescence. Surface is cold and blue to touch.
3) ***Aneamic*** especially after acute disease and have greatly depleted the patient.
4) ***Sluggish state of 'venous system'*** predominate with symptoms of imperfect oxygenation.

- Deficient capillary circulation causes *blueness* of skin and *coldness* of extremities.
- In *varicose ulcers,* varicose veins where there are blackish patches caused due to stagnation in venules.

- Frequent victims of *heamorrhoids* which turn blue and frequently suppurate.

5) *General sluggishness – physical and mental. There is dullness of mind due to inadequate oxygenation of brain.*
6) *Coldness* – Runs throughout the body. Coldness of breath, nose, face, extremities especially knee, cold sweat (imperfect oxygenation). This is accompanied by a *strong desire to be fanned* to inject oxygen into the system. *External coldness and internal heat.*
7) *Mucous membranes* break down, become *spongy, bleed*, ulcerate and become putrid. Heamorrhage of dark decomposed unclotted blood from all outlets with general *paleness*.
8) *Looseness of teeth* with easily *bleeding gums.*
9) *Weak digestion* –

- Simplest food disagrees.
- Excess accumulation of gas in stomach and intestine on *lying down.*
- Wind belched is putrid.
- Sensation as if stomach would burst.
- *Eructations give temporary relief.*
- Person craves for things that make him sick.
- Old topers crave whisky or brandy.
- Patient wants loose clothing around the abdomen.
- Desire for – coffee, acids, sweets, salt things.
- Aversion to most digestible things – milk.

Particulars :

1) MIND
2) HEAD
3) FACE
4) EAR
5) MOUTH
6) RESPIRATORY SYSTEM
7) HEART
8) G.I.T
9) FEVER
10) SKIN

MIND

- Mental *sluggishness* – Dullness of mind and patient is slow to comprehend. Patient cannot concentrate because of inadequate oxygenation of brain.
- There is *indifference* and the patient does not care whether he lives or dies. No fear of death.

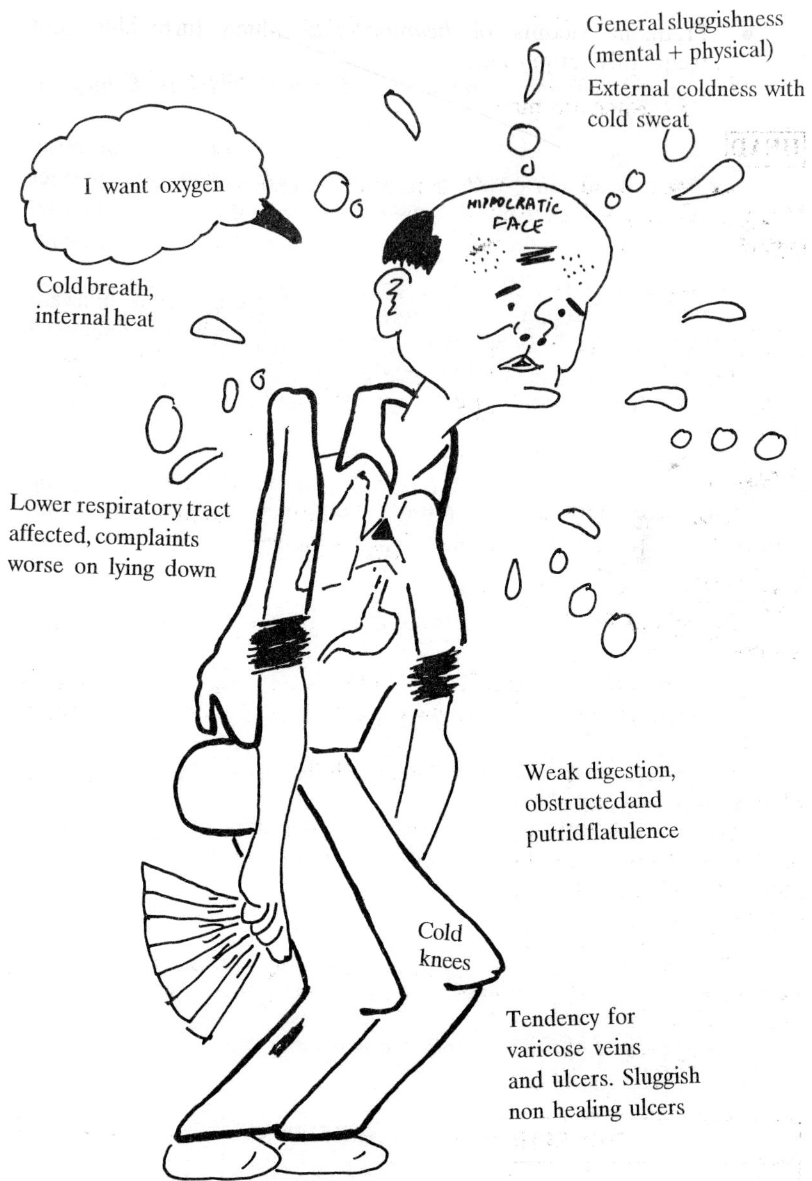

CARBO VEGETABILIS

- *Spells of loss of memory*—i.e. the patient suddenly loses his memory.
- Patient has *fixed ideas* and does not change her opinion regarding any matter.

HEAD

Occipital headaches with sensation of contraction of the scalp. Head feels heavy as lead. Sweat on the head feels cold.

FACE

Hippocratic, pale and ashy grey face. There is great *pallor and coldness* with lips pinched, nose pointed and drawn. Lips are puckered, blue, livid and deathly. Face is *cold pale and covered with cold sweat.*

Tongue is pale and cold with cold breath and yet the *person wants to be fanned*. Lustreless eyes with burning pains and pupils do not react to light.

EAR

Discharge—Offensive, watery, ichorous acrid, excoriating especially those dating back to malaria, measles or scarlet fever.

MOUTH

In typhoid fever, blood poisoning etc Carbo veg acts like a sheet anchor.

Mouth and throat are filled with black *apthous ulcers* which were little white spots to grow with but have grown *purplish* and now ooze black blood.

In low type of fever *tongue* becomes inflamed and exude a blackish bloody, offensive putrid exudate.

Gums—Scorbutic gums i.e. there is separation of gums from the teeth with bleeding of gums. Teeth decay rapidly and there is bleeding of gums while cleaning the teeth.

RESPIRATORY SYSTEM

Coryza —Cold begins in the nose and travels down the larynx. If cold goes down the chest it may have its ending in the bronchial tubes or chest.

Hoarseness and rawness in throat in evening.

CARBO VEG

	PHOSPHORUS	CAUSTICUM	EUP. PERF.
Aphonia— in evening < Damp warm weather	Aphonia in morning	Aphonia in morning < Dry, cold weather	Aphonia in morning with bodyache

Asthma – Carbo veg affects the lower respiratory tract. It becomes indicated when lung conditions have progressed to a fairly advanced state.

Asthma < Lying Down.

- Blood stagnates on lying down.
- Headache becomes intolerable.
- Respiration feels as if it has been arrested on falling asleep.
- Sluggishness marked so the usual automatic mechanism whereby circulation adjusts itself to changes of position are sluggish.
- In 'acute state' or 'state of collapse' with laboured breathing there is coldness of breath, coldness of tongue and coldness of nose. Reduced body temperature with blueness around lips and tips of fingers. Patient appears like a corpse and is very indifferent.
- Person is greatly relieved by hard fanning and belching.
- Carbo veg. is especially indicated in asthma which is reflex from accumulation of flatus in the abdomen.
- Internal burning and external coldness.

Spasmodic Cough

Carbo veg. is a good remedy for beginning of whooping cough.

Cough with gagging, vomiting and redness of face. There is mucus in the chest i.e. tough, purulent, yellow and thick and the patient cannot get it up. Patient is exhausted with cough.

Heamorrhage of lungs i.e. heamoptysis and bronchorrhoea.

Anxiety is very evident with burning pain in the chest. Pulse is intermittent and thready. Face is pale and often covered with cold sweat. Patient wants hard fanning to make up for the oxygen.

HEART

Carbo veg affects the *venous side* of the heart that is in distress. Veins are engorged with a state of relaxation and struggling.

Pulsations are felt all over the body.

Pulse is imperceptible with weakness of whole vascular system.

Blood stagnates in the capillaries with burning in chest.

G.I.T

Carbo veg is one of the most *flatulent remedies* (China, Lyc.).

- Stomach feels full and tense with great accumulation of flatus at night, lying down.
- Complaints from obstructed flatulency (may be pains in the head or heart or anywhere which are relieved by discharge of flatus).
- Flatus has a putrid and a very stinking smell.
- All food taken into the stomach turns into gas. Simplest food disagrees and still there is desire for disagreeable food.
- Patient is always belching and relieved for a while by belching.

- There are cramps and burning pains in the stomach.
- Abdominal fullness aggravates all complaints of body. Food remains a long time in the stomach, becomes sour and putrid. It passes into the bowels and ferments further finally passing off in the form of putrid flatus. There is colic, burning pains distension, constriction and cramping pains.
- Bad affects of excess indulgence in table luxuries and for too bad affect from wines and liquors.
- Flatus collects here and there in the intestine as if there was a lump. There is a sense of constriction of the intestine which holds it in one place so that it feels like a lump. There is burning in the abdomen.
- Bloatedness causes the diaphragm to press on the heart and thus causes periodic collapse.
- Great acidity of stomach with frequent eructation of wind.
- Desires – coffee, acids, salt, to be fanned forcefully.
- Aversion – milk, fat, alcohol (Contrary to the usual belief milk produces acidity in Carbo veg patient.)
- Even a sip of alcohol causes a great flushing of face.

TRIO OF FLATULENCE

CARBO VEG	CHINA	LYCOPODIUM
• Debility arises due to organic causes and there is a picture of collapse with hippocratic face and coldness of body particularly of knees.	• Functional debility due to loss of vital fluids.	
• Better from belching.	• Worse from belching.	• Belching does not relieve
• Flatulence in upper abdomen.	• Flatulence – whole abdomen.	• Flatulence – lower abdomen.
• Passage of offensive flatus with bitter taste in mouth.		• Sour taste in mouth with belching.
• Desires salt.	• Desires sour.	• Desires sweet.
• Sleeps propped up.		• Sleeps on right side
• Prefers direct wind, fanning from close distance.		Worse – Morning direct wind

Dysentry

- Abdomen is greatly distended and tympanitic.
- There are burning pains situated deep in the abdomen usually in one or other side of colon.
- Discharges from bowels are horribly offensive and brown, watery and slimy in appearance.
- Soreness in abdomen.

Cholera Infantum– Stools are mixed with mucus. The child sinks from exhaustion with coldness, pallor and cold sweat.

Gastric Ulcers– Mucous membranes break down, become spongy, bleed, ulcerate and become putrid. Carbo veg is a deep acting medicine and has cured ulceration of stomach.

Liver– Sluggish and enlarged. Portal system is engorged and hence heamorrhoids develop.

FEVER

Carbo. veg is useful in typhoid and intermittent types of fever for collapse during fever and for yellow fever.

In intermittent fever of low grade

Chill stage– marked by thirst. Feet are icy cold upto knees.

Coldness of body, cold breath, cold sweat, cold nose.

Heat stage– Comes in burning flashes.

Sweat stage– Either sour or excessively offensive.

In collapse from various causes there is lack of animal heat with cold extremities.

CARBO VEG	CAMPHOR	VERAT ALBUM
• Later stage of cholera. External coldness and internal heat.	• Early stage of cholera. Scanty discharges still causing a state of collapse.	Cramps in calves of legs with cold sweat on forehead.

UTERUS

- Metrorrhagia from uterine agony.
- Relaxed condition of mucous membrane causes continuous bleeding from one period almost to another.
  Blood– putrid, dark and incoagulable.
- Subinvolution from atonacity without contraction.
- Carbo veg prepares a woman for confinement. She is run down and relaxed. There is flatulence, offensiveness, weakness with

enlarged veins. The enlargement of veins is not from pressure but from weakness of veins itself.

- Atonacity is marked in Carbo veg. constitution. No contraction after heamorrhage.

(Bell, Ipec, Sec, Hamemelis – Contraction after heamorrhage)

SKIN

Heamorrhage :

Bleeding all through the remedy bleeding from all mucous membrane : –

- Lungs, uterus, bladder etc bleed due to relaxed conditions of mucous membrane.
- Heamorrhage causes indescribable paleness with internal heat and external coldness. Coldness especially of the knees is marked. Blood – dark, putrid and incoagulable.

There is passive capillary oozing. The arteries have all been tied and closed and the veins do not seem to have any contractility in their walls.

Ulceration :

If an ulcer is established it will not heal. Hence there are indolent ulcers with bloody, ichorous, acrid and thin discharges. Blood stagnates in capillaries. Flat ulcers that spread on the surface rather than dip deeply. Feeble parts develop gangrene. Any little inflammation or congestion becomes black or purple and sloughs easily. Discharge – offensive with burning pains at night. An ulcer once established does not heal. Blood stagnates into capillaries.

Varicose veins varicose ulcers :

Carbo veg is extraordinarily useful and there are blackish patches caused by stagnation in veins and capillaries.

Carbuncles :

Bluish and livid with offensive discharge associated with burning pains.

General Modalities :

Aggravation – FAT FOOD
ABUSE OF QUININE
WARM
DAMP WEATHER LYING DOWN.

Amelioration – BELCHING
BEING FANNED RAPIDLY.

Relations

Complements – Dros, Kali carb, Phos.

Remedies that follow well – Acid phos, Ars, Acon, Chin, Dros, Kali carb, Lyc, Nux, Puls, Sep, Sulph, Verat.

Inimicals – Carbo an, Kreos.

Antidotes – Ars, Camph, Coffee, Lach

Important Questions ?

Q.1. Give indications of Carb veg in

1. Gastric symptoms [1972, 73, 74, 76, 77, 83, 87, 90, 93]
2. Heart [1978, 83]
3. Collapse [1972, 77, 81]
4. Spasmodic Cough – [1972, 82]
5. Cholera. [1979]
6. Asthma. [1972, 82, 87, 90, 93]

Q. 2. Compare Gastric symptoms of Carbo veg, China, Lycopodium, Raphanus. [1993]

Q.3. Compare Collapse of Camphor, Carbo veg. [1993]

29. CAUSTICUM

Hahnemann

Common Name – *Potassum Hydrate.*
Miasm – antipsoric, antisyphilitic, antisycotic.

- Caustium is a *deep acting medicine*. Like Psorinum and Sulphur, Causticum can be thought of when improvement comes to a standstill.

Constitution – *Hydrogenoid* constitution (aggravation from washing and bathing; better from being warm in bed).

- Patient is *sallow, aneamic*, sick looking with dark hair and rigid fibres.
- Child is afraid to go to bed in dark.
- Suited to *old broken down* constitutions suffering from *chronic diseases.*

Relations with heat and cold – Chilly patient.

KEYNOTES :

1) *Right sided remedy* – paralysis, chorea, arthritis etc.

2) Aggravation – Dry cold weather.

   Amelioration – Damp wet weather, warm air [Nux vom, Hep. sulph, Med.]

3) *Graduality* – Complaints come on slowly.

- There is ***gradual paralysis*** following an initial state of excessive hypersensitivity and over reactivity.
- *Local paralysis* – Vocal cords, eyelids, tongue, face, muscles of deglutition, bladder, extremities.
- *Paralysis* of *single parts or single nerves* especially due to exposure to *dry cold wind.*
- Paralytic weakness of muscles from being *overstrained* and being *chilled*. (Rhus-tox).

4) *Ptosis* (drooping of eyelid – (Graph, Caul., Gelsimium)

   (Both eyes – Sepia).

5) *Suppression of skin* symptoms progresses into diseases of *nervous system* or directly into mental or emotional states.

6) ***Sympathetic person*** – Patient has extreme sympathy for others and has a strong sense of social justice. Intolerance of any kind of authority. Melancholic mood (Ign, Nat. mur, Phos. Acid).

7) Sensation of ***rawness and soreness of mucous membrane***. Burning is also present.

Arnica – Sensation as if sore and bruised in the muscles.

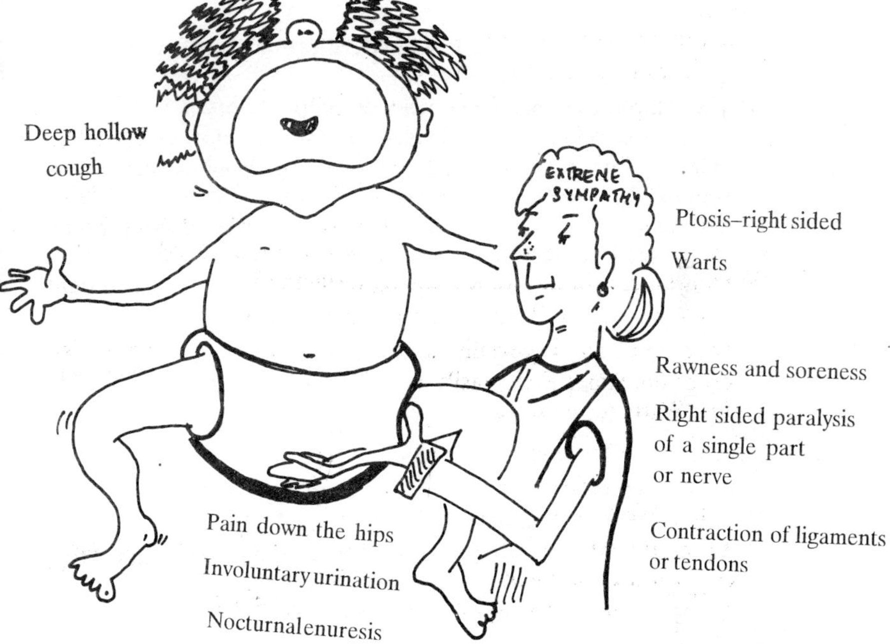
Deep hollow cough
EXTRENE SYMPATHY
Ptosis–right sided
Warts
Rawness and soreness
Right sided paralysis of a single part or nerve
Contraction of ligaments or tendons
Pain down the hips
Involuntary urination
Nocturnal enuresis
Menstrual colic. Better by bending double; menses in daytime only

CAUSTICUM

Rhus tox – Aching soreness as if sprained up in muscles, tendons and areolar tissue.

8) Tinnitus aureum – Causticum is a good remedy when sounds re-echo in the ears.
9) *Obstinate Neuralgias* – Of psoric origin which are of cramping, origin.
10) *Stammering* due to imperfect nerve control of tongue (Bar. carb, Dulc, Mu. acid, Stram).
11) *Contractions of ligaments* and *tendons* Arthritis deformens, rheumatic pains < dry cold weather > warm wet weather.
12) ***Hollow deep dry cough*** of great force which thus causes ***involuntary urination*** with the cough. Cough with *pain in the hips*. Patient tries to cough deep to get up the viscid mucus in the trachea but the mucus slips down. Aggravation – Cold, dry air.
13) Passes *stools* better while *standing* (Alumina).

    (Medorrhinum – Passes stools better by leaning backward).
14) *Warts* on skin especially nose (face, ear, neck) with moist eruption. Warts bleed easily.

Thuja – Warts on genital area.

Dulc. – Eruptions before menses.

Con – Warts on face.

Nit acid – Warts bleed easily.

15. *Menstrual colic* – Gripping pain on bending double, menses cease entirely at night.

    (After Colocynth, Caust is called for in dysmenorrhoea)

Particulars :

1) MIND
2) VERTIGO
3) PARALYSIS
4) EPILEPSY
5) FACE
6) EYE
7) EAR
8) TONGUE
9) TORTICOLLIS
10) RESPIRATORY SYSTEM
11) G.I.T.
12) G.U.T.
13) MENSES
14) ARTHRITIS
15) SKIN

MIND

- *Extremely sensitive*—People who are easily excitable, quick to react. They absorb all impressions from the enviornment and respond with hyperactivity and over reaction.
- *Strong sense of social justice*—Intolerance of any kind of authority. These people are easily and deeply hurt because injustice and oppressions can be found almost in every circumstance of life.
- This excessive sensitivity affects functions governing the CNS. Resulting pathology gradually affects the mental, physical and emotional plane. With time the patient finds himself with diminished nervous system reflexes, hardened and shortened tendons and a general state of inflexibility.
- An *intelligent analyst* at one time the person starts feeling that he is slowly *loosing his mental* power.

VERTIGO

- Weakened cerebral circulation. Patient is a great subject to vertigo which is a precursor of the oncoming paralysis. There is a tendency to fall either forward or sideways.
- Feeling of an empty space between brain and cranial bones.

PARALYSIS

- *Gradual paralysis* following an initial state of hyperactivity and overeactivity.
- Paralysis of a *single part* on a *single nerve*—facial paralysis, paralysis of oesophagus, uncontrolled drooping of eyelids, stammering from dysfunction of tongue, bladder, sphincter muscles. Worse on exposure to cold winds.
- *Suppression of skin eruption* progresses directly into nervous system. Remedy for locomotor ataxia, myopathy, multiple sclerosis.
- *Tongue*—Weakened nerve power causes stammering [Bar, carb, Dulc., Mur- acid, Stram]. *Post diptheritic paralysis*—Food goes down the wrong way.

ACONITE	RHUS-TOX.	CAUSTICUM.
PARALYSIS <Dry cold, winds Aconite suits well in the beginning and has a sudden onset.	Paralysis < Damp and cold atmosphere, overstraining >Motion	Paralysis < Dry cold winds. Causticum suits well in chronic states and has a gradual onset.

EPILEPSY

- Caused by suppression of skin eruptions.
- *Petit mal epilepsy* – Involuntary urination during unconcious state.
- *Jerking of single parts* – Chorea of one side of face.

FACE

- *Yellowishness* of face with paralysis of rheumatic or psoric origin.
- *Prosopalgia* – Exposure to cold dry air.
- *Stiffness of jaws* also of rheumatic origin.

EYE

- Gradual paralysis causing *ptosis.*
- Air seems to be full of *black insects.*
- Excellent for *cataract*.

EAR

- *Tinnitus aureum* – buzzing and roaring in the ears when sounds *Re-ECHO* unpleasantly in the ears.
- *Menieres disease* has been cured with Causticum.
- Offensive odour of ear wax.

TORTICOLLIS

- Due to contraction of muscles or tendons, head is sometimes drawn to one side.

RESPIRATORY SYSTEM

Throat – Hoarseness in evening.

(Sudden loss of voice from paralysis of vocal cords.)

Rawness, soreness and burning in the throat from cold air.

Cough :

- Weakness and paralytic tendency exhibits itself while coughing also.
- Patient is *unable to expectorate* – Person succeeds in raising the sputum so far when it slips back into the throat [Arn, Dros, Kali carb, Sepia].
- The patient *cannot cough deep enough* for relief.
- *Drinking cold water* relieves cough.
- Hollow deep cough of great force that causes *involuntary loss of urine and pain in hip* (This is also due to weakness of the sphincters due to paralysis of nerve supply to the bladder) [Apis, Nat mur, Phos, Puls, Scilla).

Hay Fever :

Cause – Cold dry winds.

- Itching inside and outside wings of nose.

- Sneezing upon waking in the morning and a viscid catarrah drops from posterior nares.
- *Obstruction of nose while lying down* especially at night.

Pthisis – Causticum is a *deep acting medicine* and cures pthisis especially quick consumption.

G.I.T.

Appetite – Patient sits down on the table hungry but the smell or sight of food takes away the appetite – [Ars, Sep, Cocc.],

- Thirst for cold drinks with aversion to water.

Stomach :

Sensation of lime being burned in stomach with rising of air.

Desires – Salt, smoked meat.

Aversion – Sweets.

Rectum :

Stools – Paralytic weakness – Rectum is inactive and fills up with hard feaces which pass involuntarily.

Constipation – Great deal of urging from defective expulsion force in the rectal muscular fibres with redness of face and fullness of blood vessels. Stools pass with less straining when the person is standing [Alumina, Med – Stools pass better when leaning backward].

Heamorrhoids – Swollen, itching, raw and sore; impede stools < walking

Fissures form on least provocation. Anal fissures itch and smart.

G.U.T.

Bladder – Two kinds of paralysis of bladder :

a) Affecting muscles of expulsion – urine is retained.

b) Affecting sphincter vesicae – urine is passed involuntarily.

Patient is unconcious of the stream as it passes.

- *Urine* escapes *involuntarily when coughing* due to paralytic weakness of muscles of bladder.
- Paralytic weakness of muscles – overstraining and being chilled (Rhus tox).

Nocturnal enuresis :

- Especially in children during first sleep in winters.
- Urine is liable to pass during the day in winters as a result of any excitement.

FEMALE SYMPTOMS

Menses – *Time* – Too early.

Character – Too profuse.

Duration – Only during day, cease on lying down.

Menstrual colic :

Gripping and cutting pains on bending double (Coloc).

ARTHRITIS

- *Right sided affections.*
- Rheumatism of joints when they get stiff and tendons become shortened drawing them out of shape.
- Rheumatism of right deltoid. [Sang]
- Contractures of muscles and flexor tendons. [F. phos]

  < Clear fine weather.

  > Damp wet weather
- Arthritis deformens – Pains and contraction of tendons and muscles force the extremities out of shape.

SKIN

Warts – Especially on wings of nose; also on face, ear, neck.

- Large jagged often pedunculated warts exuding moistures and bleeding easily.
- Itching especially on wings of nose. Warts bleed easily.

Fissures in intertriginous areas and anus.

Rawness and soreness in affected parts especially mucous membranes.

< Clear fine weather

> Damp wet weather

General Modalities :

Aggravation – CLEAR FINE WEATHER
COLD AIR.

Amerioration – DAMP WET WEATHER
WARM AIR.

Relations :

Complements – Petro, Coloc, Carb. veg.

Inimicals – Carb. An., Crcos.

Antidoes – Ars, Camph, Coffee, Lach.

Remedies that follow well :

- Acid phos., Ars, Acon, Chin, Dros, Kali, Lyc.

Important Questions ?

Q.1. Give indications of Causticum in.

1) Respiratory complaints [1973, 74, 77, 81, 82, 94]
2) Skin, Warts [1973, 75, 82, 90]
3) Paralysis
4) Arthritis [1977, 79]

5) Mentals [1973, 74, 81, 89]
6) Modalities [1972, 73, 76, 81, 86]
7) Constipation [1977]
8) Urinary Complaints [1977, 82]

Q. 2. Compare :

Arthritis – Phyt., Ledum, Abrot, Caust [1987]

PHYTOLLACA	LEDUM PAL	ABROTANUM	CAUSTICUM
Affection : • Right sided especially right shoulder.	• Rheumatism and gout both acute and chronic	• Rheumatism caused by checked diarrhoea	• Right sided affections
• Chilly patient	• Patient is cold to touch yet better by cold application.	< Night, cold > Motion	• Chilly patient <Cold, Dry wind. > Clear fine weather.
• <Motion, night, warm application	• Ascending rheumatism.	• Inflamed and painful joints	• Stiffness and contraction of flexor muscles with shortening.
• >Rest, dry weather.	• Acute – Hot, red, and swollen joints.	• Without swelling.	
• Pains flying like electric shocks.	• Chronic – nodular, formation in periosteum.	• Metastasis of rheumatism to heart is frequent.	

Q.3. Compare Paralysis of Gelsimium and Causticum.

Paralysis :

GELSIMIUM	CAUSTICUM
• Gradual paralysis	• Gradual paralysis of single part or nerve.
• Tremor	• Rawness and soreness of affected parts
• Lack of muscular coordination.	
• Patient is dull, dizzy and drowsy.	• Right side affected
• < Damp weather > Motion, profuse, urination	< Cold dry weather > Damp wet weather

30. CHAMOMILLA MATRICARIA

Hahnemann

Common Name – Matricaria Chamomilla.
Miasm – Psora in the background

A – Aconite – Turmoil in Circulation.

B – Belladonna – Turmoil in brain.

C – Chamomilla – Turmoil in temperament.

[Bell is used in disease of cranial nerves

Chamomilla is used in ailments of abdominal nerves.]

Chamomilla is used in cases spoilt by abuse of opium/morphine/coffee.

Constitution – Children who are irritable snappish with light brown hair, nervous and excitable temperment.

- One cheek red hot and other pale cold.
- Head and scalp are covered with hot sweat.

Temperament – Irritable.

Relation with heat and cold – Pains are generally relieved by warm wet weather and aggravated by cold.

(Toothache – heat, entering warm room, cold drink, cold application).

KEYNOTES

1) Chamomilla acts best on patients with a *sensitive nervous system* [Coffea, Ign., Opium, Bell, Nux vom]
2) Patient is exceedingly *sensitive to pain*. Pain drives him mad.
   Numbness alternates with pain [Aco, Rhus tox, Plat, Cocculus]
   < Heat, Evening before midnight (after 9'o clock).
3) ***Anger remedy*** – Bad affects of bad temper, convulsions, heamorrhage, biliousness etc may be brought on by anger.
4) *Cross and irritable person* – *'Cannot bear it'* child cannot bear himself, other people, pain etc. Everything is simply intolerable. *"Quiet only when carried."*
5) Used for bad affects of *narcotics, morphine or affects produced by long continued use of coffee.*
6) ***Difficult Dentition—***

- Child is very snappish and irritable.
- *Oversensitive child* – Child may get convulsions if he is reprimanded by the mother.
- *Offensive greenish diarrhoea* with dentition.

- Piteous *moaning* of child because he cannot have something he wants.
- Capriciousness – child desires something and when offered the same he refuses.
- *Insomnia* in children – Sleepy but cannot sleep.
- *Face* – one cheek red hot and other pale cold.
- *Head and scalp* are bathed in hot sweat.
- *Wants to be carried* always.

7) *Cannot stand in bed* – Burning of soles at night. Person puts the feet out of the bed (Sulphur, Puls, Med.)

8) *Rheumatic pains* drive the person out of the bed at night and compels him to walk about (Rhus tox)

9) *Cough* during nights, sleep, anger. Child does not wake up at night while coughing. Better by getting warm in bed.

10) *Pain in ends of bones of legs* while walking.

Particulars :

1) MIND

2) HEADACHE

3) FACE

4) G.I.T

5) FEMALE

6) RHEUMATISM

7) CHILD

MIND

- **Anger remedy** – Bad affects of bed temper. Nature of disease matters little – *The mentality simply shouts for Chamomilla.*
- In *acute* cases Chamomilla is simply demanded by the mental states.
- Anger can bring on convulsion in the child, threatened abortion during pregnancy, jaundice, heamorrhage etc.
- Patient is cross, ugly and snappish.

HEADACHE

- Brought on by anger.

Character of headache – Throbbing and bursting headache.

Aggravation – Thinking about complaints, after 9 o' clock and before midnight (person feels better after midnight).

FACE

- Heat of the face while rest of the body is cold.
- Head and scalp are covered with hot sweat.
- One cheek red and other is pale cold.

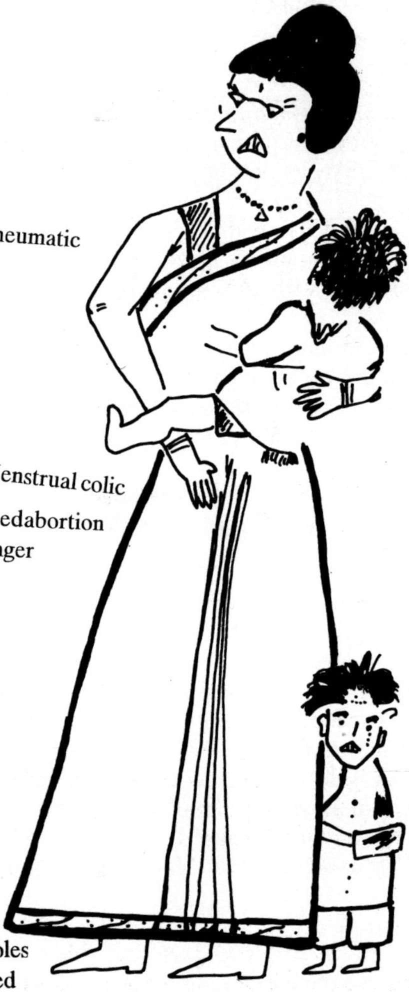

Anger remedy

Numbness with pain

Intolerablerheumatic pains

Snappish, irritable child

Desires to be carried and feels better when carried

Difficult dentition (offensive green diarrhoea duringdentition)

Menstrual colic

Threatenedabortion due to anger

One cheek red and hot, other cold and pale

Worse in heat of bed

Better in warm wet weather

Burning of soles at night in bed

Pain in end of bones of legs

CHAMOMILLA

TOOTHACHE

- Excruciating pain in teeth < Anything warm, entering a warm room, taking cold things, cold drinks.

EAR

- Violent earache – exposure to cold air.

G.I.T

Appetite :

- Unquenchable thirst for cold water and acid things.
- Aversion to coffee, warm drinks, soups – Though Chamomilla and Coffee are alike yet antidote each other.

Stomach :

- Chamomilla antidotes bad affects of morphine, coffee.
- Biliousness, gastralgia produced by anger.
- Vomiting, retching with eructation of foul gas (sulphate of hydrogen).
- Pressive pain in stomach as from a stone. Sensation of fullness and distension in hypochondria.
- Nausea and eructations of putrid gas smelling like bad eggs.
- Heat and sweat of face. Bitter taste in mouth.

Diarrhoea

- Green diarrhoea, hot, foul smelling stools looking like chopped eggs < evening before midnight.

FEMALE SYMPTOMS

- The lady is oversensitive to pain and is snappish and irritable.
- *Breast :* Nipples are inflamed and tender to touch. Milk runs out in nursing women. Infants breasts are tender to touch.
- *Menstrual colic* after a fit of anger.
- *Labor pains* – exceedingly painful. Rigidity of Os. The patient is very snappish and irritable. Pains begin in the back and pass down the inner side of thighs. After labor lochial flow is too profuse, dark, violent and intolerable.
- *In Threatened abortion* caused by anger Chamomilla is wonderful. Discharge of dark blood, frequent urination and restlessness.

RHEUMATISM

Rheumatic pains drive the patient out of the bed and compel him to walk about (Rhus tox, Zincum met, Verat Alb) < Heat ; > Warm wet weather, after sweat.

CHILD

Face – One cheek red hot and other pale cold. Head and scalp are covered with hot sweat.

Mind

- Cannot bear it – very irritable child, cannot bear himself, pain or anybody.
- Capriciousness – desires a thing and refuses when offered.
- Anger remedy – convulsion etc are brought on due to anger.
- Irritable and snappish child.
- Moaning – Child starts moaning piteously when refused something.
- Restless and sleepless.
- Wants to be carried.
- Sleepy but cannot sleep.

Dentition – Difficult, irritability during dentition.

Dentition diarrhoea – greenish, offensive, hot stools looking like chopped egg.

Cough – Night (while sleeping), anger. Child coughs during sleep. Does not wake up while coughing. Better by warmth of bed.

General Modalities :

Aggravation – HEAT
EVENING – AFTER 9' O CLOCK
BEFORE MIDNIGHT
OPEN AIR.

Amelioration – BEING CARRIED
FASTING
WARM WET WEATHER.

Relations :

Complements – Bell, Mag carb.

Remedies that follow well – Acon, Ars, Bell,Bry,Cact Calc, Cocc, Form, Merc, Nux, Puls, Rhus, Sep.,Sil,Sulph

Inimicals – Zinc

Antidotes – Aco,Alum, Borax, Camph, Chin, Coca, Coffea, Coloc, Con, Ign, Nux, Puls, Velar.

Important Questions ?

Q.1. Give indication of Chamomilla in

- Child [1974,78, 79, 81, 77, 91, 93, 94]
- Mentals [1974,79,78, 84, 87]
- Diarrhoea [1986]
- Pains [1979]
- Modalities [1973]
- G.I.T [1974, 75, 77, 82, 90]
- Rheumatism [1981]

Q.2. Compare : Child – Chamomilla/Cina. [1986, 97]

- Compare – Toothache – Chamomilla/Kreosote. [1993]

- Compare – Toothache – Chamomilla/Mag phos. [1987]

KREOSOTE	MAG. PHOS	CHAMOMILLA
• Acidity offensiveness and heamorrhage.	• Right sided affections. • Neuralgia	• Anger remedy • Oversensitiveness.
• Toothache in **carious** tooth. Pain extending to temple and left face.	• **Ulceration** of teeth with neuralgic pain < Cold things > Hot liquids	• *Intolerable toothache* < warm things, entering a warm room, evening before midnight, > cold.
• **Putrid odour** in mouth. Gums are bruised, spongy, ulcerated and scorbutic.	• **Pain** – sharp, stabbing with intermittent. paroxysm.	
• *Painful dentition* – Teeth begin to decay as soon as they appear.	• *Chilly patient* yet desires cold things.	• Slow teething • Irritable, snappish child • Dentition diarrhoea • Green, offensive and hot stools.

31. CINA

Hahnemann

Common Name – Worm seed.

Miasm – Latent psora in the background.

Santonine is the active principle of Cina which powerfully affects the *abdominal ganglia* as a reflex of which there is convulsive twitching, spasms or jerkings of limbs.

Acts powerfully in *elimination of round worms*. Acts more affectively in 200th or higher potencies than alkaloid or lower potencies.

Constitution – Adapted to children with dark hair and rigid fibres who are cross and irritable, wants to be carried without any relief. Capriciousness is marked. Pale face which is sickly white, bluish with dark rings under the eyes. One cheek red and other is pale.

Temperament – Irritable.

KEYNOTES

1) **Worm Remedy :**
   - Irritable, nervous and peevish child.
   - Pale face with blue rings around the eyes.
   - Canine hunger-hungry soon after a meal.
   - Constant digging or boring of nose.
   - Grinding of teeth during sleep.
   - Nocturnal enuresis.

2) **Touchiness** – Mental and physical; < touched or looked at. Child is peevish and snappish. Cannot bear slightest touch or even being looked at.

3) Constant *digging of nose* – child picks the nose all the time – rubs the nose on the pillow or against the mothers shoulder.

4) *Clean Tongue.*

5) *Urine* – Turbid when passed out but turns milky and semisolid afer standing.

6) Frequent *swallowing* as if something came up the throat.

7) *Desire* for *sweet and indigestible things.*

8) Child *lies* on *belly* or on *hands* and knees during sleep. Very disturbed sleep and awakes on slightest disturbance.

9) *Cough* – dry with sneezing, spasmodic. Child is afraid to speak or move for the fear of bringing a paroxysm.

10) Child *wants to be carried* all the time without any relief (Cham – relief by carrying)

11) *Complaints* come on when the patient *yawns*

Particulars (child) :

1) MIND
2) HEADACHE
3) WHOOPING COUGH
4) G.I.T
5) URINARY SYSTEM

MIND

- **Touchiness** is marked – child cannot bear anyone touching him or even being looked at or seeing strangers. Skin is sensitive to touch.
- Obstinate, willful and headstrong child.
- **Capriciousness** – Desires something and when offered the same he refuses.

HEADACHE

- *Headache* with sensitivness of eyes. Optical illusion in bright colours.
- From slight disturbance of the mind the child cannot digest food and gets on diarrhoea. **Diarrhoea** – Green slimy stools
- Brain (in a Cina patient) does not receive the messages and so the stomach develops disturbances and worms hatch out. If the patient is cured healthy gastric juice drives out the worms.

WHOOPING COUGH

- Spasmodic periodical whooping cough.
- *Cough* dry sneezing spasmodic cough. The child is afraid to speak for the fear of bringing about a paroxysm. During a paroxysm the child looks anxious and catches at her breath and gags.
- Towards the end of the paroxysm the child throws its body backwards and a **peculiar gargling** sound is heard to go down the throat (Met, Lauro, Hydrocyanic acid).
- Aphonia from exposure – (Acon, Phos, Spong)

G.I.T

When orders are not received by the brain, the stomach develops symptoms (Cina acts as a vermifuge). Characteristic symptoms due to worms.

1) Intense circumscribed *redness of cheeks alternating with paleness and coldness.*
2) *Dark rings* around the *eyes*.
3) *Dilated* pupils with dimness of vision.
4) Rolling of eyes during sleep.

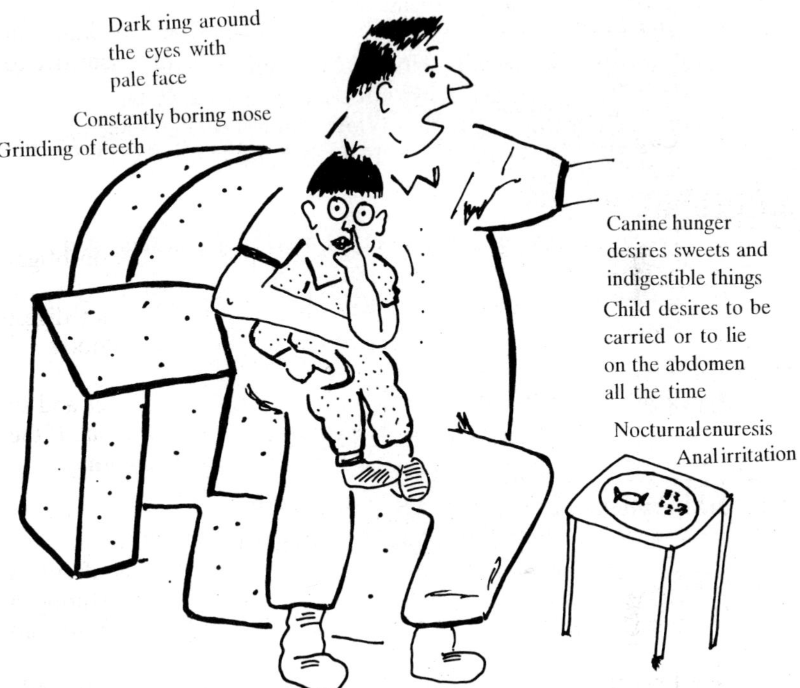

Touchiness–mental
and physical
Dark ring around
the eyes with
pale face
Constantly boring nose
Grinding of teeth
Canine hunger
desires sweets and
indigestible things
Child desires to be
carried or to lie
on the abdomen
all the time
Nocturnal enuresis
Anal irritation

CINA

5) Constant *picking and boring of nose* – child keeps rubbing his nose against the pillow or against the shoulder of the mother.
6) Alternate *canine hunger* with no appetite at all.
7) Child craves *sweet and indigestible things* and refuses mothers milk.
8) *Frequent swallowing* as if something comes up the throat.
9) *Spasmodic cough* with vomiting.
10) *Restless sleep* – desire to lie over the abdomen or in constant motion.
11) *Frequent micturition* – Nocturnal enuresis due to worm irritation; urine turns milky after standing for a while.
12) *Irritation of anus.* Stools – White thin watery looks like popped corn. Stools not copious > lying on belly.

URINARY SYMPTOMS

- Turbid urine when passed but it turns *milky and semisolid after* sometime.
- Nocturnal enuresis in children due to irritation caused by worms.

MODALITIES :

Aggravation – SWEETS
UNDIGESTIBLE THINGS
OVEREATING.

Aneuoration – LYING ON ABDOMEN OR
WHEN CHILD IS IN CONSTANT MOTION.

RELATIONS :

Remedies that follow well – Calc., Chin, Ign, Nux, Plat, Pul, Rhus, Sil, Stann.

Antidotes – Arn, Camph, Chir, Caps.

Important Questions ?

Q.1. Compare child – Cina/Chamomilla. [1986, 91, 94, 97]
Q.2. Give indication of Cina in
a) Helminth infection. [1975, 79, 93, 94]
b) Baby. [1974, 77, 78, 79, 87, 95]
c) Keynotes . [1991]

32. CINCHONA OFFICINALIS

Hahnemann

Common Name – Peruvian Bark.

China (Quinine) *prime cause behind origin of homoeopathy*. In 1790 Dr. Hahnemann tried the Cinchona Bark on himself and he discovered its power of producing intermittent fever. With this he discovered the principle of *similia similibus curantur.*

Constitution – *Broken down* constitution due to *excess loss of body fluids* like blood leucorrhoea. semen, diarrhoea, profuse sweats, suppuration. There is great DEBILITY and PROSTRATION WITH ANAEMIA due to excess loss of body fluids. Face is pale and hippocratic with sunken eyes and surrounded by blue margins.

Miasm – Psora.

Relation with heat and cold – *Chilly* patient. Sensitive to even a draft of air.

Temperament – Nervous.

Diathesis – Heamorrhagic.

KEYNOTES

1) ***Debility and anaemia*** from excess loss of fluids from the body (heamorrhage, lactation, diarrhoea, suppuration etc.).
2) ***Heamorrhage*** from every orifice of the body. Dark red clotted blood with general coldness of the body.
3) ***Oversensitive*** to external impressions like noises, bright light. Patient is sensitive to slightest touch, draft of air. Better by hard pressure, on painful side.
4) **Dropsy** following excessive loss of fluids with great debility and trembling.
5) Great *flatulence* with sensation as if abdomen was fully packed with gas. Every food particle seems to turn into gas without any relief from belching. (Carbo veg is better by passage of flatus).
6) *Painless diarrhoea* at night. **Stools** – Yellow, watery, brownish and undigested food particles.
7) *Sweat with great thirst.* Sweating during sleep and on being covered.
8) Indicated in *periodical affections* (Colic at a certain interval each day, intermittent fever with periodicity).
9) *Antineuralgic* – China is very helpful in extremely sensitive nerves. < slightest touch; > draft of air, hard pressure.

10) *Chronic affections of liver* with pain in right hypochondrium and biliousness (yellow skin, light stools, dark urine due to diminished bile content).
11) After *climacteric* there is profuse heamorrhage often resulting in dropsy.
12. Desire for sour things, sour fruits, cold water.
13. *Apathetic and indifferent,* despondent and gloomy. No desire to live but lacks the courage to commit suicide.

Particulars :

1) MIND
2) HEAD
3) FACE
4) EYES
5) RESPIRATORY SYSTEM
6) G.I.T.
7) FEVER
8) FEMALE SYMPTOMS

MIND

- *Apathetic* and *indifferent* attitude and is disinclined to think.
- *Fear* of dogs and animals especially during delirium.
- *Fixed ideas* – Person does not budge from what he thinks. Ideas in the form of persecution by enemies as if the enemies are trying to thwart him away from whatever he tries to do.
- *Nervous Erethism* – Ideas crowd on the mind in unwelcome profusion preventing sleep.

HEADACHE

Cause – Excess loss of vital fluids or sexual excess. During headache there is a great tendency to congestion of head with flushing of face and throbbing of carotids. Extremities become cold and covered with cold sweat, ringing and rearing in ears.

< Draft of air, touch, exposure to sun.

> Hard pressure.

FACE

Person is generally **anaemic and debilitated** due to excess loss of fluids. Pale and **hippocratic face** with sunken eyes and blue rings around the eyes. Post malarial *infra orbital neuralgia.*

< Slightest touch, draft of cold air.

EYES

Asthenopia, photophobia with dilated pupils. Eyes ache on attempting to use them.

Broken down constitution

Flatulence with pain abdomen, painless diarrhoea

Sweat with great thirst

BROKEN DOWN CONSTITUTION

Debility and anaemia

Intense prostration due to loss of body fluids

Oversensitive to external impressions

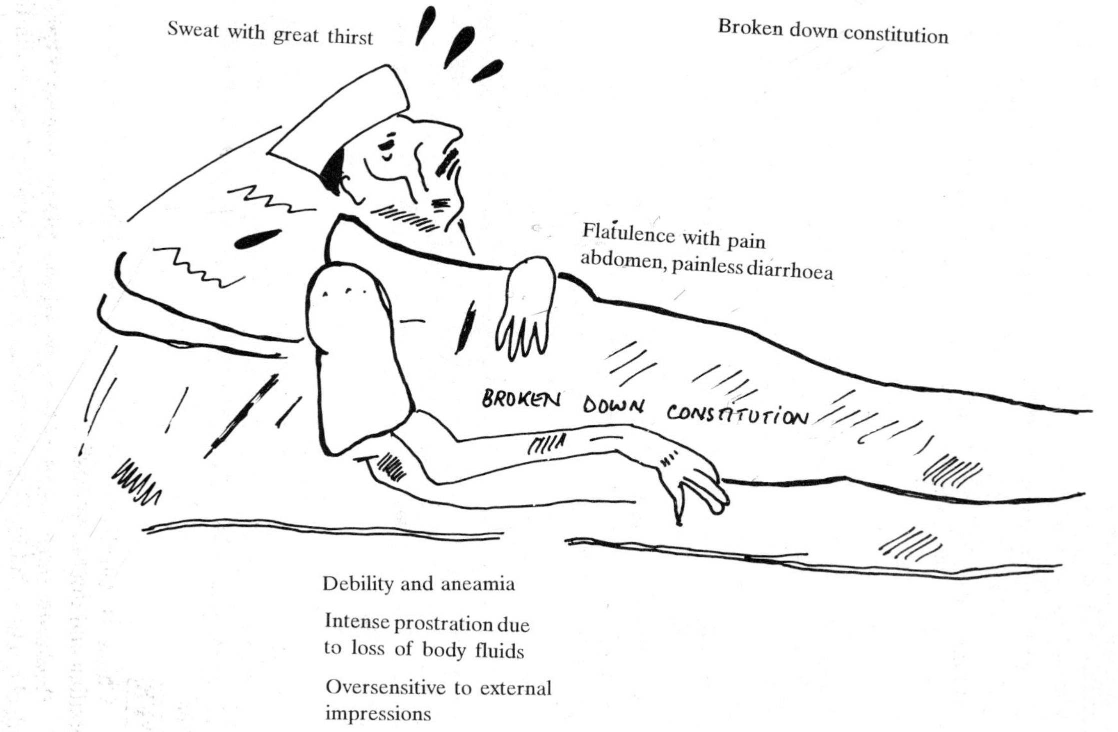

CINCHONA OFFICINALIS

This is caused generally due to *excess loss of vital fluids* or heamorrhages.

RESPIRATORY SYSTEM

China is useful in affections of lung when the sputum is retained for a long time and undergoes decomposition in lungs. As soon as the person coughs, the breath that comes out is horribly offensive.

Asthma – Rattling and filling up of the chest with mucus. Pressure in the chest as from violent rush of the blood with a dry and suffocative cough.

GIT

Teeth – Toothache worse from cold. Teeth are painful while chewing and they feel too long. Gums swell and teeth feel too loose.

Taste – Bitter taste in the mouth. Dryness in mouth and throat with difficult swallowing.

Stomach – Appetite – Canine hunger or no appetite at all. Person desires sour things and sour fruits.

Vomiting of undigested food, sour mucus, bile or blood.

Abdomen – Abnormally distended abdomen with **flatulence**. Sensation as if every food particle turned to gas. There is constant loud and strong eructation without any relief. Person can hardly breathe and still feels hungry at meal time.

Liver – China is used in chronic liver troubles. Pain in the right hypochondrium and liver may be felt below the ribs – enlarged hard and sensitive to touch. Yellow skin, dark urine and light stool (caused due to improper secretion of bile). In Splenic diseases also China is a very good remedy.

Stools – Painless diarrhoea at night after eating. Diarrhoea occurs during hot weather and after eating fruits.

Character of stools – Yellowish, watery, brown, offensive with undigested food particles. This condition is often found in children – the child is weak, pale with dark ring around the eyes (may be caused due to worms).

FEVER

China is curative in *intermittent fever* – tertian, double tertian, quotadian and double quotadian.

Prodromal stage – marked by thirst, canine hunger, nausea, anguish, headache and debility. General feeling of illness and restlessness in the prodromal stage. *Paroxysm* starts with general shaking and shivering below the legs.

Chill Stage – No thirst during chill but thirst is present before and after chill. Patient desires to be warm and wraps himself up.

Heat state – Distension of veins with congestion of head. Face becomes fiery red. Heat stage is long lasting and person prefers to rest. No thirst, stupurous condition.

Sweat State – Thirst is present. Sleep is more profound and deepened.

Apyrexia – Face is sallow with bilious complications. Enlarged spleen, liver with canine hunger or total loss of appetite. Feet become oedematous may be from disturbance in composition of blood or interference in hepatic or splenic circulation. Yellow tongue with bitter taste in mouth and ringing in ears.

FEMALE SYMPTOMS

Menses :

Time – Too early.

Character – Profuse, black and clotted.

Concomitant – Pain and convulsions, come on in the midst of heamorrhage, purulent, leucorrhoea in place of menses. Uterine heamorrhages with profound debility.

General Modalities :

Aggravation – SLIGHTEST TOUCH
DRAFT OF AIR, MENTAL
EMOTIONS, LOSS OF VITAL FLUIDS
USED IN BAD AFFECTS OF TEA ETC.

Amelioration – HARD PRESSURE, BENDING DOUBLE.

Relations :

Complements – Ferrum met.

Antidoted by – Nat mur, Carbo veg.

Antidote to – Ars, Calc, Cham, Ferr, Hell, Iod, Merc, Sulph, Verat alb.

Remedy of same family – Coffea, Ipecac.

Incompatible after – Dig, Selen.

Important Questions ?

Q. 1. Give indications of China in following conditions :

1) Fever [1993, 98]
2) Malaria [1975, 76, 79, 81, 93]
3) Diarrhoea [1973, 75, 86, 82]
4) Colic [1987]
5) Stomach [1972, 73, 74, 76, 77, 87]
6) Cough [1974]

7) Characteristic Symptoms [1986]

Q. 2. Compare Phos and China in Heamorrhage. [1994]

(a)

PHOS PHORUS	CHINA
Heamorrhage caused by degeneration of tissues and occurs from small injuries or cuts even after healing. **Character of blood** – Profuse, watery bright and non coagulable. Pours out freely and then ceases suddenly.	Heamorrhage from any orifice of the body. Coldness of surface of body and features show presence of collapse. Gasping for breath caused by insufficient supply of oxygen. **Character of blood** – Dark, profuse and clotted.

(b) Jaundice of Chelidoneum and China. [1975, 91]

CHELIDONEUM	CHINA
• Right sided affections	• Chronic liver troubles.
• Constant pain in lower angle of scapula	• Oversensitiveness marked. Complaints due to loss of vital fluids.
• Desires – hot drinks.	• Desires – sour things, cold drinks.
• Yellow grey colour of skin, yellow coated tongue with imprint of teeth. < change of weather > eating	• Yellowish skin, light stools, dark urine, bitter taste. < Slightest touch, draft of cold air. > Hard pressure.

33. COLCHICUM AUTUMNALE

Stapf

Common Name – Meadow Saffron.
Miasm – Psoric miasm.

Constitution – Adapted to *rheumatic, gouty diathesis*. Person of robust and vigorous constitution. Circumscribed redness of cheeks with marked paleness of nose.

Temperament – Leucophlegmatic, melancholic.

Diathesis – Uric Acid Diathesis.

Relation with heat and cold – Chilly patient.

KEYNOTES

1) *Chilly patient* – Very sensitive to cold damp weather.

2) *Specific for gout* – Spell of cold wet weather slacks the flow of urine, makes it scanty and decreases the quantity of solid in urine and hence intensifies the gout.

b) *Shifting/Flying pains* – Tendency to move from one joint to another.

c) *Rheumatism* with or without swelling.

d) *Dropsy* caused due to scanty urine;swellings that are inflammatory and rheumatic.

e) *Metastasis* – Gouts may leave the joints and attack the heart and stomach.

f) *Pains* < chilly wet weather
> warmth, warming up.

3) *Urine* – Inky, very dark brown sometimes almost black and loaded with albumen.

4) *Odour of cooking food cause nausea/fainting*

5) *Bad* affects of *night watching* or over study.

6) *Burning/icy coldness* of *stomach* and abdomen.

7) *Autumnal dysentry* – discharge from bowels contain white shreddy particles (scraping of mucous membrane of intestine)

8) *Abdomen* is intensely *distended with gas* with a feeling as if it would burst.

Particulars :

1) G.I.T.

2) RHEUMATISM, GOUT.

3) KIDNEY AFFECTIONS.

G.I.T

- Profuse secretion of saliva.
- *Aversion to smell/sight of food.* Odour of cooking food especially eggs, fish etc causes faintness and nausea.

Stomach – Burning or icy coldness in pit of stomach.

Abdomen – Intensely distended with gas with sensation as if it would burst.

Dysentry – Caused especially during autumn.

- **Stools** – Frequent, watery, bloody and contain shreds or portion of lining of membrane of bowels.
- Violent *tenesmus* – in the rectum followed by spasm of sphincter ani. Patient is greatly relieved of the tenesmus after stools, so much that he falls asleep on the vessels as soon as tenesmus ceases < Slightest motion, checked perspiration chilly cold wet weather; > Lying still.

RHEUMATISM AND GOUT

- *Cause* – extremes of cold and wet or warm and dry weather.
- Rheumatism with or without swollen joints. Joints are dark red or pale in colour.
- *Shifting/flying pains* – Pains in joints keep shifting from one joint to another. Joints are sensitive to slightest touch or motion.
- Parts seem to be *paralysed.*
- *Metastasis* – of rheumatism from joints to heart or stomach.
- *Urine is pale and scanty.*
- *Dropsy* caused by scanty urine. Urine that passes contains blood and is mostly as black as ink and is loaded with albumen.

  Swelling in hands and feet which pit upon pressure. Dropsy of abdominal cavity, pericardium, pleura, serous sacs with pale urine.
- Patient is extremely *irritable to slightest external impression* – light, noise, strong odour.
- In gout *great toe* is generally involved.

Torticollis – Colchicum is used with great success. Severe pain and tension in cervical muscles. Pain is so intense that even swallowing is difficult.

KIDNEYS

Inflammation of kidneys, nephritis. *Congestion in kidneys* causes rupture of fine capillaries and consequent pouring out of blood in the pelvis of kidneys.

Urine – Copious, watery dark, inky, smoky, turbid containing albumen, sugar and tube casts.

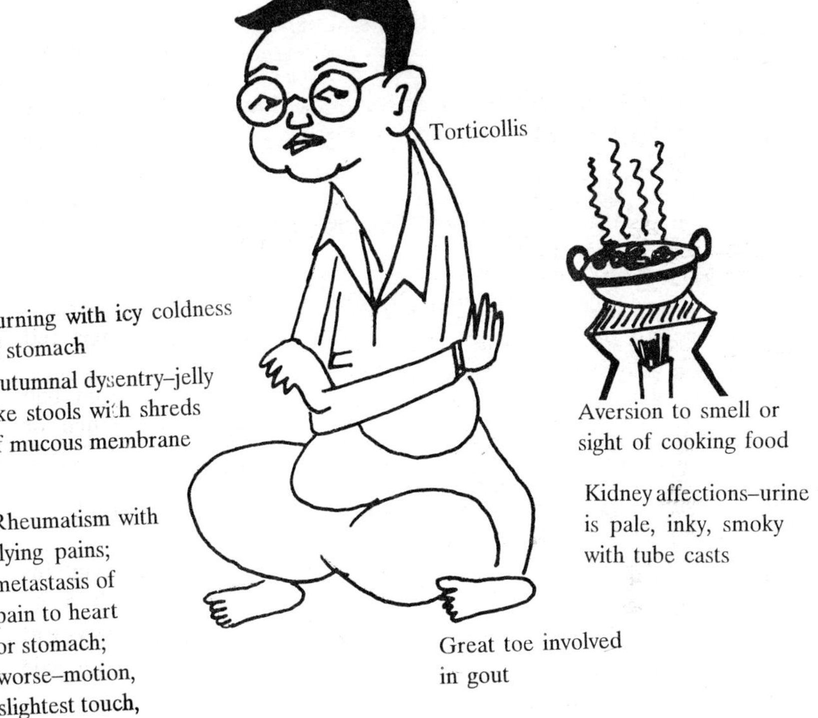
Torticollis
Burning with icy coldness of stomach
Autumnal dysentry–jelly like stools with shreds of mucous membrane
Rheumatism with flying pains; metastasis of pain to heart or stomach; worse–motion, slightest touch, cold wet weather
Aversion to smell or sight of cooking food
Kidney affections–urine is pale, inky, smoky with tube casts
Great toe involved in gout

COLCHICUM AUTUMNALE

Modalities :

Aggravation – COLD DAMP WEATHER
SMELL OF COOKING FOOD
MOTION
AUTUMN
EXERTION – NIGHT WATCHING OR OVER STUDY.

Amelioration – WARMTH
LYING DOWN QUIETLY.

Relations :

Remedies that follow well – Carbo veg, Merc, Nux, Puls, Sep, Rhus.

Antidotes – Acet. acid, Acon, Cham, Chin, Grat, Merc, Puls, Sulph.

Important Questions ?

Q. 1. Give indications of Colchicum in the following

1) Rheumatism [1977, 81, 82, 85, 86]
2) GIT Disorders [77, 79 , 83, 87]
3) Nausea [1974]

Q. 2. Compare the following

1) Colchicum/Cocculus in vomiting. [1979]
2) Colchicum/Bismuth – G.I.T Disorder [1988]

COLCHICUM	COCCULUS
• 1) Nausea and faintness from odour of cooking food especially fish, egg.	• 1) Vertigo, nausea and vomiting from motion. Sea sickness, car sickness
• 2) Burning/icy coldness in stomach.	• 2) Sensation of hollowness or weakness in various organs - stomach.
• 3) Bitter taste in mouth.	• 3) Loss of appetite and metallic taste in mouth.

COLCHICUM	BISMUTH
• Nausea and faintness from odour of cooking food.	• Vomiting of water as soon as it reaches the stomach but solid food is retained for a long time and is vomited out when it becomes decomposed and is very offensive.
• Burning or icy coldness of stomach.	• Cramping pain in stomach due to accumulation of food.

• Autumn Dysentry • Stools are frequent watery bloody and contains shreds of mucus membrane lining the intestine. • Violent tenesmus. • Abdomen is intensely distended with gas. < MOTION	• Headache alternates with gastralgia. • Solitude unbearable. > MOTION

34. COLOCYNTH

Hahnemann

Common Name – Bitter or squirting Cucurbitacea.
Diathesis – Rheumatic, gouty, nervous.

KEYNOTES

1) ***Anger and with indignation*** – Colic, vomiting, diarrhoea etc are all caused due to anger or nervous excitement.
2) *Left sided affections.*
3) *Aggravation* of complaints – 4-9 P.M.
4) ***Terrible colic*** – Pain is unbearable and the patient twists and turns about to get relief < Anger, standing still, 4-9 P.M., cheese;
> Doubling up, hard pressure.
5) *Vertigo* – on quickly turning the head especially on the left. Sensation as if he would fall.
6) *Neuralgia* – Colocynth affects the nerves causing facial, ovarian neuralgia, colic and sciatica. **Faceache** – Pains on the left side. Pains come in waves (Bell, Mag phos) > Hard pressure;
< Rest.

Sciatica – Left sided sciatica. Pains radiating down from hip joints to posterior part of thigh and further to popliteal fossa.
Ovarian neuralgia – > Hard pressure, doubling up
< Anger, rest, upright position.

7. *Dysentry* like diarrhoea renewed after least food or drinks often with characteristic colicky pains.
8. Tendency to *painful cramps* in muscles.
9. *Aggravation of complaints* from *rest, anger; amelioration* from motion, hard pressure.

Particulars :

1. HEADACHE
2. NEURALGIA – FACIAL
SCIATICA
OVARIAN
3. G.I.T

MENTAL GENERALS

Colocynth produces a state of the nervous system like that found in individuals who have for years been labouring under annoyances and relaxations.

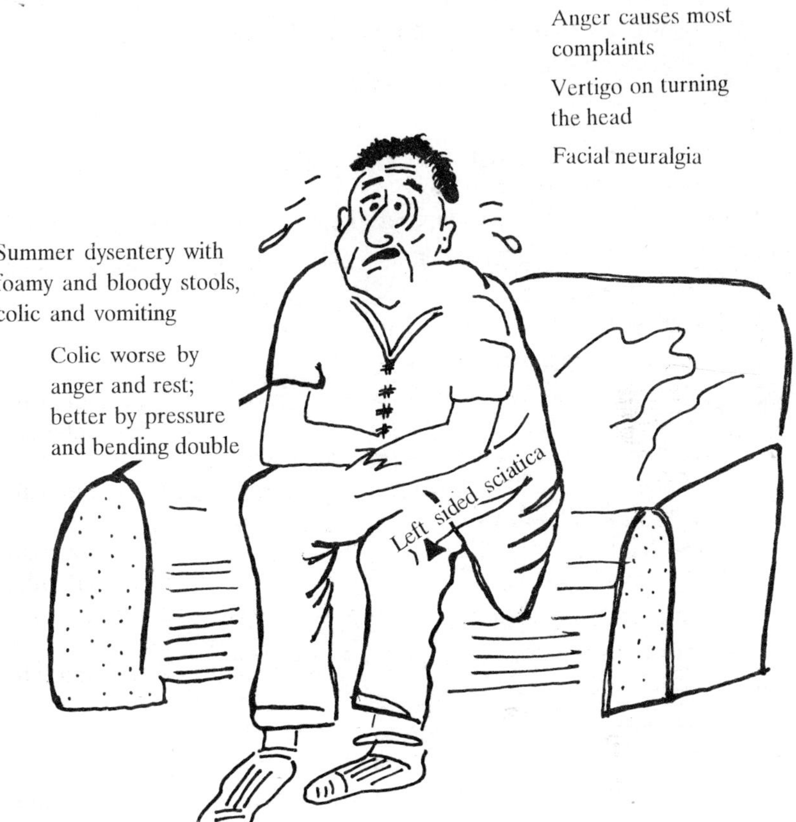
Anger causes most complaints
Vertigo on turning the head
Facial neuralgia
Summer dysentery with foamy and bloody stools, colic and vomiting
Colic worse by anger and rest; better by pressure and bending double
Left sided sciatica

COLOCYNTHIS

A man whose business affairs have been going wrong becomes irritable and nervous exhaustion follows.

A women who must watch her unfaithful husband night and day to keep him away from other women, gradually assumes a sensitive and irritable state of mind and is upset by least provocation.

HEADACHE

Cause – Anger, delayed menses
Location – Frontal region.

Character of pain – Tearing and digging pain through whole brain becoming unbearable when moving the eyes.

Concomitants – Vertigo on quickly turning the head.

Modalities > Anger, staying still
< Motion, hard pressure.

NEURALGIA

Facial Neuralgia – Left sided pain. Face is destroyed with anxious look from the severity of suffering. Finally the face becomes pale and cheeks become blue. Severe pains are brought on in waves. <Anger, vexation; > Hard pressure, motion.

[*Mag phos* – Pains <Heat, pressure]

[*Bell* – Right sided pains.]

Sciatica – Left sided sciatica extending from hip joints to posterior part of thigh and further to popliteal fossa. There is numbness and aneasthesia accompanying the pain.

Ovarian Neuralgia – Violent neuralgia such that the woman flexes the limb of the painful side hard against the abdomen
< Rest, anger
> Pressure, bending double.

GIT

Colic – *Cause* – Anger, flatus, undigested food.

Character of pains – Gripping, cramping and digging. Pains may spread all over the abdomen. Intestines feel as if they were squeezed between stones and would burst. Pain continues till the patient is nauseated and vomits.

Concomitants – Stools may be fluid, copious feacal, flatulent. Gripping pains are relieved after passage of stools.

Modalities < Rest, anger, eating, drinking
> Motion, bending double, hard pressure.

Diarrhoea

Cause – Summer, Anger.

Character of stools – White mucoid, thick and ropy with blood. Initially they are copious strong smelling and later become yellow scanty and inodorous.

Character of pains – Gripping in the abdomen forcing the patient to bend double. Relief is obtained after emaciation of stools but returns soon after and lasts till another stool.

General Modalities :

Aggravation – ANGER, REST, CHEESE.

Amelioration – PRESSURE (pressing abdomen hard against table), CONSTANT MOTION.

Concomitants – Bitter taste, violent thirst empty eructations, nausea vomiting of bitter fluid.

RELATIONS :

Remedies that follow well – Bell, Bry, Caust, Cham, Merc, Nux, Puls, Spig, Sulph.

Antidotes – Camph, Caust, Chan, Coffee, Op., Staph.

Important Questions ?

Q.1. Give indications of Colocynth in following :

a) Mental Generals . [1995]
b) Urinary Complaints. [1994]
c) Colic. [1972, 74, 76, 78, 79, 82, 87, 93, 94]
d) Modalities. [1979, 82]

Q.2. Compare colic of Chelidoneum /Colocynth. [1994]

35. DROSERA ROTUNDIFOLIA

Hahnemann

Common Name – Sundew.

Miasm – Psoric miasm.

Diathesis – Tuberculous.

Drosera is a *very deep acting remedy*, so a single dose of 30th potency cures within 7-8 days and not to repeat which spoils the case.

Relations with heat and cold – Chilly patient.

KEYNOTES

1) Drosera acts strongly on *pneumogastric nerve* – attacks of cough are of spasmodic nature.
   a) ***Deep sounding hoarse barking cough.***
   b) Paroxysms follow each other so closely that the patient gets out of breath and *vomits* large quantities of tenacious mucus.
   c) Constant *tickling* sensation in the throat as from feather.
   d) Cough < *midnight*, lying down – as soon as head touches the pillow.
   e) Due to violence of paroxysm – heamorrhage takes place from various outlets of body during such fits of coughing.
   f) Sense of *constriction in chest* and pain in hypochondrium during cough and the patient supports these parts while coughing.
   g) *Cough < laughing, singing, lying down, talking, midnight.*
2) Indicated in *T.B. of bone, joints, glands*. Indicated in scoliosis, tuberculous sinuses, spinal caries. Tuberculous abdomen with abdominal lesions in spleen, peyer's patches etc.
3) *Laryngeal Pthisis* – Aneamia, pallor of larynx, redness, swelling of mucous membrane covering arytenoid cartilage, weakness, loss of appetite with dry tickling persistent cough. Purulent expectoration and foul pus like taste in mouth.

Particulars :

1) RESPIRATORY SYSTEM

WHOOPING COUGH

Time – Night.

Sensation – Tickling sensation as from feather.

Character of cough :

- Deep sounding, hoarse barking dry cough.
- Paroxysms follow each other so closely that patient looses breath and vomits large quantities of tenacious mucus .
- Sensation of constriction in chest and pain hypochondria.
- Copious sweat all over the body with cough.
- Heamorrhage takes place from various outlets of the body during fits of coughing.
- < Night, lying down as soon as head touches the pillow, laughing, singing, drinking, talking.
- *Expectoration* – Usually dry cough with no expectoration. If present it is yellowish green.

Laryngeal Pthisis :

T.B. of lungs and larynx –

- Chronic persistent hoarseness
- Aneamia, pallor of larynx, redness and swelling of the mucus membrane covering the arytenoid cartilage.
- Weakness, loss of appetite, dry tickling persistent cough.

Character of cough – Violent hoarse barking cough, stitching pain in chest with heamorrhage from various orifices of body. During cough there is blue face with spasm of extremities.

Expectoration – Purulent with foul pus like taste in mouth.

T.B. Of Bone, Glands, Lymphatic Gland :

- Indicated in scoliosis with deformed back.
- Tubercular sinuses with discharge of pus.
- *Joints* – Occasional cases of rheumatic arthritis with swelling and deformity.
- (Prolonged use of Drosera induces *Tuberculisation of animals* – as seen after proving).

General Modalities :

Aggravation – MIDNIGHT
LYING DOWN
GETTING WARM IN BED
DURING SINGING
LAUGHING.

Relation :

Antidotes – Camphor

Complements – Nux vomica

Follow well – After Sambucus, Sulphur, Veratrum album.

Followed well by – Calc., Puls, S.

Important Questions ?

Q.1. Give indications of Drosera in :

1. Respiratory problems. [1973, 76, 79, 82, 86, 92]
2. Whooping Cough [1993]

Q.2. Compare – Spongia/Drosera in whooping cough. [1991]

SPONGIA	DROSERA
• Cough < Dry cold winds, evening	• Tuberculous diathesis Cough < Night
• **Character of cough** – Cough sounds like a saw driven through a board. Patient awakens out of sleep with a sense of suffocation.	• **Character of cough** – Loud hoarse barking cough with constant tickling sensation in larynx with continuous paroxysms that end in vomiting of tenacious mucus.
• < Talking, reading, singing, swallowing, cannot lie with head low.	• So severe is the paroxysm that heamorrhage may take place from various outlets. Dry cough and no expectoration.

Q.3. Compare Rumex, Bell, Phos, Ipecac in cough. [1973, 76]

RUMEX	BELLADONNA	PHOSPHORUS	IPECAC
• Dry cough < Inspiring cold air. • Patient covers the head in order to prevent the membrane from cold air. • Stitching pain through left lung just below nipple.	• Dry short tickling cough < Dry cold air. > Warm room. • **Larynx** : Inflamed swollen and constricted redness of face with dilated pupils. Foreign body sensation in larynx.	• Diathesis – tuberculous, heamorrhagic. Left side of chest is affected. Sharp stitching pain and congestion of lung. Sputa - rusty blood coloured or purulent.	• Spasmodic type of cough. • **Expectoration** – great accumulation of phlegm which is difficult to get rid of. • Patient. manages to get rid of expectoration by coughing or vomiting.

Q.4. Compare Ant tart, Hepar sulph and Kali carb in cough.

ANT TART	HEPAR SULPH.	KALI CARB
• Loud rattling due to accumulation of mucus in bronchi which is impossible to expel; cynosed, pale and blue face.	• Cough < cold dry weather. • Fish bone sensation in the throat. • Expectoration – Thick yellowish • Dry croupy cough with choking.	• Paroxysmal cough between 2-4 A.M. • Spasmodic with gagging and vomiting. • Sitting up or leaning forward relieves chest affections. • Great sweating, debility and backache are the key features.

36. DULCAMARA 'Autumn Remedy'

Hahnemann

Common Name – Bitter sweet.

ConstitutionAdapted to person of phlegmatic, scrofulous constitutions, restless and irritable. Sickly patient with pale yellow, pallid and sickly face.

Temperament – Irritable.

Relation with heat and cold – Affected by sudden changes in weather especially from hot to cold, exposure to cold damp and rainy weather.

Miasm – Psoric and sycotic patient.

KEYNOTES

1) ***Autumn Remedy*** – All the complaints catarrhal, rheumatic etc return when there is a sudden change in weather from hot to cold, warm days and cold nights, approach of storm, cold damp rainy weather.
2) ***Dulcamara produces a catarrhal condition with profuse secretion from mucous membranes*** from respiratory passages, diarrhoea, urine, saliva. Such a condition is produced when there is a weather change, cold wet weather and when the elimination from the skin is reduced (perspiration)
3) ***Inflammatory rheumatism*** caused by suppressed perspiration, wet weather, sudden changes in weather from hot to cold.
   - Rheumatism frequently alternates with diarrhoea.
   - Great remedy for backache caused by taking cold.
4) ***Eruptive medicine*** – Produces vesicles, dry brown and humid crusts. Produces multiple little boil like eruptions.
   - Warts on the face, back of hands and fingers.
   - Rash comes on the face before menses.
5) ***Urticaria*** over the whole body with itching and burning after scratching <warmth; > cold air.
6) Urticarea traceable in gastric disorder.
7) ***Coryza*** with profuse discharge from nose and eyes > closed room, morning; < open air.
8) ***Catarrhal ischuria*** – in grown up children with milky urine from wading with bare feet in cold water.

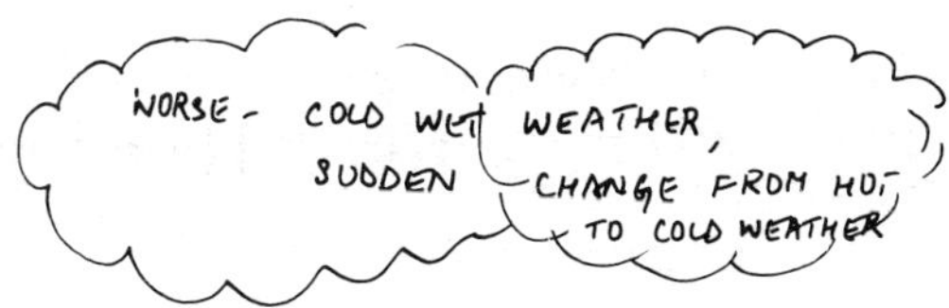
WORSE - COLD WET WEATHER,
SUDDEN CHANGE FROM HOT TO COLD WEATHER

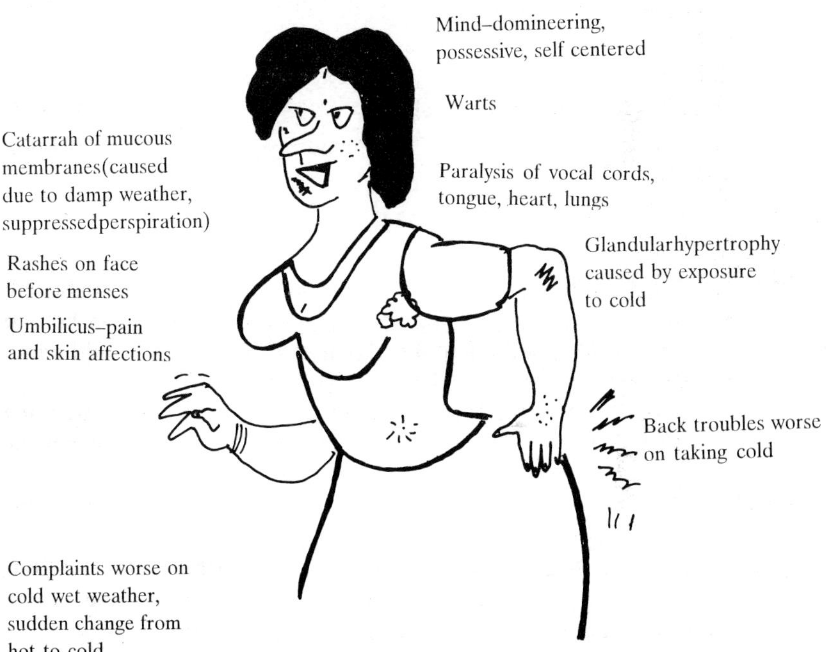
Mind–domineering, possessive, self centered
Warts
Catarrah of mucous membranes(caused due to damp weather, suppressedperspiration)
Paralysis of vocal cords, tongue, heart, lungs
Glandularhypertrophy caused by exposure to cold
Rashes on face before menses
Umbilicus–pain and skin affections
Back troubles worse on taking cold
Complaints worse on cold wet weather, sudden change from hot to cold

DULCAMARA

9) Acts on the lymphatic tissues producing *glandular enlargement* and cellular effusions. Glands swell and hypertrophy on repeated exposure to cold.

10) *Paralysis* is a common feature brought on by exposure to cold and damp weather. Any portion of the body, lungs, heart, vocal cords, tongue etc may be affected.

11) Dulcamara has a marvellous affect at or about the *umblicus*. Useful in pain, skin affections of the umblicus.

12) *Dropsy* after suppressed sweat, suppressed eruptions, exposure to cold.

Particulars :

1) MENTAL GENERALS
2) HEADACHE
3) EYES
4) RESPIRATORY SYSTEM
5) G.I.T
6) RHEUMATISM
7) URINARY SYSTEM
8) SKIN

MENTAL GENERALS

- *Domineering* and *Possessive* person— suspicious about others.
- Always insist upon their own point of view.
- *Self centered people*—it never crosses them that others also have their own rights and freedom.
- *Uptightness*—to an extent that it goes so far as to produce idiopathic hypertension.

HEADACHE

Cause—slacking up of usual catarrhal discharges causes headache. Every spell of cold, damp weather will bring on a headache.

Location—Starting from the occiput it goes to the whole head.

Modalities <Cold damp weather; >As soon as the flow from mucous membrane starts.

EYES

Everytime he takes cold it settles in the eyes producing thick yellow discharges, granular lids, eyes become red.

RESPIRATORY SYSTEM

Coryza :

Character of discharge—Bloody crusts blowing out thick yellow mucous all the time <slightest exposure to cold air, open air; > motion, warm room

Throat :

- Persons who in every cold damp spell have a sore throat from getting over heated, throwing off the wraps and getting into a cold place. These colds that settle first in the nose of every worst sort gradually creep on until the whole respiratory apparatus is in a state of catarrhal inflammation.

Cough :

Cause – Cold damp weather.

Character of cough – loose cough with free expectoration, spasmodic cough with excessive secretion.

Expectoration – Thick yellowish profuse with loose rattling cough. Patient has to get up to throw out his phlegm everytime.

< Cold damp rainy weather;
> Warm room

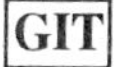

GIT

Diarrhoea :

Cause – Change of weather from hot to cold. At the close of summers. Cold damp rainy weather.

Character of stool – Yellow, slimy stool, yellow green undigested frequent stool, blood in stool and quite a mass of slime showing a marked catarrhal state.

Modalities – Night, sudden change in weather from hot to cold, cold damp weather.

RHEUMATISM

Cause – Suppressed perspiration. Brought on by sudden change in weather from hot to cold, cold wet weather.

Character of pain – Inflamed joints with sore and bruised feeling all over. Joints are red, sensitive to touch and swollen.

Modalities < Evening, night, cold damp weather
> Motion

URINARY SYSTEM

Dulcamara is useful in cystitis and other ailments of bladder particularly when a mucopurulent urine is associated with one sided sensitivness of abdomen. Urine is generally scanty, fetid, and turbid. Sometimes it contains a jelly like white mucus giving a milky apperance to the urine.

Aggravation – < damp weather, getting chilled
> becoming warm.

SKIN

- *Rash* comes on the face just before menses.

- Patients are subjected to *cold sores* upon the lips and upon the genitals. This happens everytime he takes cold.
- *Urticaria* over the whole body with itching and burning after scratching, < warm; > cold
- Thick brown yellow crusts on scalp, face, forehead, temples with reddish borders. These crusts bleed when scratched.
- *Warts* – Fleshy, large smooth or flat on the face, back of hands and fingers. (Thuja, Caust, Nit acid.)
- Great remedy for *crusta lactea.* Thick brown yellow crusts cover sores on chest, scalp and other parts of the body.
- Great remedy for retrocession of eruptions due to exposure to cold damp air.

General Modalities :

Aggravation – COLD
SUDDEN CHANGE IN WEATHER FROM HOT TO COLD
COLD WET WEATHER
COLD AIR
SUPPRESSED MENSES
ERUPTIONS AND SWEAT

Amelioration – FROM MOVING ABOUT (FERUM, RHUS. TOX)

Relations :

Complementry – to Baryta carb, Kali sulph.

Incompatible with – Acetic acid, Bell, Lachesis.

Follows well after – Calc, Bry., Lyc, Rhus, Sep.

Improtant Questions ?

Q. 1.Give indications of Dulcamara in the following

1) Cold and cough [1976, 77, 78]
2) Respiratory system [1996]
3) Urinary trouble [1977]
4) Gastric complaints [1988]
5) Dysentry [1974, 75, 88]
6) Warty Growth [1982]
7) Urticaria [1979]
8) Skin symptoms [1974, 77, 79]
9) Paralysis [1977]
10) Modalities [1976]

37. EUPHRASIA

Hahnemann

Common Name – Eyebright.

- According to Grauvogl the 'signature of a black spot in the corolla which looks like the pupil' marked Euphrasia as an eye medicine to the ancients and the Homoeopathic experiments have fully confirmed its old time reputation.
- Euphrasia is a *short acting medicine* and is useful in catarrhal inflammation with or without fever. It acts on the mucous membrane especially the conjunctiva and the nasal mucous membrane producing *profuse acrid lachrymation and profuse bland coryza.*

KEYNOTES

1) Euphrasia produces catarrhal affections of mucous membranes especially of eyes and nose producing ***profuse acrid lachrymation and profuse bland coryza.*** < Open air, windy weather;
> Warmth.

2) ***Eyes water all the time and are agglutinated in the morning.*** Margins of the lids are red, swollen and burning.

3) Profuse fluent coryza in the morning with *violent cough* and *abundant expectoration*. Expectoration is easy and almost without cough.
Aggravation of cough in *day time, open air, windy weather.*
Amelioration when *lying down.*

4) In *measles* with watery eyes, fluent coryza and cough only during day time with easy expectoration, red face, cold hands, sweat and chill Euphrasia is well indicated.

5) *Menses* are *short* and *scanty* lasting for only one hour or one day.

Particulars :

1) HEADACHE
2) EYE
3) CORYZA
4) COUGH
5) MEASLES/FEVER

HEADACHE

Headaches that occur with coryza and eye symptoms. There is profuse watery discharge from the eyes and nose.

EYES

Euphrasia cures conditions of eyes like inflammation, blepharitis, photophobia, conjunctivitis, rheumatic iritis, opacity and ulceration of cornea, ambylopia etc.

Profuse acrid lachrymation.

During *inflammation* the *eyelids* become *reddened* and injected particularly on the inner surface. They become *puffed red* or even dark. *Ulceration* takes place giving us a *discharge which is thick and excoriating. Tears* themselves are *profuse and excoriate* the cheeks. There is marked *photophobia* and the person cannot bear sunlight or artificial light. Intense *itching* with constant *rubbing* of the eyes.

Conjunctivitis – Little blisters form on or near the phlyctenule. The discharge from the eyes are acrid and purulent and a film of mucus seems to collect over the cornea causing a difficulty in vision. This blurred sight is relieved by wiping or winking the eyes. Conjunctivitis of *traumatic origin* with an acrid discharge.

Rheumatic Iritis – iris reacts very tardity to light and the aqueous humor is cloudy from the admixture of products of inflammation. Pains are burning in character with acrid lachrymation which is worse at night.

RESPIRATORY SYSTEM

Nose :

Sneezing and fluent coryza with *profuse bland fluent discharge*. Nasal mucous membrane is swollen < open air, chilly weather. After the coryza has existed for a day or two it extends into the larynx with a hard cough.

Cough :

Cough with copious expectoration along with or following coryza.

Cause – Open air, cold weather.

Character of cough – Violent cough from tickling in the larynx. Deep inspiration is difficult. Cough only during *daytime*, *ceases on lying down.* Passive pain beneath the sternum showing that trachea is especially involved in catarrhal condition.

Expectoration – *Easy* expectoration almost without cough. *Abundant secretion in the larynx causing loose cough with rattling in chest.*

Modalities – < Daytime, open air, cold weather.
> Lying down.

FEVER

Euphrasia is very useful in the first stage of measles, influenza, catarrhal fever.

- Fever occurs mostly during *daytime* with a red face and cold hands.
- Chill predominates 'there is *chill, fever and sweat'* in this remedy.

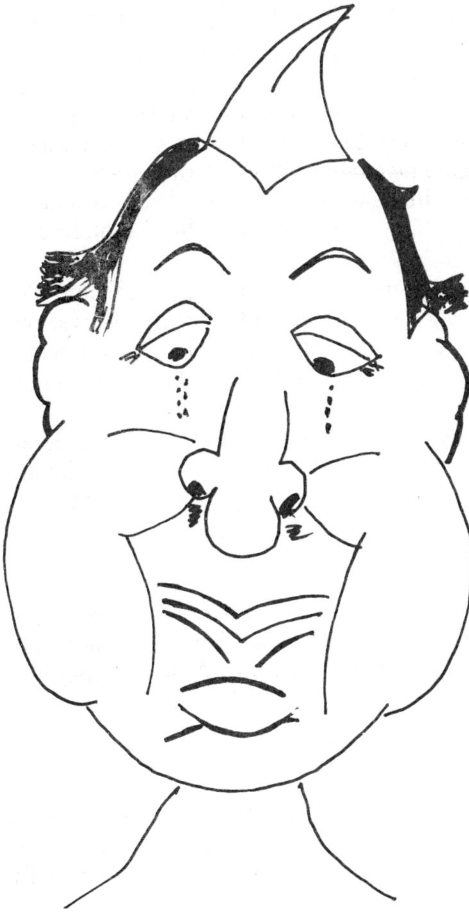

All eye troubles with profuse acrid lachrymation and bland coryza

Margins of lids are swollen and burning

Violent itching with rubbing

Cough–violent, in daytime with easy expectoration ceases on lying down.

EUPHRASIA

- Heat decends down the body. Perspiration is often confined to the front part of the body.
- Profuse acrid lachrymation and profuse bland coryza. In *measles* when the symptoms agree Euphrasia makes an attack of measles turn into simple form making the patient feel much better, brings out eruptions, controls the fever and relieves the cough, coryza and other catarrhal symptoms. Euphrasia is a wonderful medicine for measles though not as frequently indicated as *Pulsatilla* owing to the fact that this combination of symptoms does not often come true.

Important Questions ?

Q.1. Give indications of Euphrasia in :

a) Coryza [1972]
b) Eye symptoms [1979, 82]

Q.2. Compare – Euphrasia/Allium cepa in coryza. [1987 S, 86, 94]
Coryza of Euphrasia/Allium cepa/Arum triph/Silicea. [1986]
Coryza of Euphrasia/Allium cepa/Arum triph/Hepar sulph. [1987]

EUPHRASIA	ALLIUM CEPA	ARUM TRIP.	SILICEA	HEPAR SULPH
• CHILLY patient • Profuse acrid lachrymation and bland nasal discharge < Open Air > Warmth.	• HOT patient • Profuse watery acrid nasal discharge and bland lachrymation < Warmth > Open Air	• Acrid, ichorous discharge excoriating inside of nose, alae nasi and upper lip. • Picking of nose and lips until they bleed. • Cannot eat or drink on account of soreness.	• CHILLY patient • Coryza is characterised by chronacity, enlargement of lymph nodes. • Discharge is thin, ichorous and putrid. • Desire for cold food and drinks.	• CHILLY patient • Hyper-sensitive to cold • Discharge is thick, yellowish and loose. Hepar is indicated in later stages when discharge becomes thick. > Warmth, warm food and drinks.

38. FERRUM PHOSPHORICUM

J.C. Morgan

Common Name – Phosphate of Iron.

Ferrum phos is a *broad, deep acting, anti psoric medicine*.

Pathogenesis – Iron Phosphate colours the blood corpuscles red, carries oxygen to all parts of the body and thus furnishes the vital force that sustains life. Without the proper balance of iron in the blood, health cannot be maintained. When a deficiency of this cell salt occurs, the circulation is increased, for the blood tries to carry enough oxygen to all the tissues of the body with limited amount of iron in hand and in order to do so must move rapidly.

This increased motion being changed to heat by the law of conservation of energy is called fever. The interference with metabolism thus caused soon prevents the functioning of the other cell salts, with the result that they also loose their power of union with the organic matter and are thrown out of the system. A deficiency in Potassium chloride always follows a deficiency in iron. A lack of Ferrum phos. or an improper balance in blood is the cause of colds. When a deficiency of iron occurs, nature or natural law draws the blood away from the outer parts, the skin, in order to carry on the process of life more perfectly about the heart, lungs, liver, stomach, brain. This on account of closing pores of skin gives rise to accumulation of non functional matters which are thrown out by way of the mucous membranes and forms discharges of colds, catarrahs, pneumonia, pleurisy etc. Thus Ferrum phos is used in all conditions whenever there is *inflammation in the first stage before the stage of exudation.*

Ferrum molecules toughen the cellular structure in the circular walls of the blood vessels, hence a lack of iron frequently causes a breaking down of the walls of minute blood vessels producing *heamorrhages.* Ferrum phos is indicated in bright red heamorrhage from any part of the body.

Constitution – Pale and aneamic subjects who with all their weaknesses are subject to sudden and violent local congestion and inflammations.

Miasm – Predominatly Anti-psoric medicine.

Relation with heat and cold – Chilly patient.

KEYNOTES

1) Ferrum phos is the remedy for ***first stage of all febrile disturbances*** before exudations set in. Fever with pain and heat are leading indications for inflammation when Ferrum phos is to be prescribed.

2) *Bright red heamorrhages* from any orifice with a tendency of the blood to coagulate rapidly.
3) ***Aneamic and chlorotic*** people with great ***lassitude*** (lack of heamoglobin in blood).
4) *Lack of vital heat* and aggravation from cold and becoming cold.
5) *Congestion* of head and organs with fever and red face (false plethora).
6) Motion that is real exertion aggravates but slow motion ameliorates.
7) Pulsations felt all over the body.
8) Soreness all over the body with oversensitiveness to touch.

Particulars :

1) HEADACHE
2) EYES
3) EAR
4) NOSE
5) FACE
6) GIT
7) RESPIRATORY SYSTEM
8) URINARY SYSTEM
9) MALE SEXUAL SYMPTOMS
10) FEMALE SEXUAL SYMPTOMS
11) RHEUMATISM
12) TISSUES
13) FEVER

HEADACHE

Location – Temples, above the eyes, frontal headache.

Sensation – Headache with rush of blood to the head. Throbbing headache with flushing over the face. Head is sore to touch.

Aggravation – Motion, coughing.

Amelioration – Epistaxis relieves headache, cold applications.

EYES

- Acute inflammation of eyes in the first stage.
- Conjuctivitis with photophobia.
- Redness of conjunctiva, of balls and lids.
- Granulations of eyelids with feeling as if grains of sand were there.

EAR

- Inflammation of the first stage.

- Earache with beating and throbbing pain, inflammation of the external ear with redness and burning.
- Noises in the ear like running water from unequalisation of blood in the blood vessels.

FACE

- Earthy pale sallow face with circumscribed redness of cheeks. Red face alternating with paleness. Pseudo plethora with aneamia. Red face during fever, during headache.

GIT

Mouth – Inflammation of mouth. Gums hot swollen and inflamed.

Teeth – Toothache due to an inflammatory condition. For feverishness in teething complaints.

< Hot liquids, motion.

> Cold things.

Tongue – Clean and red tongue, showing an inflammatory condition. Tongue is dark red and inflamed.

Gastritis :

- First stage of gastritis with pain in the stomach from smallest quantity of food.
- Burning sore pain in the pit of the stomach.
- Headache with gastritis.
- Vomiting of undigested food or bright red blood.
- Dyspepsia with flushed face and throbbing pain in the stomach. > hot drinks
  < cold drinks

Abdomen :

First stage of inflammatory condition of the bowels, enteric fever, cholera, dysentry, peritonitis etc. when the patient complains of feeling chilly. Soreness and tenderness of bowels.

Diarrhoea :

Diarrhoea and dysentry in hot weather; chest trouble and catarrah in winters.

- Undigested, watery stools.
- Morning diarrhoea like sulphur.
- Tenesmus at stool.

Constipation :

Heat in the colon or rectum with dryness of the mucous membrane.

Piles – Bright red blood with sore painful anus.

RESPIRATORY SYSTEM

Nose :

- First or inflammatory stage of the cold in head. Takes cold easily.
- Predisposition to *bleed* in aneamic and poorly nourished subjects. Ferrum phos is excellent in epistaxis from any cause, even injury epistaxis.

Throat :

First stage of throat diseases when there is pain, redness and heat. Inflammation of tonsils when they are red and swollen. Ulcerated throat with pain and fever.

Cough :

- In the beginning of cough and cold caused by cold air.

Character of cough – short spasmodic and painful expectoration – scanty and blood streaked < Cold air; > Warmth, warm water etc.

All inflammatory condition of the respiratory tract (pneumonia, bronchitis, pleuritis, tracheitis) *in the first stage.*

- Breathing short and hurried at the beginning or during the course of the disease when there is heat and fever present.
- Cold air in the chest with hard, dry cough and soreness in the lungs.
- Scanty blood streaked expectoration.
- Heamorrhages in the lungs of bright red blood.

URINARY SYSTEM

- First stage of inflammation of the bladder causing retention of the urine with pain and smarting when urinating.
- Cystitis often caused by retaining the urine for too long which should be voided.
- Brights disease and diabetes when there is feverishness, pain or congestion in any part of the system.
- Suppression of urine through heat particulary in children.
- Wetting of bed from weakness of muscles of the neck and bladder (Kali phos). (If from worms – Nat phos).
- Constant urging to urinate if not chronic.

MALE SEXUAL SYMPTOMS

First stage of irritation and inflammation of the prostate gland, orchitis etc. when there is feverishness, pain and throbbing.

FEMALE SEXUAL SYMPTOMS

- Inflammation of womb and vagina with fever and also vomiting of undigested food.
- Spasm of vagina with excess dryness.

- First stage of gonorrhoea, metritis etc.
- Dysmenorrhoea when there is pain congestion and fever and also vomiting of undigested food.
- Menses with bright red blood.

RHEUMATISM

- Rheumatic lameness of joints when fever is present<catching cold, motion.
- Inflammation and pain in the back with fever.
- In sprains and strains of the first stage.
- Cold extremities and coldness of back.

SKIN

Inflammation stage of all skin affections, abscesses, carbuncles, boils, felons etc require this remedy with heat. pain and throbbing.

TISSUES

- In injuries of soft tissues, strains, sprains, cuts, bruises when there is inflammation pain and fever.
- *Epistaxis* in children and aneamic people.
- *Heamorrhages* in any part of the body with tendency to coagulate rapidly.
- *Aneamia* – Ferrum phos colours the red blood cells.

FEVER

Fever at the commencement of any disease (gastritis, enteritis, typhoid, rheumatism, measles, chicken pox etc.) Ferrm phos should be continued as long as fever and inflammation exist to control and subdue the heat, inflammation and pain. Intermittent fever with chill at 1 P.M.

General Modalities :

Aggravation – NIGHT, TOUCH, MOTION.

Amelioration – COLD.

(Cold should be applied directly to congestion or relief would not be felt. If inflammation is deep seated, heat should be applied to relieve the engorgement of deeper vessels.)

39. GELSIMIUM NITIDUM

W.E. Payne

Common Name – Yellow Jasmine.

Gelsimium is a *short acting remedy* with *gradual onset of symptoms.*

Constitution – It has been used mostly in *acute troubles* and hence the person does not have a definite constitution.

Temperament – Nervous and Hysterical temperament.

Relation with heat and cold – Gelsimium is a remedy for warm climates.

Miasm – Psora is in the background.

KEYNOTES

1) ***Complete relaxation and prostration of the whole muscular system with almost or entire motor paralysis.*** Eyelids droop and muscles refuse to obey the will causing – aphonia, dysphagia, trembling, great weight and tiredness of limbs, uterine atonacity, impotency etc.
2) *Gradual onset* of all symptoms.
3) ***Dullness, dizzyness, drowsiness and trembling*** are the marking features. Dullness of mental faculties with listlessness and prostration. Trembling of hands or lower extremities on attempting to move.
4) *Headache with passive congestion.* Pain begins in the nape of the neck and settles down over the eyes. The person cannot think and is listless and stupid.

   Aggravation – Mental exertion, smoking, heat, head lying low.

   Amelioration – Head held high, profuse urination.
5) *Vertigo* with blurred vision; dilated pupils; double sight; sense of intoxication.
6) *Nervous chill* – Violent shaking with no sense of coldness (chill runs up and down the back in wave like succession from sacrum to occiput; chill begins between the scapulae).
7) In **inflammation/fever** Gels. is prescribed on the following keynotes.
   - Flushed face
   - Determination of blood to head
   - Cold extremities
   - Disturbance of sensation
   - Drooping of lids with suffused red face

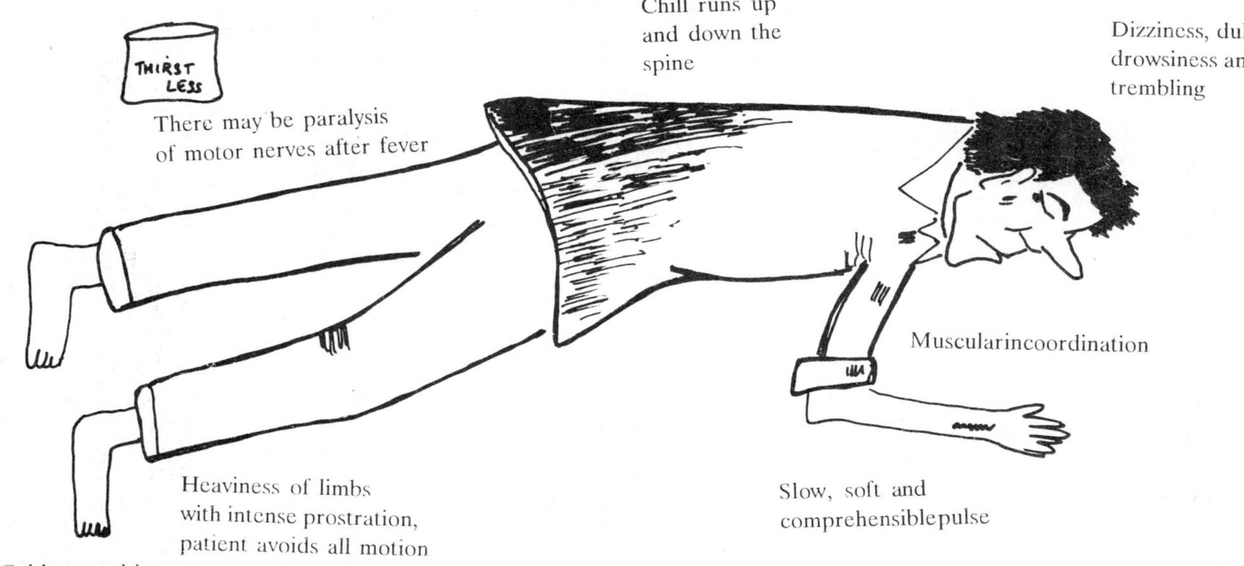
THIRST LESS
Chill runs up and down the spine
Dizziness, dullness drowsiness and trembling
There may be paralysis of motor nerves after fever
Muscularincoordination
Heaviness of limbs with intense prostration, patient avoids all motion
Slow, soft and comprehensiblepulse
Cold extremities
Worse by heat, mental exertion, emotions
Gradual onset of fever

GELSIMIUM NITIDUM

- Delirium with dullness of mind
- Paralysis/Weakness of sphincters

8) *Pulse* is slow when quite but greatly accelerated on motion. In slow pulse of old age Gelsimium is very useful.
9) Excessively sensitive condition of nerves. *Susceptibility and mental disturbance* such as a sudden excitement or emotion, bad news or fright, anticipation of an unusual ordeal brings on diarrhoea, headache etc.
10) Desires to be *quiet;* feels too weak to move.
11) Patient is generally ***thirstless.***
12) Children have *fear of falling;* seize the nurse; grasp the cradle.
13) Fears that unless constant motion is kept up,the heart would stop beating. (Dig – Heart would cease to beat on beginning to move).
14) Gelsimium is an excellent medicine for *influenza* – before, during and after.

Particulars :

1) MIND
2) HEADACHE
3) PARALYSIS
4) CORYZA
5) FEVER
6) MALE GENITILIA
7) FEMALE SEXUAL ORGANS

MIND

- Patient is in a *depressed* mood and wants solitude.
- Lacks the capacity to think or fix their attention on anything.
- Troubles brought on by *fever and dread* – nervous diarrhoea, headache, abortion etc. caused by *anticipation,* excitement, shock, fear of going before public. A person on becoming overwhelmed by some surprise becomes faint, weak and exhausted; he becomes tired in all limbs and is unable to resist opposing circumstances.

HEADACHE

Cause – Mental exertion, smoking, heat of summers. (Gelsimium causes *passive congestion* la dilated condition of both arteries and veins.)

Sensation – Gradual onset of pain. Patient becomes listless and stupid; he has dizziness with blurred sight and heaviness of the head.

Look – Face is suffused red in colour with cold extremities. Eyes grow heavy and blood shot.

Aggravation – Mental exertion, heat, head lying low.

Amelioration – Head held high, profuse urination.

PARALYSIS

Gelsimium is a great paralyser. *Gradual onset* of both mental and physical paralysis. There is *paralysis of motor nerves* thus affecting various groups of muscles about the eyes, throat, chest, larynx, sphincters and extremities. There is extreme *prostration and weakness. Tremor* is the keynote. Muscles lose the power to contract at the patients will.

Mind–*Patient is confused and has a sluggish state of mind. Lack of capacity to think or fix their attention on anything.*

Physical Symptoms :

- *Ptosis* or paralysis of the upper lid with double vision. Eyeballs feel sore.
- *Dysphagia* due to weakness of muscles of deglutition.
- *Aphonia* with want of voice.
- *Thick speech* with tongue as though unweildy. Patient answers questions slowly or imperfectly.
- *Heaviness of limbs* – painful and unable to move.
- *Weakness of heart muscle* – instinct on the persons part to move and to stimulate it to act.
- Relaxation of male genital organs with frequent *involuntary emissions*.
- *Uterine inertia* – womb becomes inert and loses all its tone and elasticity < Emotion, excitement, fear, shock,thunderstorm, warmth.
- *Post diptheritic paralysis* – Child does not possess sufficient strength to hold himself. Spine in the upper cervical region becomes bent backward. Strabismus with thick and slurred speech. Suffused red face with drooping eyelids.
- *Congestion/Inflammation* – Gelsimium produces a passive congestion of all organs with high grade inflammation.
    - There is delirium with flushed face.
    - Determination of blood to head with cold extremities.
    - Heaviness of limbs.
    - Disturbance of sensation.
    - Paralysis of sphincters.

CORYZA

Cause – Warm, moist weather, morning.

Character of discharge – Excoriating discharge from the nose making the nostrils sore.

Concomitants – Sore throat with dry teasing cough and very little expectoration. Dryness of mouth with general prostration.

FEVER

- Remittent, intermittent, bilious, eruptive fevers.

Remittent :

- Typhoid, Bilious fever, influenza.
  Cause – Heat of summer.
  Onset – Gradual onset.

Symptoms :

- Nervous restlessness with continuous tossing about.
- Suffused redness of face with drowsiness.
- Great prostration and every part of the body feels sore.
- Heaviness and redness in eyes, unable to lift the lids.
- Delirious condition with difficulty in speech. Patient answers the questions slowly.
- Full bound pulse.
- Constant trembling of muscles.
- Slight or partial sweat.
- Heaviness in limbs.
- Thirstlessness.
- Patient dreads motion – wants to be perfectly still.

Intermittent Fevers :

Chill stage – Nervous chill – running from sacrum to the nape of neck. Chill is so severe that the patient wishes to be held tightly so that he may not shake so much. Thirstlessness with profuse urination. Patient wants to be kept warm.

Heat stage – Thirstlessness with intense burning. Patient is extremely *exhausted* and is in a *semi – stuporous* state.

Sweat stage – very slight perspiration.

Eruptive fevers of children :

- Tendency to convulsions at the time of eruption.
- Restlessness with chilliness.
- Watery discharge from nose excoriating the alae nasi and the upper lip. Hard barking cough with hoarseness.

MALE SEXUAL ORGANS

Impotency :

Cause – Weakness of muscles and sphincters.

Symptoms – Frequent involuntary emissions at night with relaxation of organs, no lascivious dreams and often cold sweat on the scrotum. The sexual power is so completely exhausted that even the most powerful stimuli fail to excite the patient and bring an efflux of blood into his sexual organs.

FEMALE SEXUAL ORGANS

- *Abortion* caused by fright, mental excitement.
- *Labor* – Rigid Os uteri. Patient is hysterical and full of nervous excitement. Pains leave the uterus, fly all over the body or shoot upward and backward. It may go up to the throat and cause choking.
- Atony of uterus – Neck of the uterus is as soft as a putty. It is flabby and the bag of water bulges freely from the os but there is no attempt whatever at expulsion.

Non Pregnant State :

Reflex headaches due to ovarian irritation. Head feels enormously enlarged with temporarily blurred vision. Heaviness in the uterine region. White leucorrhoeal discharge, nervousness, excitability and backache.

Congestive Dysmenorrhoea :

Gelsimium is an excellent medicine for congestive dysmenorrhoea.

- Suffused countenance due to congestion to the head.
- Bearing down sensation in the abdomen.
- Cramps in the uterus and legs.
- General hysterical condition.

General Modalities :

Amelioration – PROFUSE URINATION
LYING STILL.

Aggravation – DAMP WEATHER
BEFORE THUNDERSTORM
COITION
EXCITEMENT
BAD NEWS
TOBACCO SMOKING
THINKING ABOUT HIS AILMENTS.

Relations :

Remedies that follow well – Bapt, Cact., Ipec.

Antidotes – Atrop., Chin, Coff., Dig.

Important Questions ?

Q.1. Give indications of Gelsimium in following :

1) Fever [1986, 93 S, 93, 94, 95]
2) Influenza [1977]
3) Typhoid [1967, 83, 91]
4) Cardiac Disease [1970, 82, 91]
5) Mental Generals [1986, 89, 90]
6) Head [1986]

Q. 2. Compare.

1) Gels/Causticum in paralysis [1976]
2) Bry/Bapt/Arnica/Gels in Typhoid [1987]
3) Gels/Digitalis – Hearts symptoms [1969]

PARALYSIS :

GELSIMIUM	CAUSTICUM
• Complete motor paralysis of functional origin.	• Paralysis from exposure to the cold of winter.
• Tremor, dullness, dizziness and drowsiness are the keynotes.	• Paralysis of single parts – face, tongue, pharynx.
• Incoordination of muscles.	• Right sided remedy.
• Aphonia, dysphagia, speech, prostration.	• Rawness and soreness in affected parts.
• Heaviness of limbs, suffused red face.	• Rigidity of flexor tendons.

TYPHOID :

GELSIMIUM	BRYONIA	BAPTISIA	ARNICA
• Gradual onset.	• Gradual onset.	• High fever with sore bruised feeling all over.	• Sore, lame and bruised feeling.
• Fever brought on by warm relaxing weather	• Fever brought on by taking cold in hot summer, exposure to cold wind.	• Offensiveness of all discharges.	• Restlessness
• Languor, muscular weakness and heaviness of limbs.	• Dry and coated tongue.	• White coated tongue with red-papillae.	• Stupor with involuntary discharges of stool and urine.

• Suffused face.	• Patient avoids motion – wants to lie down quickly.	• Delirium – Body is scattered into pieces and he is unable to keep them covered.	• Delirium – Patient answers correctly, in full and then delirium returns.
• Dullness of mind, dizziness and drowsiness.	• Low muttering delirium	• Flushed, dusky, red face	
• Thirstlessness	• Profuse perspiration	• Bradycardia	
• Partial chill with full flowing pulse	• Tachycardia	• Low muttering delirium that returns in the middle of the answer.	
• Tachycardia			

HEART SYMPTOMS

GELSIMIUM	DIGITALIS
• Patient is aroused out of sleep feeling that the heart will stop beating. He is impelled to move about to keep the heart going.	• Heart symptoms are just opposite. Heart feels as if it stood still. Patient feels as if blood stood still. Patient fears that the heart will stop beating if he should make any motion.

40. GRAPHITES NATURALIS

Hahnemann

Common Name – Black lead.

Graphites is a *deep acting remedy.*

Constitution – It is a remedy for *crude and coarse people* who do a lot of physical work like labourers.

- Patient is *fat, chilly and costive* with swollen lymphatic glands.
- Patient is *stout and aneamic with a tendency to skin affections and constipation.*
- Tendency towards *obesity is marked. This is due to malnutrition and imperfect assimilation.*
- Hair is blonde with pale face and a low spirited person.
- In women *obesity* is associated with *habitual constipation* and history of *delayed menstruation.*

'What Pulsatilla is to puberty, Graphites is to climacteric.'

Temperament – Irritable.

Relation with heat and cold – Very chilly person.

Diathesis – Scrofulous diathesis.

Miasm – Powerful anti-psoric remedy

KEYNOTES

1) ***Fat but unhealthy individuals*** – There is deficient animal heat owing to deficient oxygenation of blood.
2) Tendency to *rush of blood to the head with flushing of face.* Circulation is at first excited followed by loss of energy and consequent venous hyperemia. Slight *erethism* followed by weakness, aneamia and *chlorosis*.
3) *Craving for open air* (in all carbon groups).
4) ***Blandness*** – lack of sensitivity to any stimulus – body, emotions and intellect. Mind is dull and lethargic. Poor memory for recent events. Anxieties, fears and irresolution.
5) Women with tendency to ***obesity, constipation and delayed menstruation.***
6) ***Sadness*** is a general state of mind – listening to *music makes him worse.*
7) ***Unhealthy skin*** – Every injury *suppurates with discharge of watery, transparent and sticky* fluid looking like semen; offensive. Rough hard dry skin with very little tendency to sweat.

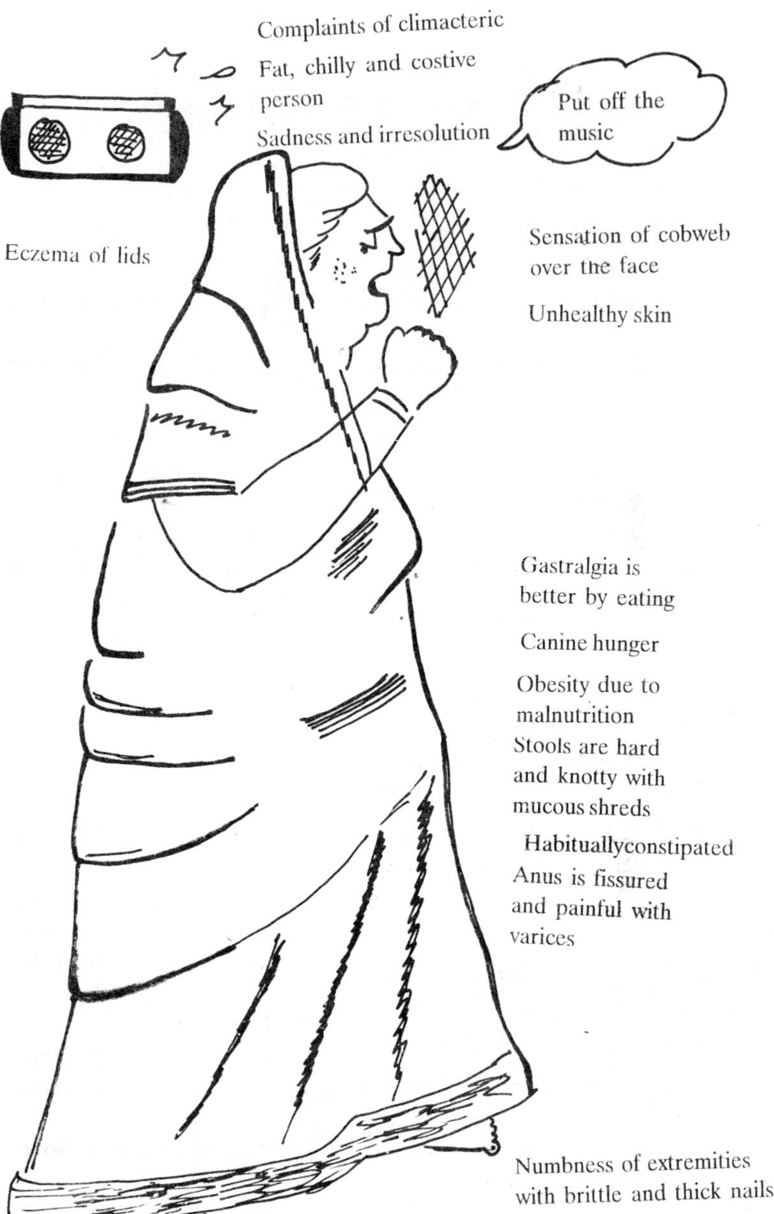
Complaints of climacteric
Fat, chilly and costive person
Sadness and irresolution
Put off the music
Eczema of lids
Sensation of cobweb over the face
Unhealthy skin
Gastralgia is better by eating
Canine hunger
Obesity due to malnutrition
Stools are hard and knotty with mucous shreds
Habituallyconstipated
Anus is fissured and painful with varices
Numbness of extremities with brittle and thick nails

GRAPHITES

- *Old hard cicatrices soften up* and go away under its action especially those left by abscesses of mammae.

8) *Nails* grow thick, *cracked* and out of shape.
9) *Mucous outlets* – Scanty secretion with tendency to cracks and fissures.
    - *Eyelids* inflamed with pustules.
    - *Ears* discharge; moist sore places behind the ears.
    - *Mouth* cracked in corners.
    - *Anus* – eruptions, itching with fissures.
10) Strong tendency to *constipation*. Stools – knotty, large lumps united by mucus threads.
11) *Hears better when in noise* – whenever there is rumbling sound – eg. while riding in a car.
12) *Numbness of extremities* – tips of fingers.
13) Sensation of *cobweb on face*, tries hard to brush it off.
14) **Aggravation** – Morning, cold air, during and after menses.
    Amelioration – Open air, eating.

Particulars :

1) MIND
2) HEAD
3) EYES
4) EAR
5) FACE
6) RESPIRATORY SYSTEM
7) GIT
8) MALE SEXUAL ORGANS
9) FEMALE SEXUAL ORGANS
10) SKIN

MIND

- *Sadness and despondence* are their ever present companions.
- *Sadness is worse during music.*
- *Blandness* in all spheres – mind, emotions and intellect. Mind is dull and lethargic.
- Irresolution with emptiness of thinking.
- Poor memory for recent events.
- Mind is dull as if there are callouses on his mind preventing anything from penetrating.

HEAD

Graphites is peculiar in headaches of fat, aneamic women with disordered menses.

Cause – Becoming cold, looking at bright light.

Location – Occiput.

Sensation – Heavy weight in the occiput. Numb and heavy feeling in the head.

Modalities – < Warm room, morning, bright light.
> Open air.

EYES

Graphites is an **excellent** remedy for the affections of eye.

- *Eczema of lids* – eruptions moist and fissured, margins of the lids covered with scales and crusts.
- Graphites leads all remedies for *eczematous eruptions of lids* (Staph, Sulph).
- Scrofulous opthalmia – Cornea is apt to be covered with superficial ulcers.
- Blepharitis – worse in the angles of the eyes in the **canthi**. Mucopurulent discharge from the eyes is thin and excoriating.
- If there is tendency for the edges of the lids to crack and bleed Graphites is the sure shot remedy.
- *Hardened styes* – may appear along the edges of lids.
- *Vision* – letters appear double when writing and run together when reading. He also sees fiery zig-zags around his field of vision.
- *Intense photophobia* – in the sunlight with copious lachrymation. No remedy has photophobia more marked than Graphites.

EAR

- *Tinnitus aureum* – Lot of humming, hissing, crackling sounds heard; sensation as if skin were before the ear, obstructing sounds. These patients hear better in noise.
- Eczema behind the ears; discharge is sticky, viscid pus and offensive.
- Discharge from the ear – sticky, viscid, bloody and offensive.

FACE

- Pale, waxy and sticky face.
- Tendency to falling of hair and whiskers and in consequence there are nude spots on the scalp which look bald and shiny at places.
- Sensation of *cob-web* over the face and the patient constantly keeps wiping his face to remove it.
- Submaxillary gland is swollen and indurated.

RESPIRATORY SYSTEM

Nasal catarrah – Extreme dryness of nose alternates with discharge of lumps or clinkers. Discharge is offensive and bloody. Border of the nostrils are sore, scabby and crack easily. *Person cannot bear the odour of flowers.*

Sore Throat – Sensation of lump in the throat < empty swallowing.

Cough – Characteristic dry cough with great deal of strangling making the face red and eyes water < deep inspiration.

GIT

Mouth – Disagreeable smell in the morning as if he had been eating eggs.

Stomach – Gastralgia, chronic gastric catarrah and gastritis.

- Burning and colicky pain in the stomach.
- *Relief* is obtained by *eating* (Petr., Chel., Anac.).
- Patients suffer from excessive canine hunger.
- *Aversion to sweets*, very thought produces nausea.
- Desire for chicken.
- Graphites has great value in *gastric and duodenal ulcer.* Base of the ulcer is hard, indurated with burning pains. Pains > eating.

Abdomen :

- Abdomen is greatly distended with flatus with rush of blood to the head. Abdomen is full from accumulation of old feaces and incarcerated flatus, such that they cannot tolerate anything tight about their waist.
- Dyspepsia of a chronic form mostly seen in old people and it is brought by over indulgence in strong spirituous liquors, debauchery, rich foods.

Diarrhoea :

Stools – Brown fluid, mixed with undigested substance and of an intolerable fetor.

Constipation – Person is habitually constipated.

Stools – Large hard, knotted joined together with mucus shreds.

Anus – As a result of such passage of large hardened feacal matter anus becomes fissured and varices make their appearance. Anus is extremely sore and the patient is very much annoyed when sitting.

MALE SEXUAL ORGANS

Graphites acts prominently in impotency.

Impotency – Want of sensation during coition with no discharge of semen. It also relieves hydrocele with herpetic eruptions.

FEMALE SEXUAL ORGANS

Menses :

Time – Delayed.

Quantity – Scanty.

Concomitants – Constipation, chilliness with co-existent eruptions.

- Violent itching in vulva before menses.

Graphites is indicated in *displacement of uterus* – anteflexion, anteversion with bearing down extending into hypogastrium.

Leucorrhoea :

Watery and profuse coming out in gushes day and night.

SKIN

- Graphites is very useful when eruptions or discharges have disappeared suddenly from any cause and grave chronic phenomenon have followed.
- Every injury suppurates.
- Skin is *dry parchment like – absolutely devoid of moisture. (Graphites pictures more of herpes; Petroleum of eczema).*
- Characteristic *glutinous eruptions* which are apt to occur on flexor surfaces in elbows, groins, popliteal fossa, ears, corners of mouth and in canthi.
- Tendency to *eczema* with glutinous sticky discharge.
- Eruptions on the skin oozing out a thick honey like fluid.
- *Itching* in the skin with or without eruptions – itching worse at night in warm bed.
- *Fissures* at the end of fingers, on nipple, labial commisures, at anus, vulva, between toes.
- *Recurrent herpes* upon all parts of the body especially about the anus. Burning in all parts of the body.
- *Old hard cicatrices soften up* and go away under its action especially those left by abscesses of mammae.
- *Lumps* in the breast of suspicious appearance go away under the action of Graphites.
- Erisipelas with burning and stinging pains. *Crusta lactea* – Crusts ooze a liquid fluid that lifts them up.
- Little pimples with or without pus appear and are apt to be worse at the menstrual periods.
- Induration and burning at the base of ulcers.
- Cancerous development in old cicatrices is a strong feature of this remedy.
- *Brittle nails* crumble on slightest excuse.

General Modalities :

Aggravation – SKIN AFFECTIONS – MORNING
NIGHT
COLD AIR
BEFORE AND
DURING MENSES.

Amelioration – OPEN AIR
GASTRIC COMPLAINTS > EATING.

Relations :

Complementry – Hepar, Lycopodium.

Follows well – Lyc, Puls

Obesity – Calc.

Skin affections – Sulph

Gushing leucorrhoea – Sep.

Similar to – Lyc, Puls in menstrual troubles.

Important Questions ?

Q.1. Give indications of Graphites in :

1) Skin [1975, 77, 85, 86, 91, 99]
2) Stomach [1977, 78, 82]
3) Mental Generals [1972]
4) Female Complaints [1973, 79, 88, 88, 90, 91]
5) Leucorrhoea [1974, 79, 81, 90]
6) Constitution [1973, 76]
7) Peptic Ulcer [1977]
8) Contipation [1982]
9) Drug Picture [1974, 92]

Q.2. Compare :

1) Constipation of Alumina/Graphites [1995]
2) Female of Helonias/Graphites [1995]

CONSTIPATION :

GRAPHITES	ALUMINA
• Dry hard knotty stools combined with mucus threads causing fissures in ani.	• Paresis of rectum – dry hard knotty stools or soft stools. Even a soft stool, like putty and sticking to the anus requires great straining.

FEMALE SYMPTOMS :

GRAPHITES	HELONIAS
• Complaints of *climacteric*. Sadness with tendency to obesity, habitual constipation, history of delayed menses, tendency to skin affections.	• Uterine tonic especially at *puberty, pregnancy* or after *labor*.

• Fat, chilly and costive women.	• Suits women worn out with hard work or those who are enervated by indolence and luxury and consequently have atony of pelvic organs and tissues.
• Erethism followed by chlorosis.	• Pain existing from back to uterus.
• Obesity due to malnutritum – labourers remedy.	• Conciousness of womb – sore, aching, tired feeling.
• Menses – delayed and scanty.	• Menses – Frequent, too profuse with dark red, coagulated and offensive flow.
• Leucorrhoea – watery and thin in gushes.	• Leucorrhoea – Dark, offensive and flows on every little exertion.
	• Abortion from slightest exertion.
	• Patient is better if she can keep her mind off herself.

41. HELLEBORUS NIGER

Hahnemann

Common Name – Christmas Rose.

Constitution – Weakly delicate, psoric children prone to brain troubles with serous effusions.

Temperament – Irritable.

Relation with heat and cold – Chilly patient.

Miasm – Psora in the background.

KEYNOTES

1) ***Weakly delicate, psoric children : prone to brain troubles; with serous effusions.***
2) *Young girls* at *puberty* become *melancholic,* woeful when menses fail to return or after typhoid.
3) ***'Blunt sensorium'***
   - Diminished power of mind – Patient does not comprehend anything and has a vacant and thoughtless look with staring eyes.
   - Sees or hears imperfectly.
   - Taste is absent.
   - Muscles do not obey will readily unless mind is strongly exerted.
   - Slow action of heart muscle with feeling of heaviness in the entire body.
   - Headache of stupefying character.
   - Face expressive of stupidity.
4) Face is pale, almost cold with small weak and imperceptible pulse.
5) Brain symptoms during dentition.
6) *Convulsions* with extreme *coldness* of body.
7) Acute *cerebro spinal meningitis* with exudation paralysis and cri-encephalique.
8) ***Hydrocephalus*** – Post scarlatinal or tubercular which develops readily – automatic motion of one arm and leg.
9) *Fever* generally corners on in afternoon from *4 – 8 P.M.*
10) Boring head into the pillow; rolling from side to side or beating head with hands.
11) *Diarrhoea* during acute hydrocephalus, dentition, pregnancy.

Stools – Contain jelly like mucus like frog spawn.

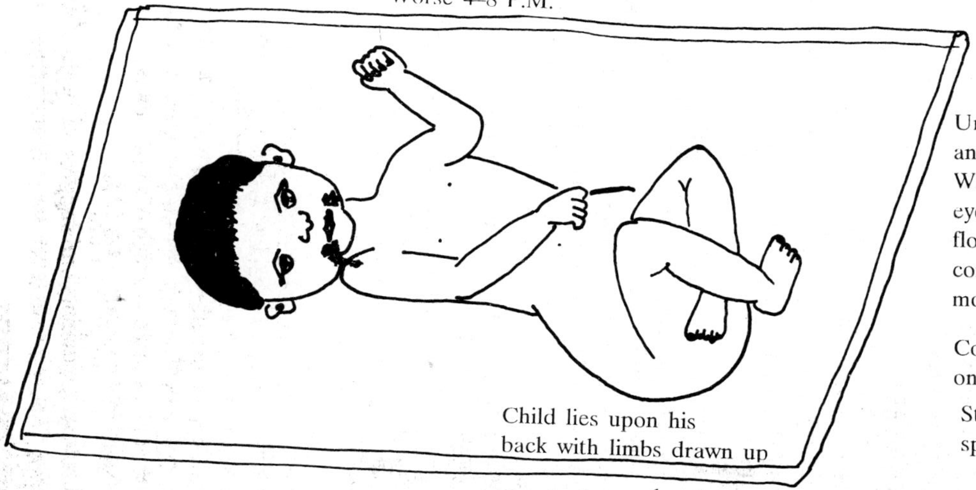

Brain troubles

Convulsions with coldness of body and intense thirst
Worse 4–8 P.M.

Urine is scanty and coffee ground
Wide open staring eyes with saliva flowing down the corners of the mouth

Constant motion of one arm and leg

Stool – frog spawn, jelly like

Child lies upon his back with limbs drawn up

Constantsomnolence

Blunt sensorium

HELLEBORUS NIGER

12) ***Dropsy*** of brain chest, abdomen after scarlatina, intermittent fever, debility, suppressed urine.

13) *Urine* – Dark, black, scanty, coffee ground sediment; suppressed in brain toubles and dropsy; albuminous. (Increase in urine is first sign of improvement).

Praticulars :

1) BRAIN TROUBLES
2) DIARRHOEA OR DYSENTRY
3) TYPHOID FEVER

BRAIN TROUBLES

Helleborus is indicated in acute cerebro spinal meningitis with or without exudation; post scarlatinal or tubercular hydrocephalus. Brain troubles during dentition.

Symptoms :

- *Blunt sensorium.*
- *Constant somnolence* out of which the child may be aroused with great difficulty.
- In case of a child there is *cri-encephalique*. Sudden screaming or crying due to sharp shooting pains.
- Child *bores its head into a pillow* and rolls the head from side to side.
- Automatic motion of one arm and one leg which occur at regular intervals.
- *Eyeballs are turned upwards* such that the cornea is scarcely visible.
- When offered a glass of water the child siezes the glass as if it were very *thirsty* – this is on account of intense thirst and nervousness.
- Water drunk decends audibly into the stomach.
- Child lies upon his back with limbs drawn up.
- *Convulsions* with *extreme coldness* of body.
- Bowels are usually constipated with jelly like *frog spawn stools*.
- *Urine is dark scanty* with *coffee ground* sediment (Increase in quantity of urine is a sign of improvement).
- Aggravation occurs – 4-8 P.M.

(Helleborus is indicated in dropsies of brain, chest and abdomen, post scarlatina nephritis with fever, debility and suppressed urine).

DIARRHOEA/DYSENTRY

Caused during dentititon, hydrocephalus, pregnancy.

Stools – White jelly like mucus, like frog spawn and involuntary.

TYPHOID FEVER

Symptoms :

- Blunt sensorium.
- Constant somnolence.
- Dark soot about the nostrils.
- Dark and yellow tongue with red edges.
- Horribly offensive breath.
- Pale and almost cold face.
- Faint and weak pulse.
- Scanty urine.
- Complete muscular relaxation.

Aggravation – 4-8 P.M.

General Modalities :

Aggravation – 4-8 P.M., UNCOVERING.

Important Question ?

Q.1. Give indication of Helleborus in :

a) Mental Symptoms [1973, 74, 87]
b) Typhoid Fever [1977, 79]
C) Meningitis [1975, 79, 81]

42. HEPAR SULPHURIS CALCAREA

Hahnemann

Common Name – Sulphate of Lime.

Symptoms of Hepar sulph can be summarized under the term *'H'*.

- Hypersensitive
- Hyperimpulsive
- Heavily sweating
- Hasty in speech and drinking
- Hoarseness in morning
- Hepar hastens suppuration and cure
- Amelioration by heat, hot fomentation and covering.

Constitution – For torpid, lymphatic constitutions; persons with light hair and complexion, slow to act, muscles soft and flabby stands half way between Sulphur and Calcarea.

Relation with head and cold – Very chilly patient.

Miasm – Powerful antipsoric but covers all the miasms.

Diathesis – Lymphatic and scrofulous.

KEYNOTES

1) ***Oversensitive*** both mentally and physically. *Hypersensitiveness of nervous system* – an inflamed part feels sore and bruised and cannot bear slightest touch. **Mind** – Slightest cause irritates him.
2) ***Slightest injury causes suppuration*** with oversensitiveness of parts. Unhealthy skin with thick and offensive discharge.
3) ***Cold air and cold applications increase sufferings.*** Cough, croup, bronchitis, consumption , exposure to least cold air.
4) *Splinter* sensation in *throat* (Arg nit, Nit acid,).
5) Hepar is indicated in *glandular* diseases in the stage of *suppuration* when inflammation has gone on to formation of pus.
6) *Hyper – sweating* day and night without any relief.
7) *Sour taste* in mouth. Longing for acids, alcohol, condiments.
8) *Atony – stools* passed with great difficulty even when soft.

   *Bladde*r – Atony of muscular coats hence urine passes slowly in drops.
9) *Marasmus* – Sour smelling child with weakness of digestion; diarrhoea with undigested white and sour stools.
10) *Syphilitic ulcers* – Formed after abuse of mercury. Ulcers are very sluggish, indolent and very slow to heal. Discharge is bloody, purulent and has an odor like that of cheese, extreme sensitiveness of border of ulceration.

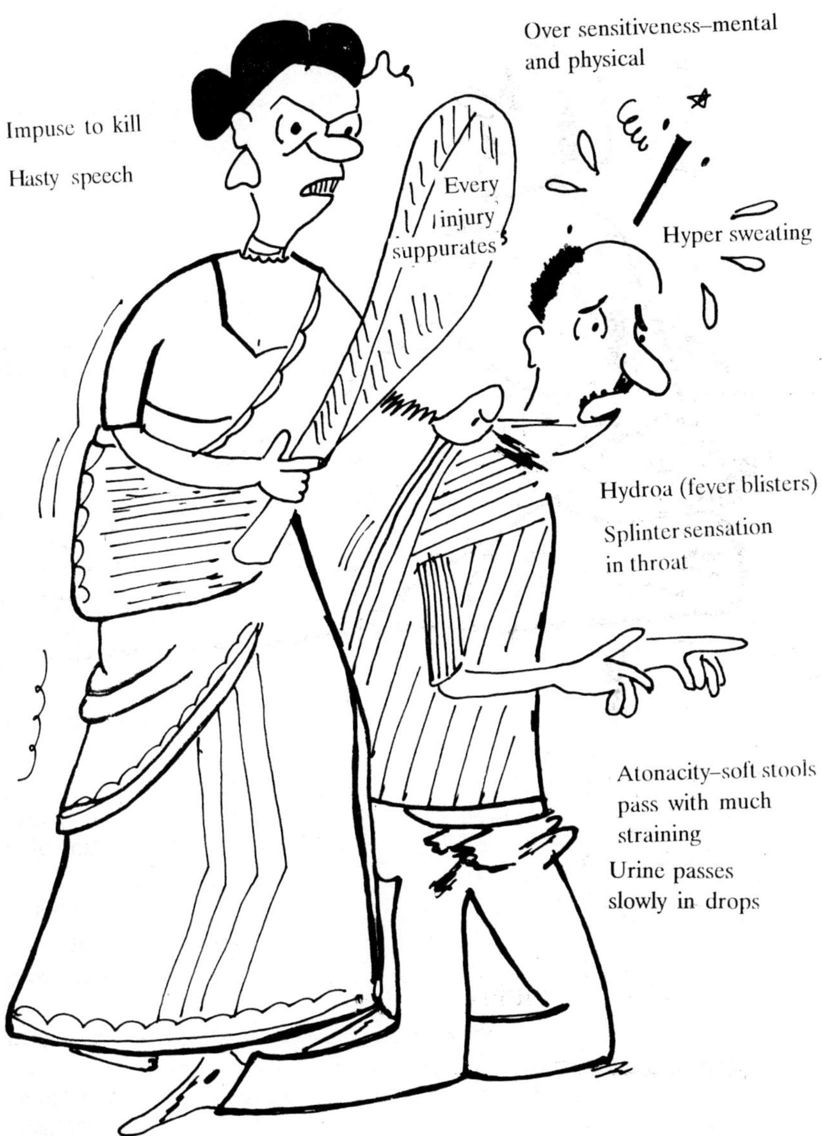

HEPAR SULPHURIS

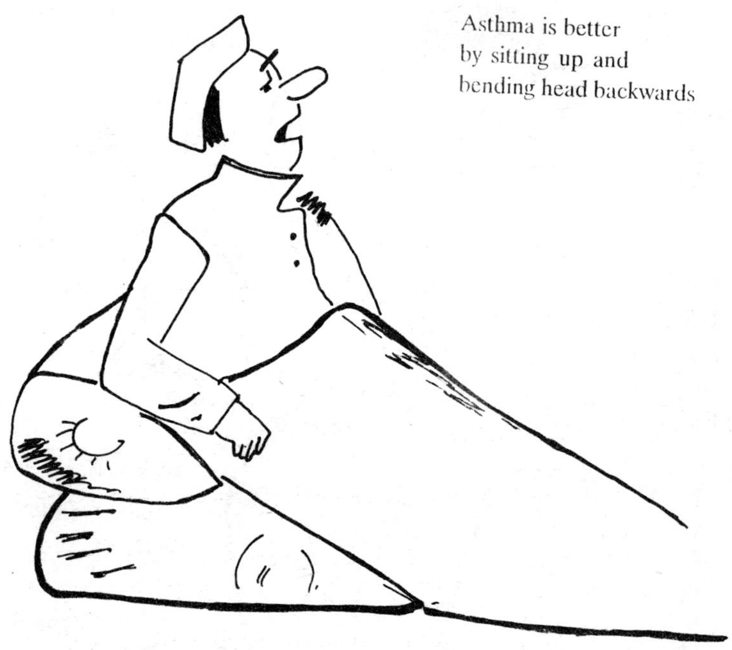

Asthma is better
by sitting up and
bending head backwards

HEPAR SULPHURIS

11) *Sad and low spirited* person with an impulse to kill the dearest person, to do violence, to burn, to commit suicide.

13) *Fever with icy coldness of body*, nettle rash during chill, fever blisters around the lips (*Hydroa*).

14) Modalities :

< Cold air, cold applications, dry cold weather, putting hand or foot outside bed.

> Damp wet weather, warmth.

Particulars :

1) MIND
2) EYE
3) EAR
4) RESPIRATORY SYSTEM
5) GIT
6) URINE
7) SKIN
8) MARASMUS
9) FEVER

MIND

- *Oversensitive and abusive*—Patients become angry, nasty vicious and abusive of others.
- *Intolerance to suffering*—Hepar patients abuse other people because of their own intolerance to pressures, stresses or suffering.
- *Destructive impulses*—A women may have a strong desire to kill her child, desire to set things on fire.
- *Suicidal thinking*—Hepar patients in later stages constantly start dwelling upon suicide.

EYE

- Inflammation of eye or eyelids with swollen and oedematous eyelids, suppurating styes.
- *Oversensitiveness*—Patient cannot bear to have his eye touched.
- Little pimples surround the inflamed eye <cold air, cold applications.
- Ulcers of cornea with granulations, bloody and offensive discharge from the eyes, profuse lachrymation, redness of cornea.

EAR

Inflammation of the external or internal auditory meatus with increased sensitiveness to touch. Inflammation of the middle ear with formation of an abscess; ear drum ruptures and there is bloody purulent thick, offensive discharge with tearing pains in the ears.

RESPIRATORY SYSTEM

Catarrah of the nose, throat, larynx, chest. Hepar is indicated in *later stages* when exudation becomes *purulent* especially in *chronic form*.

Cold – Hepar patient is subject to coryza especially in dry cold wind. Least exposure causes cold. Used in *advanced stages of cold.*

Character of discharge – Watery discharge followed by thick, yellow and offensive discharge.

< Dry cold air, uncovering.

> Damp wet weather.

Throat – Throat has a catarrhal condition with *oversensitiveness*. Pain as if *splinter* is lodged in the throat. *Hoarseness* is worse in *morning*.

< Cold dry air.

Cough – 'Moist cough'.

Character of cough – Hard barking cough with rattling of mucus.

Character of expectoration – Thick yellowish and offensive discharge.

Modalities :

< Least exposure, even uncovering arm or foot excites spells of coughing.

> Damp wet weather.

Concomitants – Much sweating with cough. Patient sweats whole night without relief. Weeps during or before cough.

Croup :

- Croup is accompanied with loose cough, wheezing and rattling of mucus.
- *Early morning aggravation.*
- Sensation as if *fish bone* were lodged in *throat*.
- As the croup travels downwards the larynx is attacked, then the bronchia and even the lungs. Breathing becomes rattling, anxious and wheezing with threatened suffocation.
- Respiration is so difficult that the child throws its head far back in order to straighten the air passages.
- So *sensitive* is the child to cold that least exposure – even uncovering an arm or a foot excites a spell of coughing.

Cough < Morning, cold dry air, uncovering.

> Wamth, damp wet weather.

Tonsillitis – Hepar is indicated in the stage of suppuration with throbbing pains. Hypersensitive to touch, swallowing liquids and solids, cold air.

Asthma – *Cause* – Suppression of skin eruption.

Character – Chronic asthma. Cough when any part of body is uncovered.

Modalities :

> Patient must bend head backward and sit up which gives him temporary relief, damp wet weather.

Pneumonia :

- Hepar is indicated in stage of resolution. It comes late in disease during resolution with pus formation.

T.B. (tuberculosis) :

Oversensitiveness. Hepar is indicated in harsh, croupy cough with production of tenacious mucus in chest < Morning.

According to Dr. Kent – "Deposits of tubercular character are often located in a place that can easily be suppurated out and the action of this remedy on them could establish suppuration at that vital area which could be very dangerous. Sometimes caseous deposits in lungs become encysted which then become safe. If they are touched by medicines hastening suppuration (Hepar, Silicea, Sulph) it would become extremely dangerous – hence great caution has to be administered while prescribing these remedies. An encysted tubercle might become an open abscess again after their administration."

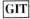

GIT

Mouth :

- Sour taste

Stomach :

- Desires acids, alcohol, condiments.
- Atonic form of dyspepsia.
- Hunger; gnawing empty feeling in stomach; eating any kind of food provokes indigestion.
- Can bear no pressure about epigastrium.
- Constant sensation of water rising into oesophagus.

Constipation :

- **Stools** – Soft but passed with great difficulty.

Diarrhoea :

Stools – Undigested, thin papescent, whitish sour smelling.

URINARY SYMPTOMS

Catarrah and atony of bladder.

Urine – Walls of the bladder become hardened so that it has no power to expel its contents and the urine passes in a slow stream or drops. Unfinished sensation even after passing urine. Copious mucopurulent discharges in urine.

SKIN

- All injuries tend to *suppurate* with *oversensitiveness* of parts.
- Patient is extremely sensitive to slightest touch.
- It is indicated in *eczema, crusta lactea, and intertrigo* which spread by means of new pimples appearing just beyond old parts.
- It produces moist eruptions in folds of skin.
- Eruption < Morning with itching.
- *Ulcers* bleed easily, are extremely sensitive and emit odor like old cheese.
- *Sweating* all night without relief.
- *Suppuration around foreign bodies* – A needle point may break off against the bone of the finger, or small portions of needle may exist where they cannot be found – Hepar will remove it. A little abscess will form and the little needle would be discharged.
- Syphilitic ulcers of bone, throat, soft palate, osseous portion of roof of mouth, chancre etc. Hepar is indicated where there is extreme tenderness, offensiveness, stick sensation. Bloody and purulent discharge with odor of old cheese. Extreme sensitiveness of border of ulcers.

(If Hepar is given in a *high potency* with throbbing, stabbing pains in the affected part and general rigor showing the *onset* of *inflammation* – it will *abort* the whole trouble. In other cases where *suppuration* is *necessary*, Hepar given in *low potency hastens* the process).

MARASMUS

Hepar is used in complaints of children with weakness of digestion. Diarrhoea with white and sour stools < morning. Child smells sour.

FEVER

- Paroxysm is generally around 6-7 P.M. Patient is susceptible to cold and feels extremely chilly and wants to be near a warm stove.
- Icy coldness of hands and feet.
- Nettle rash during chill.
- Hydroa – Fever blisters around mouth (Nat. mur.).

General Modalities :

Aggravation – COLD DRY WEATHER
UNCOVERING
TOUCHING AFFECTED PART
ABUSE OF MERCURY

Amelioration – DAMP WET WEATHER
WARMTH

Relations :

Complementy to – Calendula in injuries.

Antidotes – Bad affects of metals and mercury.

Remedies that follow well –

Nit acid, Abrotanum, Acon, Arum triph, Bell, Bry, Calend, Iod., Lach, Merc, Nux, Rhus, Sep., Spong, Sil, Sulph.

Antidotes – Acetic acid, Ars, Bell, Cham, Silicea.

Important Questions ?

Q.1. Give indications of Hepar in following :

1) Eye Affections [1974, 81]
2) Respiratory Symptoms [1966, 76, 86, 87, 96]
3) Suppuration [1993]
4) Skin [1973, 75, 76, 79, 81, 85, 90]
5) Tonsillitis [1975, 76, 76 S]
6) Characteristic Symptoms [1974, 76, 77]
7) Bone Affections [1970]
8) Otorrhoea [1987]
9) Injuries [1995]
10) Modalities [1972, 77]

Q.2. Compare Sulph and Hepar sulph – [1987]

Compare Silicea/Hepar sulph – skin symptoms

SULPHUR	HEPAR SULPH.
• SKIN – Dry itching and hot; very sensitive.	• SKIN – All injuries suppurate; oversensitive to touch.
• Redness of all orifices.	• Hypersweating
• Burning everywhere < warmth	• > Warmth
• Ragged philosopher	• Destructive impulse

SILICEA	HEPAR SULPH.
• < Warm Wet Weather	• > Warm Wet Weather
• Profuse head sweat at night. Intolerable offensive foot sweat.	• Sour profuse general sweats.
• Slow glandular suppuration that is also very slow to heal.	• Sudden and rapid gland suppuration.
	• Promotes and regulates suppuration.
	• Required at an eariler stage than Silicea.

43. HYOSCYAMUS NIGER

Hahnemann

Common Name – Henbane.

Constitution – Suited to weak, debilitated, nervous and hysterical people.

Temperament – Sanguine temperament.

Relation with heat and cold – Chilly patient.

Miasm – Psora in the background.

KEYNOTES

1) ***Extreme excitation of sensorium without any evidence of inflammation.*** Hyoscyamus occupies a place midway between Belladonna and Stramonium. It lacks the constant cerebral congestion of the former and the fierce rage and maniacal delirium of the latter.

   Hyos – Nervous irritation without congestion.

   Bell – Congestion/inflammation of brain.

   Stram – Congestion with more cerebral excitement and *violence*.

   The patient has strange notions arising from abnormal impulses.

2) In Mania – the person is *weak and debilitated* and is preoccupied with an internal state sitting and *muttering to himself.*

   - ***Jealousy and suspicion*** – Paranoid state when the person is convinced that the people are trying to poison him. He refuses food and drink in fear of poison. Jealousy motivates the behaviour including the violent outbursts.
   - ***Obsessive character*** – Person imagines a queer kind of paper on the wall and he keeps imagining strange things about the figures. He talks of imaginary things. Illusion of vermin, rats, mice in the room. Picks up bed clothes; makes no complaints.
   - ***Erotic mania*** – The person becomes shameless and exposes his/her genitals to anyone, plays with his genitals ceaselessly. Increased sexual desire and behaviour.
   - ***Unconscious*** – The unconscious which was previously governed by obsessive and paranoid ideation finally erupts – unconscious affects the lower limb, functions of defeacation and urination – involuntary loss of stool and urine.

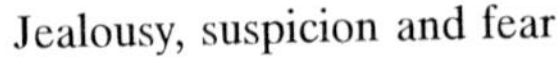
Jealousy, suspicion and fear

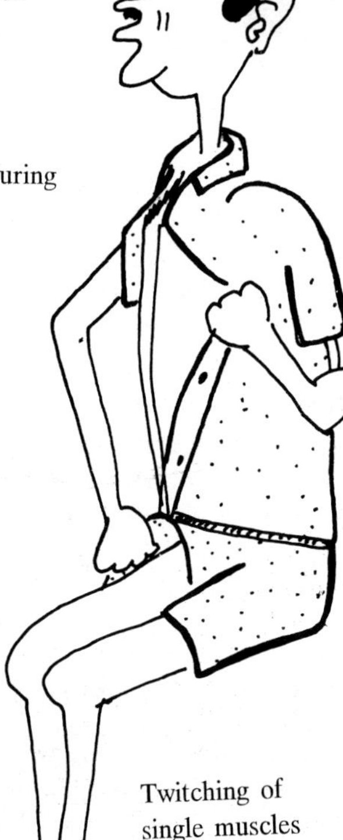
I am sure
my wife wants
to kill me
Sleeplessness in
irritable and nervous
persons
Dry hacking cough
better by sitting
Sordes on teeth
with dry and
red tongue
Dark red face
with debility during
fever
Erotic mania–
desire to uncover
Incontinence of
stool and urine
Twitching of
single muscles

HYOSCYAMUS NIGER

- In acute delerium there is ***twitching of every muscle*** from eyes to the toes.

3) *Convulsions of children* from fright or irritation of intestinal worms; during labor, during puerperal state.
4) *Incontinence after labor* – No desire to urinate in lying in women.
5) *Intense sleeplessness* of irritable excitable persons from business embarrasment.
6) *Cough* – Dry, nocturnal and spasmodic < Lying down, eating, drinking, night.
> Sitting up (Dros. Phos.)
7) In *later stages of typhoid* – Hyoscyamus is indicated when the stupor becomes more marked, dry and cracked tongue, difficult speech, sordes on teeth, involuntary stool and urine and drooping of lower jaw.

Particulars :

1) DELIRIUM
2) CONVUISIONS
3) TYPHOID

DELIRIUM

Increased cerebral activity of non-inflammatory type. Delirium occurs in the following stages –

The person is *not active, energetic* and violent. He is more pre-occupied with internal state, sitting and muttering to himself, or talking to absent or dead people. This is generally seen in elderly senile people muttering to themselves, picking at their clothes, oblivious to surroundings.

Jealousy and suspicion run through the sickness. Suspicion that his wife is going to poison him. Imagines that his wife is not faithful etc. *Loquacity* due to excessive anemation. Visualises a *queer kind of paper* on the wall and he lies and looks at it and if possible tries to turn the figures into rows. Imagines vermin, rats, cats, mice etc. He is in alternate states – one minute he raves and another he scolds in delirium. Finally he passes into *profound stupor* with complete unconciousness – even in this state when he realises nothing he makes passive motions, mutters, talks to himself and once in a while utters a shrill scream if he is aroused. He picks at his bed clothes. Both urine and stool are passed involuntarily. Pulse is irregular without good volume. Patients are silly and laugh in a flippant manner.

- *Fear of water*/running water (Stram, Bell, Hyos.).
- *Erotic mania* – Hyoscyamus has such sensitive nerves all over his body in the skin that he cannot bear the clothing to touch

the skin and he takes it off. This occurs in insanity and delirium and he has no idea that he is exposing his body. There is another phase running through the insanity which is salacity or nymphomania – the person exposes his/her genitals to the view of everybody coming in the room.

Violent sexual excitement and nymphomania. He/she is violent, strikes and bites, sings amorous songs, lies in bed naked. (Complaints come on from disappointed love, fear etc. – it drives her insane and she may take on any of these phases.

(Hyos. is used extensively in insane assylums for acute non – inflammatory mania. Eating is at once followed by exaggeration of symptoms.)

CONVULSIONS

Hyos. is useful in convulsions, hysteria and mania. Convulsions begin with twitchings of mouth, face and especially of muscles about the eyes. Spasms are clonic in nature (Bell – convulsions are tonic). Movements are mostly angular, face is dusk red and bloated. Angular motion is *provoked by eating*. (It is used commonly in convulsions of children especially after fright and from intestinal worms.) It is also used in epilepsy, when before the attack the patient complains of vertigo, sparks before the eyes and ringing noise in ears. The convulsions are so violent that it seems that the joint and spine will be broken into pieces. After an attack the patient falls into deep sleep with continuous fever for several hours.

TYPHOID FEVER

Hyoscyamus is indicated in later stages of typhoid (Bell earlier stages) when *stupor* is more marked.

- *Brain is active but wanders* – He labours under distinct hallucinations and he is centered in a desire to escape from the room. He is excessively loquacious and laughs, sings, swears and prays in same breath.
- Patient picks at the bed clothes or his fingers in a *somnolent* sort of way and occasionally reaches out as if grasping something in air.
- Mouth remains open and lower jaw hangs down.
- Face is dusky red and hot.
- Tongue is red and dry with difficult speech.
- Sordes on teeth with involuntary stool and urine and drooping of lower jaw.
- Muscles all over the body twitch intermittently.
- He is disturbed with dry nocturnal cough which prevents sleep.
- Sphincter muscles of both anus and bladder are paralysed with involuntary passage of stool and urine.

General Modalities :

Aggravation – LYING DOWN, NIGHT, EATING MENTAL AFFECTIONS, DURING MENSES, JEALOUSY.

Amelioration – COUGH IS RELIEVED BY SITTING UP.

Relations :

Remedies that follow well – Bell, Puls, Stram.

Antidotes – Acet acid, Citric acid, Bell, Chin, Stram.

Important Questions ?

Q.1. Give indications of Hysocyamus in :
1) Mental symptoms [1974, 78, 77, 81, 90, 91, 93]
2) Typhoid [1971, 77]
3) Cough [1974, 77, 79, 82]
4) Meningitis [1979]

Q.2. Explain the 'trio of delirium' with their keynote symptoms. [1997]

BELLADONNA	STRAMONIUM	HYOSCYAMUS
• Congestion – Constant cerebral congestion.	• Congestion with violence	• Non inflammatory cerebral excitement
• *Light and company* – Desires.	• Desires	• Aversion
• *Spasms* – Tonic	• Tonic	• Clonic
• *Choreic movements* – Tonic	• Gyratory	• Angular < Eating.
• *Fever face* – 'High grade fever with red and hot with throbbing of carotids.	• Red face and cold body	• Low grade fever. Dusky red
• *Mania* – Violent.	• Violent and religeous	• Lascivious. Before the fit there is vertigo, ringing in the ears.
• *Epilepsy (during)* – Spasms of larynx and clutching of throat during fit.	• Risus sardonicus and quick thrustings of head to right.	• Sparks before the eyes, gnawing hunger; during the fit – purple face, eyes projecting, shrieks, grinding teeth, enuresis, followed by sopor and snoring.

44. IGNATIA AMARA

Hahnemann

Common Name – St. Ignatius Bean.

Ignatia is a womens remedy, is a Feminine of the masculine Nux vomica. Both are chemically and botanically similar and are *spinal* remedies. Under Nux – over excitability is exhibited by anger and vehemence. In Ignatia by melancholy and tendency to weeping. *Ignatia is acute of Natrum mur* and hence mostly used in acute or recent cases. When Ignatia fails to remove the symptoms Nat-mur frequently comes in to complete the cure.

Dr. Clarke says – Ignatia is applicable and curative in sudden and acute attacks. It is best to administer the dose in the *morning* if there is no occasion for hurry.

Constituion – Suited to women of sensitive, easily excitable nature with dark hair, dark skin but mild disposition, quick to percieve and rapid execution. Ignatia is not suitable in persons in whom anger, eagerness and violence is predominant. It is suitable in nervous women who are burdened with grief particularly when they dwell upon their troubles in secret.

Temperament – Nervous.

Relation to heat and cold – Remedy of paradoxicalities and hence changes with the situation.

Miasm – Psora in the background.

KEYNOTES

1) Ignatia is a great remedy of ***moods and contradictions of mental stress and strain*** connected with shock, bereavement, disappointment or distress.

- Ignatia patients keep their annoyance to themselves – they have no tendency to break out violenty – *silent grieving.*
- *Intelligent and sensitive* patient with a forbearing nature.
- Ignatia is used for *recent grief* – Suppressed or deep grief with *long drawn sighs*. (Nat. mur generally finishes up the case that Ign. starts).
- Thinks she has neglected her duty.
- *Changeable mood* – the patient is at one time full of merriment and joy, to be followed suddenly with the other extreme of melancholy, sadness and tears – these states of mind rapidly alternate.
- *Indifference* during menses.

- Ignatia at a point may break down and become *hysterical*—she goes *sighing*, cries so much that she goes into a spasm, disturbance in hormonal system—growing hair etc, paroxysms of cough without any time to breathe etc.
- *Easily frightened.*

2) ***Remedy of contradictory symptoms/paradoxicalities***. In Ignatia symptoms that are most *unnatural and unexpected* are found.
    - An inflamed part with heat, redness and throbbing but without pain.
    - Inflamed throat is better by swallowing of solids.
    - Head is better by lying on the painful side.
    - Red face with thirst during chill.
    - Empty feeling in the stomach not better by eating.
    - Cough getting worse on more coughing.
    - Noise in ears getting better by noise.
    - Piles feeling better by walking.
    - Prolapsus ani worse during soft stools.
3) Ignatia is a *'spinal remedy'*—Its tendency to produce increased excitability renders it useful in *spasms* of hysterical origin or in delicate women who are not hysterical; in children spasms brought on by fright, after punishment, teething, worms etc.
4) *Oversensitive to pain* (Acon, Cham, Coff.).
5) *Aversion to tobacco*.
6) Fever (Intermittent)—

Contradictory Symptoms :

a) Red face during chill
b) Chill with thirst
c) Chill better by external heat.
d) Heat without thirst <covering.

7) Ignatia is an excellent remedy for *anal* troubles with *pains shooting upwards into the rectum*.

Particulars :

1) MIND
2) CHOREA
3) TOOTHACHE
4) HEADACHE
5) GIT
6) FEVER
7) FEMALE SYMPTOMS

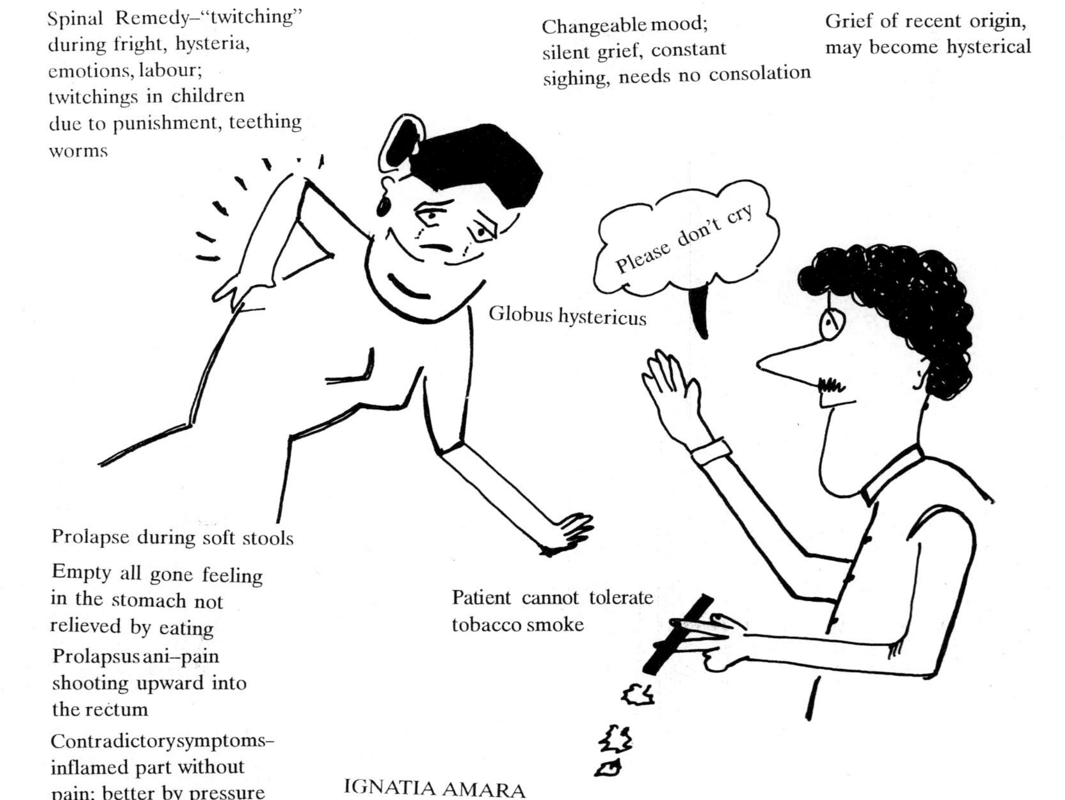

Spinal Remedy–"twitching" during fright, hysteria, emotions, labour; twitchings in children due to punishment, teething worms
Changeable mood; silent grief, constant sighing, needs no consolation
Grief of recent origin, may become hysterical
Please don't cry
Globus hystericus
Prolapse during soft stools
Empty all gone feeling in the stomach not relieved by eating
Prolapsus ani–pain shooting upward into the rectum
Contradictory symptoms–inflamed part without pain; better by pressure
Patient cannot tolerate tobacco smoke

IGNATIA AMARA

MIND

- *Bad affects of grief of recent origin* (for chronic and long lasting affects – Nat. mur, Acid phos.)
- Grief caused due to disappointed love, controversy at home, losing someone etc.
- *Nervous and sensitive* person – Too sensitive to be scolded or punished – develop spasms.
- *Silent grief* – The patient does not share her problems with anyone. She keeps sobbing all alone in a room. (Puls – women is tearful and melancholic like Ignatia but she makes her grief known to everybody. She seeks sympathy and consolation).
- Ignatia *does not seek consolation.* (Hell, Nat mur. Lil tig, Sil).
- *Changeable mood* – Joy changes into sorrow, laughing into weeping, mental calm into furious rage.
- The patient does most unaccountable and most *unexpected things* – have no rule to work, no philosophy, no judgement – patient feels better by lying on the painful side etc.
- She has headaches, trembles, is excited, weeps, is sleepless, unable to control herself.
- Ignatia patient is not the one that is sluggish or idiotic but the one that has been brought into such a state from *overdoing, overexcitement,* becoming tired.
- Sighs much with weakness in pit of the stomach.

CHOREA

Ignatia is a *nervous remedy* – it acts on the spine affecting both the nervous and motor nerves. *Twitchings* arising from grief, fright, punishments of children, worms. Face is distorted, convulsed, pale and sickly. Shock seems to produce a cramp in the whole system – may affect the vagus nerve.

Hysteria :

- Unable to breathe properly.
- Unlimited crying such that the whole system goes into a spasm.
- Paroxysm of cough with face turning blue and no time to breathe.
- Globus Hystericus – sensation of lump in the throat.
- Cannot digest simplest food but feels better with heavy food.
- Affects hormonal system with growing hair etc.
- Sudden momentary paralysis.
- Torticollis.

TOOTHACHE

Pain is worse between than during the acts of eating <Smoking tobacco, lying down.

HEADACHE

Cause – Grief, sorrow, tobacco, coffee, bad news, suppressed emotions.

Location – pain over a small spot that can be covered with the tip of a finger.

Sensation – As if nail were sticking into the side of the temple, better by lying on it. Changeability of pain – sometimes it comes gradually and abates suddenly, at other times it comes on suddenly and goes similarly.

Relief – Heat, pressure on painful side, profuse flow of colourless urine.

Worse – Cold, turning head suddenly, stooping, changing position, noise, light.

GIT

Mouth – Bitter or sour taste in the mouth with copious salivation.

Stomach – Gastralgia.

- Patient has *aversion* to fruits, tobacco and warm foods.
- Empty all gone feeling in the stomach not relieved by eating.
- Vomits everything taken in.
- Hysterical stomach – Gentle/simple food disagrees; feels better with heavy or raw food.

Abdomen – Excess of flatulence which leads to protrusions on various parts of the abdominal wall. Bowels are inclined to be loose with a tendency towards heamorrhoidal knobs in rectum. Heamorrhoids < soft stools.

Constipation :

Cause – Constriction of rectum.

Stools – Hard or soft stool requires severe straining with certain amount of procidentia recti.

Sensation – Pressure as if a sharp instrument from within outward. In consequence of this straining, he becomes an easy victim to heamorrhoids.

Prolapse Of Rectum :

Cause – Straining at stool, stooping, lifting.

Symptoms – Sharp pains shooting upwards into the rectum. Prolapse becomes worse when stool is soft. (Ignatia is an important remedy for anal and rectal complaints).

Itching and creeping at the anus as from *'ascarides'* or *'threadworms'* (Ignatia is an excellent remedy).

FEVER

Ignatia is an excellent remedy for fever. Symptoms are paradoxical –

1. Thirst during chill.

2. Chill relieved by external heat.

3. Heat aggravated by external covering.

4. Red face during chill.

There are the four legs to the stool on which Ignatia can be prescribed with confidence.

FEMALE

Dysmenorrhoea – 'Hysterical symptoms' during menses – labor like pains during menses with great deal of bearing down in the hypogastric region. There is constant *sighing* and sobbing with a *faint* feeling in the stomach.

General Modalities :

Aggravation – TOBACCO, BRANDY, CONTACT MOTION, MENTAL EMOTIONS GRIEF, COFFEE, STRONG ODOURS.

Amelioration – WARMTH, HARD PRESSURE, SWALLOWING, WALKING.

Relations :

Complements – Natrum mur.

Remedies that follow well – Phos. Ac, Ars, Bell, Calc, Chin, Cocc., Lyc, Puls, Rhus, Sep, Sil, Sulph.

Inimicals – Coff, Nux, Tabac.

Antidotes – Acetic acid, Arn, Cocc, Cham., Puls.

Important Questions ?

Q.1. Natrum mur is chronic of Ignatia. Justify ? [1997]

Q.2. Describe why Ignatia and Nux vom are called woman's and man's remedy – [1987]

Q.3. Justify Ignatia as the 'Remedy of great contradiction'. What are its mental symptoms ? What relation has it got with Nat. mur. – [1981]

Q.4. Give indications of Ignatia in :

a) Heamorrhoids [1986, 70]

b) Hysteria/Mental symptoms [1973, 74, 82, 83, 88, 89, 91]

c) Intermittent fever [1975, 82]

d) Rectal Prolapse [1976]

e) Labor [1977]

f) Colic [1979]

g) Drug Picture [1975, 74, 77, 79, 83, 93]

h) Characteristic symptoms [1969]

Q.5. Compare Ignatia/Pulsatilla in Hysteria. [1987 S, 88]

PULSATILLA	IGNATIA
• Ladies usually fair and beautiful looking but inclined to be fleshy with fine hair and blue eyes, soft and lax muscles, aneamic and chlorotic with pale face at puberty.	• Dark looking lady with dark hair and complexion. Grief may even bring on troubles on the physical plane – choreas, torticollis, headache, hysteria.
• Seeks sympathy, tearful, sad and melancholic. Makes her grief known to everyone.	• Sensitive and excited. Quick in perception. Solitary patient. Reserved person, does not seek sympathy. Dwell upon their troubles in secret.
• Craves consolation.	• Consolation aggravates troubles.
• Changeability is marked.	• Remedy of contradiction. Sighing with hysteria.
• Stomach complaints aggravated after fatty food.	• Stomach is better by fatty or heavy food.
• Silicea is chronic of Pulsatilla.	• Nat. mur is chronic of Ignatia.

45. IPECACUANHA

Hahnemann

Common Name – Ipecac.

Constitution – Adapted to cases where gastric symptoms predominate. Pale face with blue rings around the eyes.

Relation with heat and cold – Chilly patient.

Temperament – Irritable temperament.

Miasm – Psora in the background.

Diathesis – Heamorrhagic diathesis.

KEYNOTES

1) *Persistent* ***'nausea'*** *which nothing relieves* – not even vomiting. (Active principle emetin gives to the drug its power of producing vomiting).
2) Ipecac affects the vomiting centre in medulla which may account for a *clean tongue* and *profuse salivation*.
3) ***Heamorrhage*** from all natural orifices of the body – mouth, nose, lungs, bowels, uterus, bladder etc. *Bright red flow* of blood with heavy breathing and nausea. Deathly pale face with blue margins about the eyes.
4) Chief action is centered around the pneumogastric nerve producing *spasmodic irritation* in *chest* and *stomach*.
5) Great accumulation of mucus in the respiratory tract causing danger of suffocation and exciting a *spasmodic, dry cough with vomiting. Difficult* and *scanty expectoration* with epistaxis. (Ipec is used in *early* stages while *Ant. tart* is used in *later* stages).
6) Violent degree of dyspnoea, great weight and anxiety about the precordia.
7) In *acute gastritis caused by rich food* (pastry, pork, fruits, ice, creams etc) with nausea and vomiting (Puls, Ars alb, Ant crud).
8) Fermented or grass green stools with colic and nausea.
9) ***Thirstlessness*** is marked with all complaints.
10) Pains as if bones are all torn to pieces.
11) Ipec. is useful in intermittent fevers with persistent nausea, backache and occipital headache. Short chill stage with thirstlessness : long heat stage with thirst.

Aggravation – Warm room, external heat.

Amelioration – Open air.

Blue margins around
the eyes with
pale face
Clean tongue

Profuse bright red
heamorrhagesfrom
natural orifices
especially the uterus

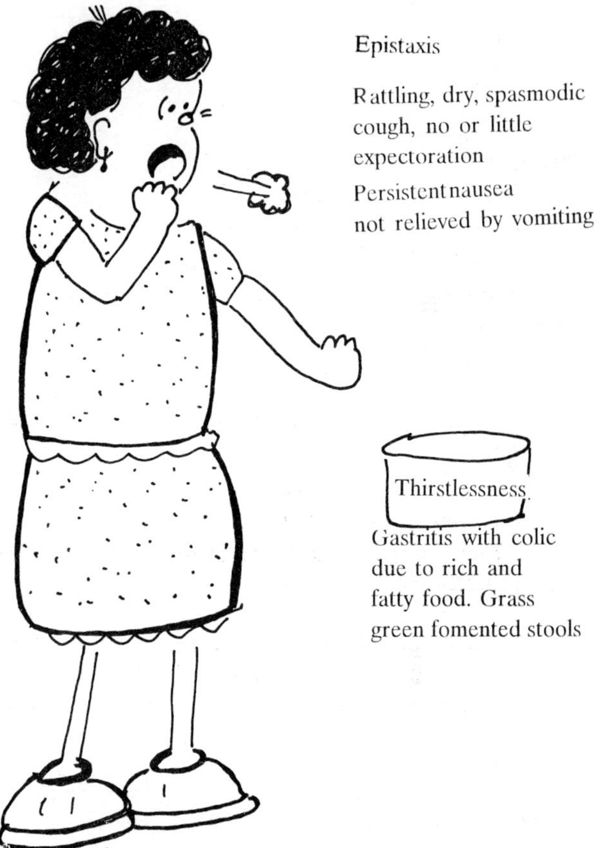

IPECACUANHA

(Ipec. is used in intermittents after abuse of Quinine).

Particulars :

1) MIND
2) HEADACHE
3) HEAMORRHAGE
4) RESPIRATORY SYSTEM
5) GIT
6) INTERMITTENT FEVER

MIND

Irritable patients full of desires but do not know what they want. Children scream continuously. As an adult he is irritable, morose, holding everything in contempt.

HEADACHE

Headache of rheumatic origin.

Sensation – Bruised or crushed feeling of the head seeming to go down the root of the tongue. Headache is accompanied by constant nausea not relieved by vomiting.

Modalites – Aggravation – Warm room.

Amelioration – Open air.

Concomitant – face is pale with blue rings around the eyes.

HEAMORRHAGE

Ipecac is a great heamorrhagic remedy. Heamorrhage from almost every organ – lungs, bowels, uterus, bladder etc.

Character of blood – Profuse, bright red foamy blood associated with nausea, thirstlessness and clean tongue.

*Conc*omitants – Face is deathly pale with blue margins about the sunken eyes. Mentally irritable and taciturn.

Uterus – Gushing flow of bright red blood with a fainting feeling.

Menses – Character of blood – Bright red and copious flow with fainting sensation. Flow may continue for many days with weakness. (Ipec. would help to cure and end the menstural flow normally).

Vomiting – Vomiting clots of blood in connection with ulceration. Ipecac controls the heamorrhage when symptoms agree.

Kidneys – Urine is extremely red with blood which settles to the bottom of the vessel. Every attack of pain in the kidneys is attended with that condition of urine.

RESPIRATORY SYSTEM

The inflammation that comes upon the mucous membrane in Ipecac is violent. The inflammation comes on suddenly and the mucous membranes inflame so rapidly that the parts become purple and bleeding seems to be the only natural relief.

Coryza :

Stuffed feeling in the nose with loss of smell, epistaxis and nausea. Colds often begin in the nose and spread to the chest.

Bronchitis :

Symptoms – Colds have a tendency to settle down in the chest.

- Great accumulation of mucus which loads up the air cells and bronchi until there seems to be a danger of suffocation.
- Violent dyspnoea with suffocation and great weight about the precordia.
- *Dry, spasmodic and rattling cough* caused by accumulation of mucus in the bronchi.
- Persistent *nausea* with *vomiting* following an attack of cough.

Character of expectoration – Difficult and scanty discharge.

Concomitant – Pale face with sunken eyes. Constant nausea with thirstlessness and clean tongue.

Whooping Cough :

- Spasmodic cough caused by tickling in larynx.
- Cough is so suffocating that the child turns, blue, faint and stiff.
- Paroxysm may be so strong so as to bring about an attack of *epistaxis* as well as bleeding from mouth.
- *Nausea and vomiting* usually follow an attack of coughing.
- *Red face, thirstlessness, violent whooping* with convulsions and vomiting of all that he eats.

Asthma :

Cause – Damp weather, sudden changes in weather, cold air, warm moist weather.

Symptoms – Sensation of constriction in the chest worse from least motion. Dyspnoea with wheezing, great weight and anxiety about the precordia.

Character of cough – Spasmodic cough with rattling of mucus and no expectoration. Relief from sitting up.

Pneumonia :

Chest loaded with mucus, rapid and wheezing respiration, surface blue with pale face.

GIT

Gastritis :

Cause – Indulgence in rich food – pastry, pork, fruits, candy, ice-cream etc.

Symptoms – Constant nausea. Vomits just after eating. Vomiting of foods and drinks taken in followed by bile, mucus with morning sickness. Clean tongue, with thirstlessness and distress in stomach. Loss of appetite with disgust for food, coldness of extremities, imperceptible pulse, profuse discharges of cold and clamy sweat. *Coli*c of gripping character about the umblicus.

Stools – Grass green fermented stools. Diarrhoea may be associated with tenesmus indicating catarrah of the lining of membrane of bowels.

Dysentry :

Character of stools – Patient is compelled to sit almost constantly upon the stool and passes little slime or a little bright red blood.

Conc. – Awful tenesmus with smarting, burning and constant nausea. While straining at stool the pain is so great that nausea comes on and he vomits bile.

Cholera Infantum :

Symptoms :

- Nausea and vomiting.
- Child immediately vomits all what he eats and drinks.
- Child passes copious green, fermented stools like molasses.
- Pallor of the face with blue rings about the eyes and fontanelles remain open showing defective nutrition with frequent attacks of nose bleed.
- Frequent long drawn sighs, a distressed feeling in the abdomen with a constant gripping colic.

INTERMITTENT FEVER

Persistant Nausea

Chill stage – Short; patient is thirstless, has a clean tongue with redness of one cheek and paleness of other > Warm room, external heat
< Open air.

Heat stage – Long lasting with thirst, nausea and vomiting. Oppression of breathing with dry hacking cough.

Sweat – Patient is worse at this stage and better after it. Sour sweat with turbid urine. (Ipec. is useful in those cases of Malarial fevers which have been tempered with by mal administration of clinic.)

Modalities :

Aggravation – WINTERS
DRY WEATHER
WARM MOIST WEATHER
SLIGHTEST MOTION

Relations :

Complementry – Cuprum.

Followed well by – *Ars.* in influenza, chills, croup, debility, cholera, infantum.

Ant. Tart – foreign bodies in larynx.

Similar to – Puls, Ant crud, in Gastric troubles.

Important Questions ?

Q.1. Give indication of Ipecac in the following :

1) Cough [1973, 74, 78, 79]
2) Asthma [1995]
3) Respiratory symptoms [1986]
4) Cholera [1993]
5) Diarrhoea and vomiting [1973, 79, 82]
6) Nausea [1974]
7) Menstrual Symptoms [1973]
8) Heamorrhagic symptoms [1975, 82]
9) Dysentry [1977]
11) Drug Picture [1983]

Q.2. Compare Ant tart/Ipec. in respiratory symptoms. [1983, 88, 90, 91]
Camphor/Ipec. in Cholera [1996]
Bromium/Ipec in Asthma [1995]
Drosera/Rumex/Bell./Phos/Ipec in cough [1973]

RESPIRATORY SYMPTOMS

IPECAC	ANT. TART.
• Symptoms come on rapidly.	• Symptoms come on slowly.
• Stage of irritation.	• Stage of relaxation.
• Difficult expectoration, still the patient manages to get rid of a portion of accumulated phlegm either by means of coughing or vomiting.	• Patient fails in every attempt to overthrow the phlegm.
• Due to suffocation the child turns blue, pale and stiff.	• Great exhaustion, deathly pallor of face, sooty nostrils.

CHOLERA

CAMPHOR	IPECAC
• Scanty discharges.	• Profuse discharges with intense nausea, vomiting and tendency to heamorrhage.
• Intense prostration, bluish, icy cold face, cold body, weak and squeakly.	• Vomits all what he eats.
• Coldness, dryness and blueness are marked.	• Grass green like fermented stools with colic.
• Relief by warmth.	• Aggravation by warmth. Better in open air.

ASTHMA

BROMIUM	IPECAC
• Much rattling of mucus during cough.	• Dry spasmodic cough that may end in vomiting with persistent nausea.
• Dyspnoea – patient cannot inspire deep enough.	• Suffocation with dyspnoea great weight and anxiety in precordia.
• Stony hardness of glands	• Difficult and scanty expectoration.
• No expectoration	
• **Aggravation** – Hot weather.	• **Aggravation** – Warm moist weather.

COUGH

DROSERA	RUMEX	BELL.	PHOS.	IPEC.
• Crawling sensation in larynx as from feather.	• Dry cough from tickling in supra – sternal fossa	• Used in first stage when cough comes on suddenly.	• Cough from irritation in trachea.	• Tickling sensation in the larynx with dry spasmodic cough.

● Nocturnal hoarse barking cough with vomiting of water, mucus, bleeding from nose and mouth. Face turns purple with copious sweat. No-expectoration	● Soreness behind the sternum with tough mucus in the larynx which cannot be hawked up.	● Dry cough with intense soreness, tenderness and fever	● Dry cough followed by constriction across the upper part of the chest. Desires cold things	● Rattling caused by accumulation of mucus in bronchi with scanty expectoration
● < Lying down, midnight	● <Cold air >deep inspiration, warmth	● <Lying down, sensitive to draft of air. >Covering, head high	● <Cold air >Warmth	● Persistent nausea not relieved by vomiting <Warmth, moist Air >Open air

46. KALI BICHROMICUM

Drysdale

Common Name – Potassium Bichromate.

Constitution – Fat, light haired persons or children disposed to catarrhal, croupy, scrofulous and syphilitic affections.

Relation with heat and cold – *Chilly* patient.

Miasm – Prominence of syphilitic miasm (Tendency to formation of syphilitic ulcers).

Diathesis – Rheumatic Diathesis.

KEYNOTES

1) ***Rheumatic pains alternate with catarrhal symptoms.***
2) ***Spottiness*** – Sharp stitching pains in small spots that can be covered with the tip of a finger.
3) ***Wandering pains*** – Pains wander from one place to another.
4) *Pains appear and disappear rapidly*. Burning is marked with pains.
5) Affections of mucous membranes with discharge of *tough, stringy, adherent mucus* that can be drawn into long strings.
6) ***Yellowness*** of discharges is marked – yellow discharge, yellow vomit, yellow sputum etc. Thus one spots Kali bich by its ***spottiness, stringiness and yellowness***.
7) *Syphilitic or non syphilitic ulcerations* – Ulcers occur in mucous membranes – *round, deep, punched out with regular edges* and are very red.
8) *Chronic ozeana* – Pressing pain in the root of the nose – *discharge of 'clinkers' plugs*.
9) *Blinding headache* caused by suppressed catarrhal affections with aversion to light and noise.
   (Blinding headache – Iris, Nat mur, Psor : Caust – Blinding does not diminish with pain: Sil – Blinding after headache.)
10) *Yellow coating at base of tongue*, dry smooth, glazed and cracked tongue during dysentry.
11) Kali bich is one of the best remedies for chronic affects of indulgence in *'beer'*.
12) Kali bich caused violent inflammation of mucous membrane with much redness and swelling and produces an excessive amount of mucous rapidly turned into fibrinous exudate tending to formation of false membrane – hence it is useful in *'croup with tough stringy discharges'*.

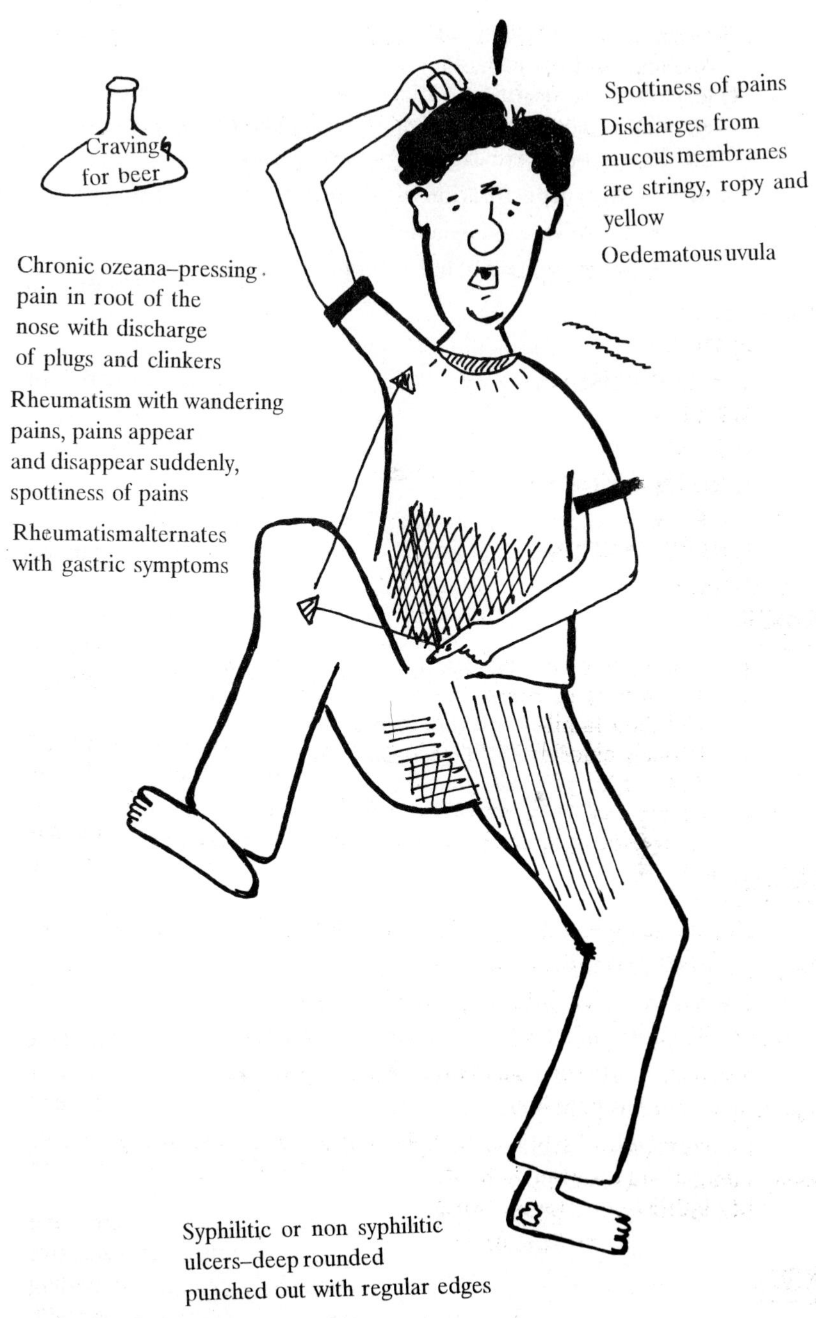
Craving
for beer
Spottiness of pains
Discharges from
mucous membranes
are stringy, ropy and
yellow
Oedematous uvula
Chronic ozeana–pressing
pain in root of the
nose with discharge
of plugs and clinkers
Rheumatism with wandering
pains, pains appear
and disappear suddenly,
spottiness of pains
Rheumatismalternates
with gastric symptoms
Syphilitic or non syphilitic
ulcers–deep rounded
punched out with regular edges

KALI BICHROMICUM

13) *Oedematous*, bladder like appearance of *uvula* with much swelling but little redness.
14) Kali bich is useful in affections of *eye* with indolence of ulceration, absence of deficiency of inflammatory redness and the disproportionate absence of photophobia.
15) *Asthma* with expectoration of tough and stringy mucous

< 3-4 A.M., cold weather

> Sitting up and bending forward, warmth.

Particulars :

1) MIND
2) HEADACHE
3) EYE
4) EARS
5) RESPIRATORY SYSTEM
6) GIT
7) RHEUMATISM
8) SKIN

MIND

- Closed, reserved, rigid and very proper people.
- *Narrowness of mind* – Conserved nature, like to spend time with their family, closed in their own world.
- Though emotionally closed and antisocial they still perform their duties quite adequately.
- Because of their narrowness and lack of social contact they seem to be excessively conscientious in explaining every detail.

HEADACHE

Cause – Suppressed catarrhal affections – Coryza, gastritis etc. Stoppage of discharge brings on the complaint.

Location – Supra orbital headache around the eye that can be covered with the tip of a finger . Spottiness is marked.

Sensation – Blinding headache – Pain is preceded by blinding and vision gets better as pain increases.

Concomitants – Aversion to light and noise; sallow and yellowish face, retching and vomiting of food.

Modalities – < Light, Noise

> Pressure

EYE

Kali bich cures conditions of eyes like conjunctivitis, trachoma, pannus, syphilitic iritis, corneal ulcers etc when the symptoms agree.

Conjunctivitis :

Inflammation of indolent character – Eyelids are swollen and agglutinated especially in the morning with a thick, stringy, yellow matter and very little photophobia. In chronic cases there is a tendency to formation of ulcers which progress slowly.

Syphilitic Iritis :

Kali bich is indicated in later stages when there has been exudation posterioly between the iris and crystalline lens causing adhesions of these structures to each other. Little or no redness and no photophobia.

Keynotes :

- Indolence of ulceration.
- Absence of redness and photophobia.
- Ulceration of cornea that looks deep and punched out.

Kali bich helps to absorb the exuded matter.

EARS

Otitis Media, ulceration of membrana tympani.

Character of pains – pains of sharp stitching character which shoot up into the head and down into the neck. Glands of neck become swollen with pains shooting from ear to the parotid.

Character of discharge – Tenacious, stringy and purulent discharge. Tendency to ulceration of membrana tympani and mucous surface of the middle ear.

RESPIRATORY SYSTEM

Nose :

Catarrah – There is dryness of nasal mucous membrane with tickling in the nose and sneezing.

Character of discharge – Tough, ropy and stringy secretion which often collects in the posterior nares < going in open air.

Chronic Ozeana :

Character of discharge – "Plugs or clinkers" hard green lumps of mucus are hawked up from the posterior nares particularly in *morning.*

Symptoms – Pressure at the root of nose due to affection of frontal sinus. The process of chronic inflammation may go on from bad to worse causing *sinusitis* and later ulceration sets in and the whole septum ulcerates – "punched out ulcers". Little pieces of caried bones come out with these discharges. Nose feels unnaturally dry due to obstruction caused by hardened masses of fetid clinkers.

- Loss of smell.
- Violent shooting pains extend from root of nose to external angle of the eye and are accompanied with dimness of sight. A cold may progress to sinusitis, bronchitis and asthma.

Throat :

Kali bich strongly affects the mucous membrane of the throat causing inflammation with a tendency towards exudation.

Croup :

Membranous croup suited to light haired, fair complexioned children who are fat and chubby.

Symptoms :

- Membranous deposit of pearly white fibrinous consistency extending downwards to larynx, trachea and bronchi.
- Enlarged glands of neck, tonsils with excessive production of mucous in throat.
- Uvula becomes oedematous and bladder like.
- Laboured breathing with smothering sensation and tight feeling in epigastrium.
- Tongue coated dirty yellow.

Bronchitis :

Bronchitis with involvement of glands on either side of spinal column and there is dullness on percussion.

Character of cough – Violent rattling hoarse and metallic *expectoration* – Tough, stringy and ropy. < Eating, sitting up.
> Lying down.

Conc. – Pain in the chest in small spots, appears and disappears suddenly.

Asthma :

Asthma dependent upon bronchiectasis.

Expectoration – Tough, stringy and ropy.

Aggravation – Midnight, 3-4 A.M., winters, lying down.

Amelioration – Sitting up and bending forward, raising of mucus.

GIT

Mouth :

- Great dryness of mouth.
- Ropy saliva and mucus.
- Deep punched out ulcers with apthous patches at the roof of the mouth through the soft palate into the posterior nares and the whole palate looks as if it would be destroyed by ulcerative process.

Tongue :

- Broad and flat with imprint of teeth.

- Thick *yellow coated tongue more towards the base with large insular patches. In typhoid and malignant dysentry tongue becomes glossy, smooth, red and cracked.*

(Kali bich has produced and cured ulceration of tongue even when syphilitic)

Stomach :

Gastric complaints from chronic effects of excess "indulgence in beer".

Gastritis :

Cause – Beer, overeating.

Symptoms :

- Vomiting of sour and clear mucus (overproduction of mucus).
- Vomiting is renewed at every attempt to eating and drinking.
- Violent pains that can be spotted with a finger.
- Burning and rawness in stomach.

Concomitants – Dyspepsia is accompanied by supra orbital headache preceded by blinding. There is aversion to light and noise. Face is apt to be pale and bloated. Kali bich is excellent in gastric and duodenal ulcers with punched out perforating ulcer with regular edges. Pains in spots that can be covered with tip of a finger and shifting in nature.

Dysentry :

(Diarrhoea and dysentry alternate with rheumatism).

Character of stools – brown watery stools with jelly like mucus and blood.

Before stools – Pain in abdomen – shifting pains with spottiness.

During and after stools – Cramping and tenesmus

Conc. – Tongue is dry smooth glazed, red and cracked.

Modalities < Hot weather.

RHEUMATISM

Rheumatism alternates with gastric symptoms.

Cause – Syphilitic rheumatism.

Character of pains

- Smaller joints suffer considerably-fingers, wrists, shoulders etc.
- Spottiness can be covered with the tip of a finger.
- Wandering and shifting pains keep moving from one joint to another.
- Pains appear and disappear rapidly.

< Summer weather, motion.

> Rest

(Kali bich has cured deep punched ulcers of legs and heels).

SKIN

Kali bich produces hard *papules* that tend to develop into *pustules* and even into *deeply eating ulcers* with severe burning pains (syphilitic in character).

General Modalities :

Skin and Rheumatism > HOT WEATHER, MOTION
< COLD WEATHER

Cough and other complaints > COLD WEATHER
< HEAT

Relations :

Compare – Brom, Hep., Iod in croup. After Canth and Carb. acid. has removed the scrapings in dysentry. After Iod in croup when hoarse cough with tough membranes, general weakness and coldness are present. After Calc. in acute and chronic nasal catarrah. Ant. tart follows well in catarrhal affections and skin diseases.

Complements – Ars.

Remedies that follow well – Ant. tart, Berb. Puls.

Anti dotes – Ars, Lach., Puls.

Important Question ?

Q.1. Give indications of Kali bich in following.

1) Rheumatism	[1975, 77, 85]
2) Diptheria	[1986, 88]
3) GIT	[1974, 77, 83, 87]
4) Respiratory symptoms	[1986, 93, 94, 95]
5) Throat	[1996]
6) Bronchitis	[1987 S]
7) Sinusitis	[1987]
8) Dysentry	[1972, 76, 77]
9) Asthma	[1977]
10) Keynotes	[1977, 79]

Q.2. Compare :

Respiratory symptoms – Kali bich/Kali carb.	[1988, 90, 91]
Catarrah – Puls/Kali bich	[1990]
Bronchitis – Phos/Kali bich	[1994]
Syphlitic Ulcers – Nit-acid/Kali bich	[1981]

RESPIRATORY SYMPTOMS

KALI BICH	KALI CARB
• Asthma dependent upon Bronchiectasis.	• Asthma with sensation as if no air in the chest. Expectoration-*blood streaked, thick yellow.*
• Bronchial tubes are filled with tough tenacious exudation.	• Constant *backache* with perspiration on the upper part of the body.
• Expectoration *yellow stringy and ropy mucus.*	• Increased saliva with scanty urine.
• > Sitting up and bending forward. > 3-4 A.M.	• >Bending forward. < 3-4 A.M.

GASTRIC CATARRAH

PULSATILLA	KALI BICH
• **Cause** – Fatty food.	• **Cause** – Beer, overeating.
• Pains are changeable, shifting in character, appear and disappear suddenly.	• Rheumatic symptoms alternate with gastric symptoms.
• Sensation of food lodged under the sternum.	• Tenesmus in stomach with pain in 'spots'. Pains appear and disappear suddenly.
• Absence of thirst with bad taste in mouth.	• Dyspepsia is accompanied with supra orbital headache preceded by blinding.
• Vomit – greenish, yellow bilious matter.	• Vomit – sour clear, ropy mucus.
• Aggravation – Evening.	• Aggravation – Morning.

BRONCHITIS

PHOSPHORUS	KALI BICH
• Subacute lingering cases in tall, slender and overgrown pthisical subjects.	• Bronchitis lingers long in subacute condition.
• Discharge – Bloody and mucoid sputum with salty or sweetish taste.	• Discharge – stringy and ropy with involvement of glands.
• Cough – Paroxysmal with pain under the sternum and embarrassed respiration < After meals, going in open air.	• Cough – troublesome towards the morning with tightness of epigastrium. < Eating, cold air. > Warmth

SYPHILITIC ULCER :

KALI BICH	NITRIC ACID
• Ulcer with deep, punched out and regular edges.	• Ulcer with zig-zag irregular edges.
• Tendency to penetrate and tenacious exudation. Pains are in 'spots'.	• Bleed easily, sensitive and splinter like pain.
• Base hard corroding with blackish spot in centre.	• Base looks like raw flesh.

47. KALI CARBONICUM

Hahnemann

Common Name – Potassium Carbonate.

Kali-carb is a *deep and long acting remedy* and indicated more in *chronacity of complaints.*

Constitution – Patient has a tendency to *obesity* with profound *aneamia, debility and backache*. Especially helpful in diseases of *old people* who are fleshy with *dropsical condition*. Puffiness of upper eyelids and paretic tendencies.

Relation with heat and cold – *Very chilly* patient (on account of aneamia) least draught of cold air makes them shiver.

Miasm – Anti psoric remedy.

DIATHESIS – Tubercular diathesis.

KEYNOTES

1) Profound ***aneamia with debility***. The skin is milky white with tendency to dropsical effusions.
2) Very *chilly patient* – On account of aneamia the patient becomes very susceptible to cold; least draught of air makes him shiver.
3) *Intense debility* and *weakness*. The patient always wants to lie down. This weakness and exhaustion gradually grow in intensity till at last they amount to a state of paresis.
4) ***Touchiness*** – The patient is oversensitive to touch particularly about the *soles of feet.*
5) *Sharp stitching and wandering pains* – Worse from rest and better on motion. Pains fly from place to place (Bry – stitching pains worse motion; better-rest).
6) *Aggravation* of complaints *2-4 A.M.*
7) ***Bag like swelling between the upper eyelids and the upper eyebrows*** (Lower eyelids – Apis; both eyelids – Phos.)
8) *Backache* (golden sign) – accompanied by great weakness and debilitating sweat. The patient constantly speaks of his back giving out. It is so bad that the patient feels like lying down on the street while walking. Backache < eating.

Sweat, backache and weakness – The trio are marked keynotes for Kali carb.

9) *Dyspepsia in aged* with empty weakness in stomach before eating and bloatedness after eating.

10) State of anxiety felt in the stomach as though from fear, apprehension etc (Mez.).
11) *Asthma* < 3 A.M., Lying down
> Sitting up with head bent forward with hands on knees.
12) *Urine* is loaded with *urates* as an evidence of exhaustion.
13) *Fishbone or splinter sensation* in the throat from becoming *cold*. (Arg nit, Dol, Hep, Nit. acid, Sil).
14) Heart has a tendency to fatty degeneration with stitching pains and slow weak pulse.

Aggravation – Taking cold, rest, 2-4 A.M., slightest draught of air.

Amelioration – Motion, Warmth.

Particulars :

1) MIND
2) ANEAMIA
3) HEADACHE
4) RESPIRATORY SYSTEM
5) HEART
6) GIT
7) KIDNEY
8) SPINE
9) FEMALE SYMPTOMS
10) RHEUMATISM

MIND

- *Desires company* (Bism, Ars, Lyco, Stram).

(Desire to be alone – Bell, Ign, Nat mur, Nux vom., Sepia)

- The patient is *uptight and proper*. His mind maintains an iron control over behaviour and emotions.
- Mind is systemic, proper and routine oriented.
- The patient may appear to be devoid of emotions but is quite sensitive emotionally. He may appear to be devoid of emotions because of his controlled expression of them, but he may well feel things quite strongly.
- The person tends to ignore the problems until they have taken a serious stage.
- The exaggerated mental control drives the symptoms expression more characteristically into *solar plexus* – A state of anxiety, fear and apprehension felt in the stomach (Mez.). A Kali carb patient maintains tight control over expressing his sensitivity and for this reason he develops *sleeplessness* – sleep is a time in which mental controls are naturally relaxed, something which is difficult for a Kali carb patient and hence the patient develops extreme sleeplessness.

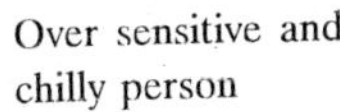

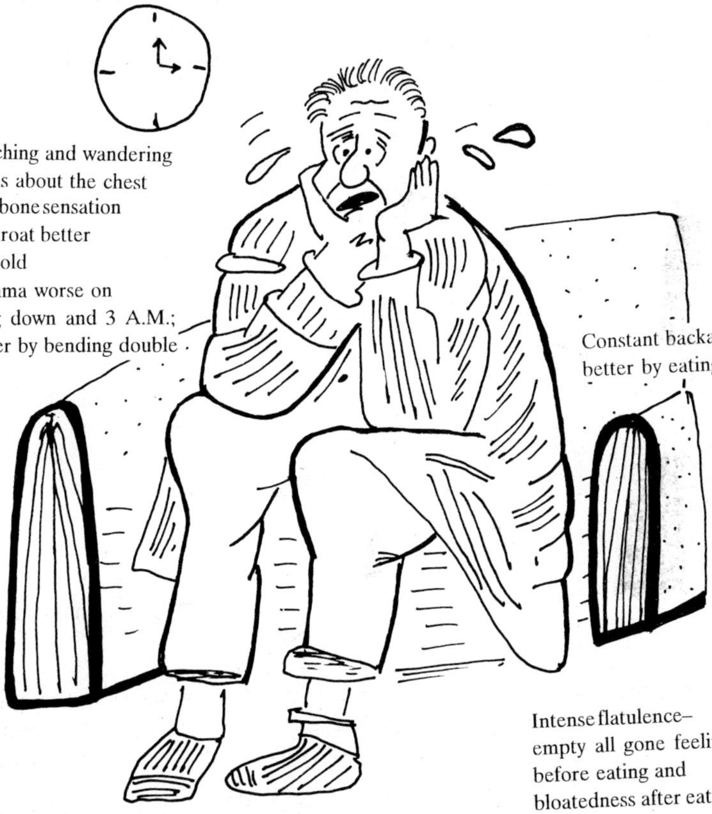

Over sensitive and
chilly person

Aneamia with intense
debility
Cold sweating

Worse – 2–4 A.M.

Stitching and wandering
pains about the chest
Fishbone sensation
in throat better
by cold
Asthma worse on
lying down and 3 A.M.;
better by bending double

Constant backache
better by eating

Intense flatulence–
empty all gone feeling
before eating and
bloatedness after eating

Anxiety felt in pit
of stomach
Swelling in the upper eyelids

Touchiness–especially about
the soles of feet

KALI CARBONICUM

- As the pathology progresses there is an *irritability* arising from the sense of dogmatism, duty and correctness.
- As pathology progresses there is prominence of many *fears and anxieties* – Fear of dark, fear of future, fear of impending disease, fear of ghosts (*desire for company* owes its origin to fear of being alone).
- Unlike many other remedies the stages of mental pathology rarely progress to insanity.

ANEAMIA

Kali carb exerts a profound influence over the blood making process. The blood lacks the red corpuscles. *Patient is aneamic with great debility, skin watery or milky white. Pseudo plethora* – Flushing which is not fulbloodedness but local influx of blood. Flushing is one sided and partial. One cheek is red hot and the other pale and cold. This condition is especially found in young girls at the age of puberty – *amenorrhoea* because of poor quality of blood and general weakness. Due to aneamia the patient is very *chilly* and is sensitive to slightest draught of air. The person inclines to *bloat* especially about the face on the upper eyelids with backache and weakness. Aneamia with *throbbing* all throughout body. Aneamia at *menopause* and old age is found with *dropsy*; bag like swelling over the upper eyelids; weak heart with irregular pulse; *backache* with intense *weakness* and patient throws herself on the bed completely exhausted. Aching down the hips into the gluteal muscles. *Cold sweat* upon the slightest exertion particular combination of sweat, backache and weakness.

- *Vertigo,* weakness of sight from sexual excess.
- *Urine is loaded with urates* on account of exhaustion.
- Kali carb is eminently useful in *convalescence form* of disease when there is great weakness, profuse sweat and a mental state of abject hopelessness.

HEADACHE

Cause – exposure to cold, sexual excess.

Location – both temples and occipital region.

Sensation – Loose feeling in the head. Stitching pains through the eyes, scalp, cheek bones.

Modalities – < cold air (cessation of discharges), 2-4 A.M.
> warmth.

Concomitants – Yawning during headache, great dryness with falling of hair.

RESPIRATORY SYSTEM

Catarrah – "Acute and Chronic catarrah".

Cause – Slightest draft of cold air.

Sensation – Dryness in the nose alternating with stuffing up.

Discharge – Thick fluent yellow discharge. In the morning the patient blows out and hawks up dry hard crusts that fill the nasal passage. These dry crusts when blown out cause bleeding.

Concomitants – Sensation as if there was a lump or fish in the throat which must be swallowed < cold air.

Cough :

Cause – Slightest draft of air.

Character of cough – Dry hawking cough with morning expectoration spasmodic cough with gagging and vomiting.

Expectoration – Tenacious, copious, offensive, lumpy blood streaked expectoration when it becomes warm. Expectoration relieves the person.

Concomitants – Face becomes puffed with swelling between the eyelids and eyebrows.

Modalities – < Cold weather, eating and drinking, 2-5 A.M.

(Dr. Kent has written that Kali carb has given excellent results in an epidemic of whooping cough with the striking keynote of bag like swelling below the eyebrow and above the eyelids).

Lung :

Affections of lungs – pleurisy, pneumonia, bronchitis, pthisis pulmonaris.

Symptoms – the disease is located mostly in lower right lung with profuse expectoration of matter of pus like appearance, great emaciation, no appetite.

- Cough is difficult and the patient cannot get up the sputum. He raises it partly when it slips back into the pharynx.
- Coldness of chest.

character of pains – Wandering stitching pains in chest aggravated by rest, cold, pressure, lying on painful side. Pains that extort are between breaths independent of respiration (Bry – stitching pains worse on motion, slightest movement, heat).

Concomitants – Puffiness of the upper eyelids. Backache with debility and sweating.

Asthma :

Cause – cold weather, humid air.

Symptoms – Patient cannot lie down, must sit up bent forward. Must lean forward with head on knees. Wakes up at 3 A.M. with difficult wheezing breathing and suffocation.

Character of cough – Dry and hard hacking cough with difficult expectoration of yellowish green lumpy blood streaked mucus. Expectoration relieves the patient.

Concomitants – Fish bone sensation in the throat brought on by taking cold.

HEART

- Kali carb is indicated late in heart troubles when there is deposition in cardiac valves.
- Tendency to produce fatty degeneration of heart with great influence in insufficiency of mitral valve.
- Pulse is intermittent, slow and weak.
- Stitching pains in chest aggravated between acts of breathing (3 A.M.).
- Dyspnoea is better by leaning forward.
- Easy choking – food gets easily into the wind pipe and is followed by severe paroxysm of coughing.
- Sweat, backache and weakness.

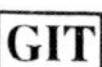

Teeth :

- Gums seperate from teeth and teeth decay, become discoloured and loose so that they have to be extracted early in life; offensive smell from teeth, pus oozing out from around the teeth.

Stomach :

- "*Anxiety felt in stomach*". The patient when frightened, apprehensive or anxious has a strange feeling of emptiness, gone feeling in the pit of the stomach.
- *Dyspepsia* particularly in *old persons with empty, weak feeling in the stomach before eating and bloatedness after eating.*
- There are sour eructations, heart burn and an easy nervous feeling when hungry.
- Great flatulence – everything seems to be converted to gas – belches wind upwards and flatus passes downward < eating.
- Cutting pain in the abdomen better by doubling up, a chronic coldness felt in the abdomen externally and internally.

Stools – Diarrhoea alternates with constipation.

Constipation – Hard and knotty stools that require great straining.

Diarrhoea – Painless diarrhoea with rumbling in abdomen and burning at stool. "Chronic cases with puffiness under eyebrows."

Piles – Externally sensitive to touch, bleed copiously and cannot be put back. There is great aggravation from stool < During and after stool.
> Sitting on cold water.

KIDNEY

Acute Nephritis with puffiness of face and bag like swelling on the upper eyelids. Abdomen feels distended and feels as if it would burst.

Severe backache, profuse perspiration and weakness. Nausea and vomiting of sour fluid. Nausea better when lying down. Complaints are worse between 2-4 A.M., lying on left and painful side, cold weather.

SPINE

Kali carb causes spinal irritation hence causing backache with pressure in the small of the back. Backache is worse when the patient is exhausted while walking and is better by lying down. *Backache worse on eating.* Backache frequently occurs with uterine symptoms, labor pains, dyspepsia, respiratory symptoms. Patient is so exhausted that she drops herself into a chair or may even lie down to obtain relief.

Backache is accompanied by great weakness and profuse sweating. Sensation of *heavy weight* in the pelvis and pain may shoot down the gluteal muscles into the buttock to thigh and thence to knees.

RHEUMATISM

Cause – Change of temperature, cold weather.

Character of pains – Sharp stitching and wandering pains.

Modalities – Worse – Rest, lying on painful side.

Better – Moving about, lying on painless side, warm, weather.

Concomitants – Severe backache, profuse perspiration, weakness, great flatulence, feeling as if abdomen would burst.

FEMALE SYMPTOMS

Puberty :

Amenorrhoea with pale waxy look. False plethora due to local congestion. Girls do not menstruate at puberty due to aneamia. Chilly girls with bloated faces.

Labor :

Pains not sufficiently expulsive to make progress in labor with intense backache, sweat, water in urine, debility etc.

Uterine Heamorrhage :

After abortion, labor, metrorrhagia, uterine fibroids, in incessant pale, waxy and heamorrhagic women. Flow is copious with intense backache, sweat and debility.

Menopause

Dropsical tendency with bag like swelling about upper eye lids. Weak heart with sweat, debility and backache extending down the hips and gluteal muscles. Flushing of face, false plethora due to local congestion.

General Modalities :

Aggravation – 2-5 A.M., SLIGHTEST DRAFT
REST, COLD AIR, COITION

Amelioration – MOTION, WARMTH
LYING ON PAINFUL SIDE.

Relations :

Complementry – Carbo veg.

Compare – Bry, Lyc, Nat mur, Nit acid, Stan.

Follows well – Kali sulph, Phos, Stann. in loose, rattling cough.

Will bring on menses when Nat-mur though apparently indicated fails.

Important Questions ?

Q.1. Give indications of Kali carb in the following :

a) Respiratory system [1976, 76 S, 79, 82, 87 S, 91]
b) Pneumonia [1979]
c) Mind [1970]
d) Female [1995]
e) Asthma [1993]
f) GIT [1983]
g) Rheumatism [1981]
h) Modalities [1969]

Q.2. Compare :

1) Respiratory symptoms of – Kali carb/Kali bich [1988, 90, 91]
2) Rheumatic pains – Kali carb/Ranunculus bulbosus [1988]
3) Female – Kali carb/puls [1994 S]
4) Bronchitis – Kali carb/Phos [1994]

RHEUMATIC PAINS

RANUNCULUS BULBOSUS	KALI CARB
• Intercostal rheumatism with neuralgia and myalgia of chest.	• Stitching and wandering pains in the chest; worse rest and better by motion.
• Sore bruised sensation of chest with sensitiveness to touch.	• Puffiness of the upper eyelids with coldness of chest.
• Muscular pains about the margins of the shoulder blade.	• Backache, debility with sweat.
< Touch, motion, during inspiration, wet stormy weather	< Slightest draught of air, rest, between breaths, 3 A.M.
> Warmth rest	> Lying on right side, warmth.

FEMALE SYMPTOMS :

PULSATILLA	KALI CARB
• Ladies who are fair, beautiful looking but inclined to be fleshy with fine hair and blue eyes.	• Dark skinned people inclined to obesity and dropsical conditions. Puffiness of upper eyelids with paretic conditions.
• Aneamic and chlorotic with pale face at puberty.	• Aneamic and cholorotic with pale milky white face, false plethora.
• Weeping disposition	• Chilliness – wants to be covered all the time. Sensitive to slightest draft of air.
• Patient has constant chilliness with aversion to cover.	
• Changeability of symptoms both mental and physical.	• Backache, debility, weakness and sweat accompany all complaints.
• Delayed and scanty menses.	• Wandering and stitching pains, < Rest ; > Motion.
• Irregular and sluggish labor pains.	• Difficult and delayed menses; uterine heamorrhage with constant backache better by pressure.
• Wants door and windows open.	
• Dry tongue with absence of thirst.	

BRONCHITIS :

PHOSPHORUS	KALI CARB
• Suited to subacute and lingering cases in delicate tall, slender overgrown and pthisical subjects.	• Suited to dark skinned people inclined to obesity and dropsical effusions.
• Puffiness of both eyelids.	• Puffiness of the upper eyelids with dropsical tendencies and aneamia.
• Chilly patient but desires cold things. Restlessness is marked.	• Chilly patient sensitive to slightest draft of air.

• Burning and empty all gone sensation in chest. Paroxysmal cough with pain under the sterum and suffocation in the upper part of chest.	• Stitching and wandering pains in the chest (lower part).
• Expectoration – salty, sweetish and purulent.	• Expectoration of lumpy green blood streaked mucus that gives relief.
• < After meals, open air, lying on left side. > After sleep.	• Coldness of chest. < 2-4 A.M., Rest > Motion.

48. KALI MURIATICUM

Common Name – Chloride of Potassium.

Pathogenesis – *Without the inorganic salt Potassium Chloride no fibrin can be made.* Normal amount of fibrin cannot be held in proper solution in the blood without the proper balance of the cell salt. Fibrin is created by the action of chloride of Potash with assistance of oxygen, on certain albuminoids. In inflammatory exudations fibrin is found on mucous membrane such as croup, diptheria, catarrah, serous cavities such as pleura and peritoneum.

(Dr. Carey has said that in all inflammatory conditions Ferrum phos should be given in alternation with Kali mur, for iron molecules carry oxygen which becomes deficient when the proper balance is disturbed by the outflow of fibrin.

KEYNOTES

1) Kali mur is used in ***second stage of inflammation***.
2) Applicable in catarrhal affections and subacute inflammatory stages which give rise to *fibrinous exudations.* These fibrinous exudations are sticky and cause swelling of interstitial connective tissues due to resulting inflammation. (Thus Kali mur is used in dysentry, diptheria, laryngeal croup, pneumonia when acute infiltrations are suspected). Kali mur caused diminution of secretion and gradual going down of swelling).
3) ***Whiteness of secretions and tongue*** is a marked feature.
4) *White coated tongue*, mucous lining or tonsils (Fibrin becomes non-functional because of deficiency in Potassium Chloride and Oxygen).
5) *Thick white slime like expectoration* and discharges from mucous membranes.
6) *Flour like scaling of skin* – Eruptions, pustules, pimples discharge a whitish mattery substance.
7) Kali mur has a particular affinity to *middle ear* and *eustachian tube* where it sets up *chronic inflammatory condition* with earache, deafness and *thick white exudations* from the ear. Swollen glands of the ear with noises in the ear, snapping and cracking from unequalisation of air in eustachian tubes.

8) Kali mur relieves the effects of *burns* because fibrin in the tissue first succumbs to effects of heat.

(Chloride of potash by its union with albuminous substance produces new fibrin and supplies the deficiency).

9) *Acute and chronic rheumatism* when there is *swelling* of parts or white coated tongue (rheumatic fever of IInd stage when exudations take place with swellings around the joints).

10) Indigestion due to *sluggish action of liver* with white coated tongue. Fatty food and hot drinks disagree.

Particulars :

1) EYES
2) EAR
3) RESPIRATORY SYSTEM
4) GIT
5) FEMALE SYMPTOMS
6) MALE SYMPTOMS
7) RHEUMATISM
8) SKIN
9) TISSUES
10) FEVER

EYES

Inflammation, pustules, granulations with *discharge of thick white mucus*.

EAR

Catarrhal conditions of middle ear and eustachian tube.

- *Thick white exudations* from the ear.
- Earache with swelling of glands and grey or white furred tongue.
- Deafness from swelling of internal ear, cracking noises in the ear on blowing nose or swallowing (cracking noises in the ear from unequalisation of air in eustachian tube).

RESPIRATORY SYMPTOMS

Nose – Stuffy nose with thick white discharge and grey white coated tongue.

Throat – Ulcerated sore throat, inflammation of tonsils, mumps with greyish white patches and white coated tongue.

Croup – In diptheria Kali mur is well indicated with thick viscid milky white mucus. *IInd stage of all inflammatory conditions* of the respiratory tract.

- *Characteristic indication* – Thick tenacious white phlegm or milky sputa.
- Pneumonia, pleurisy in second stage with thick white viscid expectoration.
- Asthma from gastric derangement with white tongue, mucus white and hard to cough up.

GIT

Mouth – Canker of lips or mouth with swollen gums or glands, white ulcers (thrush) in the mouth of little children with much saliva.

Tongue – Coating of greyish white, dry or slimy.

Gastric Symptoms :

- Sluggish action of the liver.
- Fatty greasy food disagrees.
- White coating of tongue.
- Indigestion with vomiting of greasy white opaque mucus.

Abdomen :

Second stage of inflammatory diseases of the abdomen and bowels, peritonitis, enteritis etc.

Diarrhoea :

Cause – After fatty food.

Stools – Pale yellow, clay coloured stools.

FEMALE SYMPTOMS

Menses – Time – Too late/too scanty.

Duration – Long lasting

Quantity – Excessive discharge.

Character of blood – dark clotted tough black blood.

Leucorrhoea – Milky white thick, non irritating mucus.

MALE SYMPTOMS

Principal remedy in gonorrhoea or syphilis with characteristic white discharges, greyish tongue.

URINARY SYSTEM

Cystitis in second stage with swelling and discharge of thick white slimy mucus.

RHEUMATISM

- Rheumatism of any part of the body when there is swelling of parts or white coated tongue.
- Rheumatic fever, second stage, when exudation takes place; swelling around joints.
- Ulcers of extremities with characteristic fibrinous discharge.

SKIN

Eruptions filled with white fibrinous matter or when there exists white flour like matter on skin.

- Characteristic white coating of tongue.
- Eruptions acne, pustules, pimples with thick white content.
- Abscess, boils, festers, carbuncles etc. in their second stage with swelling before pus forms.

Tissues :

Burns of all degree – fibrin in tissues first succumb to heat. Fibrinous thick white slimy exudations from tissues.

- Useful in glandular swelling before formation of pus.

FEVER

Second stage of gastric, typhoid and enteric fever to restore integrity of affected tissue.

General Modalities :

Aggravation – Stomach and bowel symptoms are aggravated after eating fats, pastry, rich food. Pains are aggravated by motion.

49. KALI PHOSPHORICUM

H.C. Allen

Common Name – Phosphate of Potash.

Kali phos is a *long acting, anti psoric biochemic remedy.*

Pathogenesis – Grey matter of the brain is controlled by the inorganic cells salt, Potassium Phosphate. This salt unites with albumin and by the addition of oxygen creates nerve fluid or the grey matter of brain (with trace of other salts). The *nervous symptoms* that arise are due to the fact that nerve tissue has been exhausted of the phosphate of potassium from any cause. The potassium salt largely predominates in nerve fluid and that a deficiency produces well defined symptoms. It restores the equillibrium in overworked people both mentally and physically *(want of nerve and brain power).*

Miasm – Anti psoric remedy.

Relation with head and cold – Very chilly person.

KEYNOTES

1) ***Brain fag from overwork*** – Kali carb is an excellent remedy for disorders arising from *want of nerve or brain power.*
2) ***Nervous exhaustion with intense weakness,*** emaciation, aneamia and tubercular tendency.
3) ***Very chilly person*** – Takes cold easily, slightest draft of air aggravates. Aversion to open air.
4) *Aneamic and chlorotic* persons with extreme debility and exhaustion.
5) ***Aggravation*** of complaints from rest and rapid exertion; *amelioration* by gentle motion and slowly walking about.
6) Emaciation, wasting diseases with putrid stools. Ulcers with *putrid discharges, offensive catarrhal discharges.*
7) *Headaches* of students worn out with *mental work* and loss of sleep. Pains are generally relieved by gentle motion.
8) *Toothache* after exhaustion, mental labor or from loss of sleep; better by gentle motion.
9) *Tongue – Excessively dry* – coated stale brown, liquid mustard.
10) *Rheumatic pains* worse from violent exertion and rest; relieved by gentle motion.
11) Symptoms are often *one sided – one sided paralysis* from gradually increasing weakness.

12) *Neuralgia* – Occuring in any organ with depression, failure of strength, sensitiveness to noise and light, improved during pleasant excitement and gentle motion but most felt when quite and alone.

13) *Sleeplessness* from nervous causes often after worry or excitement.

14) *Gangrenous conditions* with characteristic discharge of offensive pus. Septic heamorrhages.

Particulars :

1) MIND
2) HEAD
3) EAR
4) EYES
5) RESPIRATORY SYSTEM
6) GIT
7) CIRCULATORY SYSTEM
8) URINARY SYSTEM
9) MALE SEXUAL SYMPTOMS
10) FEMALE SEXUAL SYMPTOMS
11) NERVOUS SYSTEM
12) TISSUES

MIND

- Mental disorders arising from nervous exhaustion, overwork, worry and anxiety.
- Brain fag from overwork.
- Depressed spirits, impatience and nervousness.
- Extreme lassitude and depression.
- Slightest labour seems a heavy task.

HEADACHE

Cause – Taking cold, mental exertion, overwork, headache of students, businessmen etc. those worn out by fatigue.

Location – Temples, occiput.

Sensation – Pain with intense weakness.

Modalities – < Rest, mental and physical overexertion.
> Gentle motion, eating.

Concomitants – Vertigo, empty all gone sensation in the stomach.

EAR

- Humming and buzzing in the ears.

Brain fag

Nervous exhaustion
from overwork

Worry with debility
and exhaustion

Aggravation of
complaints from
rest, exertion
Amelioration from
gentle motion

Chilly patient

Putrid discharges

Excessively dry and
brownish tongue

All gone sensation
in stomach

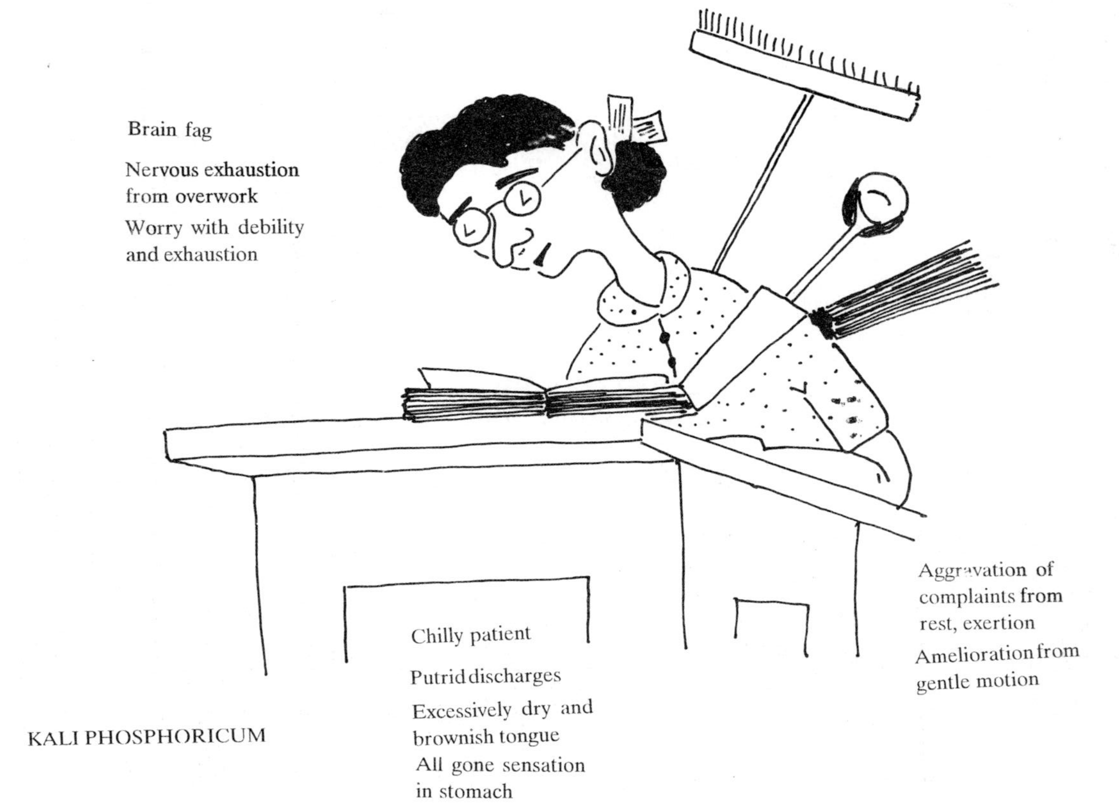

KALI PHOSPHORICUM

- Discharge from the ear – offensive, putrid and purulent.
- Deafness from exhaustion of nervous symptoms.

EYES

Weakness of sight from exhaustion. Drooping of eyelids.

RESPIRATORY SYSTEM

Nose :

- Catarrah from taking cold.

Discharge – Fetid discharge with offensive odour.

Throat :

- Throat diseases with mental or nervous prostration. (Gangrenous condition, croup with foul odour and discharges).
- Hoarseness from overexertion.

Asthma :

Shortness of breath with exhaustion and want of nerve power. Aggravation on motion, exertion, cold and open air.

GIT

Mouth :

- Stomatitis, ulcers of mouth – with very fetid offensive breath and bad taste in the mouth.

Tongue :

- Excessively dry tongue with brownish, liquid mustard coating.

Stomach :

- Desires cold drinks, sour things.

Gastritis –

Cause – Exhaustion, depression, grief, mental strains, worry.

Symptoms :

- All gone sensation in the stomach.
- Weakness, debility with nervous exhaustion.
- Excessive hunger with unnatural appetite, hunger soon after eating.
- Extreme thirst for cold water.
- Flatulence with distress about the heart or on left side of stomach.

Abdomen :

- Sensation of emptiness.
- Pain in the abdomen worse after eating, before and during menses.

Diarrhoea :

Character of stools – Putrid foul eructations, profuse and rice watery stools.

- Depression and exhaustion of nerves.

Dysentry :

- Stools consist of pure blood and have a foul and putrid odour.

Concomitants – swollen abdomen, dryness of tongue, delirious person.

CIRCULATORY SYSTEM

Irregular and intermittent pulse with weak heart after violent emotion, grief or care. Poor circulation with dizziness and fainting sensation about the heart.

URINARY ORGANS

- Inability to retain urine from nervous debility.
- Enuresis of children.
- Cystitis with weakness and prostration.

FEMALE SEXUAL SYMPTOMS

Menses – Irregular due to worry, anxiety and mental strain.

Time – Too late or too early.

Quantity – Scanty or profuse.

Character of blood – Deep red thin and non coagulating with offensive odour. Amenorrhoea from depression, nervousness and general debility.

- Tedious labour from constitutional weakness.

MALE SEXUAL SYMPTOMS

- Nocturnal emissions.
- Sexual power diminished.
- Utter prostration after coitus.

RHEUMATISM

Rheumatic pains with lameness and stiffness

< Violent exertion, rest, rising from sitting position, cold and open air.

> Gentle motion.

NERVOUS SYSTEM

Exhaustion and weakness from any cause which has lowered the standard of nervous system.

Paralysis – Paralysis of any part of the body, one sided paralysis – hemiplegia, paralysis of vocal cords, vital powers are reduced, stools have a putrid and fetid odour.

Spinal aneamia from exhausting diseases.

Neuralgia – Neuralgic pains in any organ with depression of strength.

> gentle motion, pleasant excitement, when attention is occupied.

< noise, light, quiet and when alone, rest, violent exertion.

TISSUES

- Wasting diseases when putrid conditions are present.
- General debility and exhaustion.
- Gangrenous condition with putrid discharge.
- Heamorrhages or septic heamorrhages with thin dark putrid and non coagulating blood.

SKIN

Itching of skin with crawling sensation. Felon or any other disease when matter discharged becomes fetid.

General Modalities :

Worse – COLD, OPEN AIR, EXERTION
AFTER REST, NOISE
RISING FROM SITTING POSITION
WHEN ALONE.

Better – GENTLE MOTION
PLEASANT COMPANY.

50. KALI SULPHURICUM

H.C. Allen

Common Name – Sulphate of Potash.

Kali sulph is a *deep acting remedy. It helps to finish up with a case as a complement of Puls. when Silicea is not indicated.*

Pathogenesis – Kali sulph is an *oxygen carrier*. Oxygen in the lungs is taken up by the iron in the blood and carried to every cell in the organism. A deficiency of oxygen in the skin and epithelial cells, will give rise to symptoms of chilliness, heaviness, weariness, palpitation of the heart, anxiety, sadness, headache and pain in the limbs. Kali sulph is also applicable in the ailments accompanied by *profuse desquamation of skin* including stage of desquamation following scarlet fever, measles, erisipelas etc.

Relation with heat and cold – Hot patient.

Diathesis – Tubercular diathesis.

KEYNOTES

1) ***Catarrhal affections with —thin watery yellow discharges.***
2) *Desquamation* of cells of the epidermis and epithelium (caused due to lack of Kali sulph when oxygen is not transferred to the cells). ***Kali Sulph assits in formation of new skin.***
3) *Tongue – Yellow coated* – yellow mucus with yellow slimy secretion.
4) ***Wandering pains*** in limbs, bones and glands. Pains keep shifting from one place to another.
5) *Aggravation* from *warmth*. *Amelioration* from *cold things* and open air.
6) *Pulsation* all over the body.

Particulars :

1) HEAD
2) EAR
3) FACE
4) GIT
5) RESPIRATORY SYSTEM
6) CIRCULATORY SYSTEM
7) URINARY SYSTEM
8) MALE SEXUAL SYMPTOMS
9) FEMALE SEXUAL SYMPTOMS

10) RHEUMATISM
11) SKIN
12) FEVER

HEAD

Headache caused in a heated room; rheumatic headache.

Location – Occiput, sides of head, temples.

Sensation – Heat in the head with constriction. Sensation of movement in head.

Character of pain – Boring in sides of head.

Modalities – Aggravation – Morning on waking, draft of air, warm room

Amelioration – Cool air.

Concomitants – Yellow coated tongue.

Dandruff on scalp with secretion of decidedly yellow thin matter.

EAR

- Catarrah of the ear and throat involving the eustachian tubes with a yellow slimy discharge.
- Earache with yellow watery discharge.
- Deafness from swelling of the internal ear.

Concomitants – Yellow coated tongue.

FACE

- Neuralgia of face < evening, warmth; > cool, open air.

GIT

Tongue :

- Yellow slimy coating of the tongue.

Stomach :

- Gastric catarrah with *yellow coated tongue*.
- Indigestion with sensation of pressure and fullness.
- Dread of hot drinks.
- Fasting ameliorates symptoms.

Abdomen :

- All abdominal troubles with yellow coating of tongue.
- Colicky pains – abdomen feels cold to touch.
- Evening aggravation of complaints.

Diarrhoea :

- Yellow slimy purulent stools. Sulphurous odour of gas from bowels.

Piles :

- Heamorrhoids with external and internal bleeding. Violent itching and burning pains in the anus. Characteristic yellow coating of tongue.

RESPIRATORY SYSTEM

Inflammatory conditions of the respiratory tract when the *expectoration* is decidedly *yellow, greenish and slimy* – bronchitis, pthisis, pneumonia, whooping cough, asthma etc.

Nose :

Catarrhal conditions with discharges of slimy yellow or watery greenish matter.

Cough :

Cause – Heated room.

Character of cough – Dry hoarse, croupy cough at night with difficult expectoration.

Expectoration – Purulent, yellow or greenish, slimy, watery which is difficult, must be swallowed or slips back.

Aggravation – Night, morning, evening (in bed) warm room.

Amelioration – Cool air.

Concomitants – Yellow coating of tongue.

Asthma :

- Dyspnoea with cough. Rattling short and suffocative breathing.
- Expectoration – Yellow greenish or slimy.

Modalities – Aggravation – Warm Room.

Amelioration – Open air.

CIRULATORY SYSTEM

Pulsation all over the body with hot, dry and harsh skin.

Pulse – slow and sluggish.

URINARY SYSTEM

Cystitis with characteristic discharge of *yellow slimy matter* from the urethra (Third stage of inflammation).

FEMALE SEXUAL SYSTEM

- Excoriation of genitilia with itching.
- Kali sulph builds up a woman who has been subject to abortion.

Leucorrhoea – Thin watery yellow discharge with characteristic yellow coating of tongue.

MALE SEXUAL SYSTEM

- Gonorrhoea, slimy yellow or greenish discharge.

- Syphilis with gleet when yellow and slimy.
- Evening aggravation.

RHEUMATISM

- Wandering and shifting rheumatic pains.
- Coldness of extremities.

  < Evening, warm room.

  > Cool, open air.
- Desquamation of skin of legs.

SKIN

- All sores on skin when exude a *thin yellow watery matter.* Sometimes with *dryness and desquamation* of the surrounding skin.
- Skin is hot, dry and burning with lack of perspiration.
- Eczema, dandruff, psoriasis, epithelial cancer with discharge of thin yellow purulent matter.
- Kali sulph greatly aids desquamation in eruptive diseases and assists the formation of new skin.

FEVER

- Temperature rises in evening.
- Characteristic yellow coating of tongue.
- Assits promotion of perspiration (can be used in alternation with Ferrum phos in fevers).
- In eruptive diseases Kali sulph aids desquamation.

General Modalities :

Aggravation – HEATED ROOM
EVENING

Amelioration – COOL OPEN AIR

51. LACHESIS MUTA

Hering

Common Name – Derived from Surukuku snake poison.

Lachesis was proved by Dr. Constantine Hering with some great risks to his life.

Lachesis is a *long acting, deep acting, polycrest remedy.*

Constitution – Suited to old topers, subjects of broken down constitution and in troubles incident to the climacteric age. Circulation of Lachesis subjects is very uncertain causing sudden attacks of giving away of strength, fainting, vertigo, rush of blood to the head causing apoplectic seizure, sudden flushes during climacteric period. Lachesis is suited to thin emaciated persons who have changed physically and mentally through their illness. Complexion is sickly. Women of choleric temperament with freckles and red hair. Drunkards who suffer from bad head, heamorrhoids and are prone to erysipelatoid infection.

Relation with heat and cold – Hot patient.

Diathesis – Heamorrhagic.

Temperament – Choleric.

Miasm – Greatest anti psoric remedy.

KEYNOTES

1) ***Aggravation of complaints from sleep.*** Patient sleeps into aggravation, unhappy, distressed and anxious. "Wakes up in panic".
2) ***Oversensitive to touch*** – Intolerance to touch and slightest pressure. Person cannot tolerate collars around the neck or even bed clothes to be touched.
3) *Aversion to tight clothes* around the neck, waist, everywhere. Wants loose clothing everywhere.
4) ***Left sided remedy*** – *Symptoms go from left to right (right to left – Lyc.).*
5) *Aggravation* of symptoms from *heat, warm drinks and spring.*
6) Amelioration from onset of discharges. *Feels better when menstrual flow begins.*
7) ***Sense of constriction everywhere*** – throat, heart, stomach etc. Patient cannot bear slightest touch of even bed clothes. Feels suffocated always.
8) Lachesis is full of inflammation of glands and cellular tissues with ***a purple and mottled appearance.***

9) Climacteric ailments – "Have never been well since that time" says a Lachesis patient suffering from menopausal period. Ailments caused due to suppression of menstrual flow with hot flushes, headache, mania etc. Burning *vertex* headache especially at or after menopause.

10) Cardiac affections along with other ailments causing cold extremities and hot head, feeble heart, skin covered with sweat, sense of constriction and suffocation everywhere.

11) *Desire for open air* – Great desire for *fanning* but slowly from a distance (Med.). (Rapidly from near – Carbo veg.)

12) *Throat* complaints *beginning from left side and going to right*; aggravation by warm drinks, slightest touch; liquids more painful than solids. (Bell, Bry, Ign) (Lyco – Symptoms go from right to left, better by warmth)

13) *Rush of blood to head*; after alcohol, mental emotions, suppressed or irregular menses, at climaxis, left sided apoplexy. Weight and pressure on the vertex.

14) Great physical and mental exhaustion causing trembling in the whole body aggravated in morning after waking (Gels). Would constantly sink from weakness.

15) *Trembling tongue* – Difficult to protrude. Trembles like that of a snake. Bluish black in appearance.

16) *Heamorrhagic diathesis* – Small wounds bleed easily and profusely. (Crot, Kreos, Phos). Blood is very dark and non coagulable (Crot, Sec.).

17) Boils, carbuncles, ulcers, malignant pustules with intense pain dark bluish purple appearance tend to malignancy.

18) Sensation of a *ball rolling* in the *bladder*.

19) *Mental excitability* with great loquacity (Agar, Stram.). Jumps from one idea to another. Ailments from long lasting grief, sorrow, fright, jealousy or disappointed love (Aur, Ign., Ph. Ac.).

Particulars :

1) MIND
2) EYES
3) EARS
4) FACE
5) RESPIRATORY SYSTEM
6) GIT
7) FEMALE SYMPTOMS
8) SKIN
9) NERVOUS SYSTEM

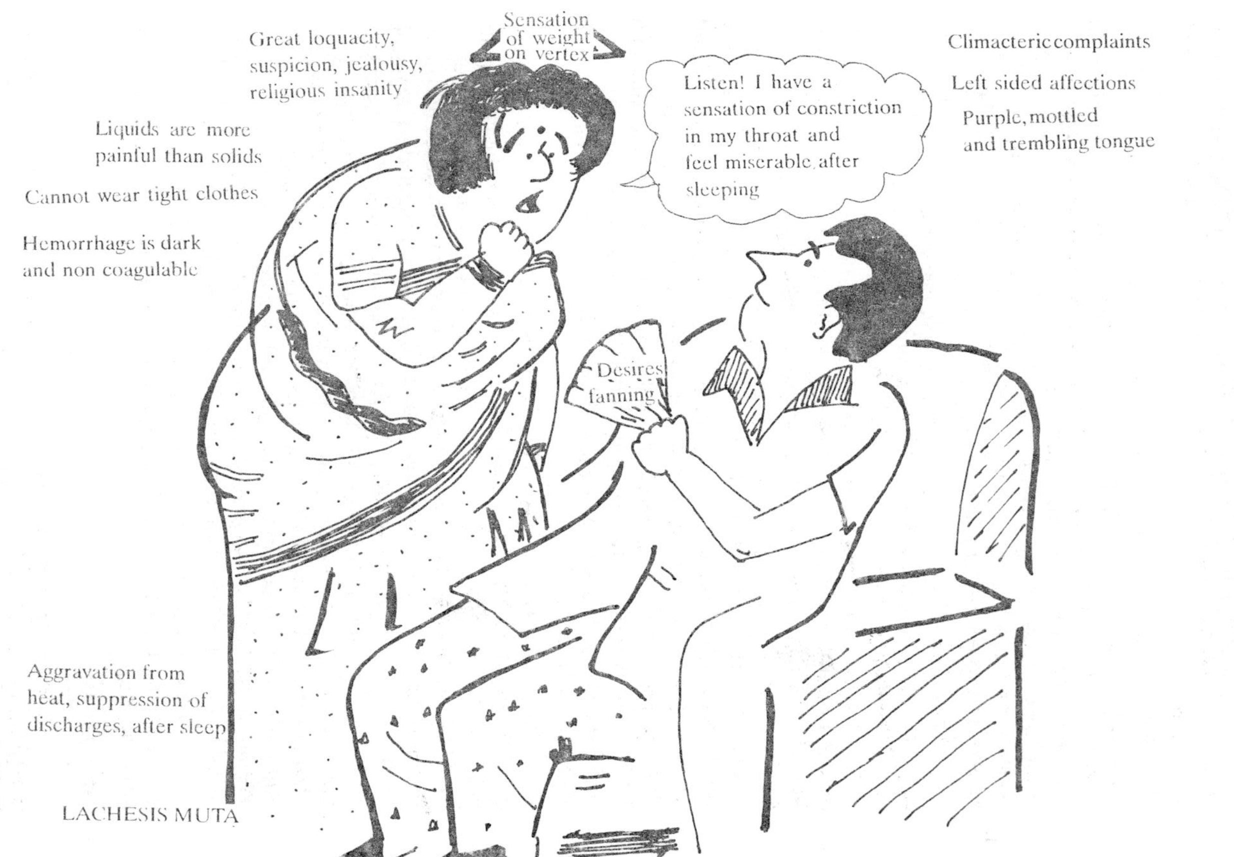
Sensation of weight on vertex
Great loquacity, suspicion, jealousy, religious insanity
Liquids are more painful than solids
Cannot wear tight clothes
Hemorrhage is dark and non coagulable
Listen! I have a sensation of constriction in my throat and feel miserable, after sleeping
Climacteric complaints
Left sided affections
Purple, mottled and trembling tongue
Desires fanning
Aggravation from heat, suppression of discharges, after sleep
LACHESIS MUTA

MIND

Cloudy state, sadness, melancholy, insane notions, jealousy and suspicion. Chronic complaints from depressing cause like long lasting grief and sorrow.

Great loquacity—Patient constantly keeps talking and changing ideas. Easy flow of ideas. Jumps from one subject to another. When taking a warm bath or after getting warm, mental symptoms are aggravated. Emotions are quite strong, quite attached to people and objects. Attachment is so strong that the patient gets pathological conditions of *jealousy* or *lasciviousness* (over indugence in sex). This *jealousy* can progress to suspicion and further progress to paranoia.

Suspicion—Patient imagines that people are cooking things against him; his family is scheming to put him in an insane asylum. Apprehension of future. Thinks or dreams of snakes, that she is dead, can go into deep states of anxiety worrying about health; especially the heart. *Paranoia* with fear of insanity at a certain stage (Hyos., Kali brom, Tarent, Stram, Plat, Ver. alb.). Thinks that she is somebody else under super human control. She is compelled to do things by spirits. Sometimes she takes form of voices in which she is commanded to steal, to murder, to confess things she never did and she has no piece of mind until she makes a confession of something she has never done. The state of torture is dreadful until it goes into delirium with muttering. Patient seems to be intoxicated with whisky—he stumbles while speaking, hardly finishing words, face is purple and head is hot. There is choking and the collar is uneasy about the neck with confusion of mind.

Religeous insanity—A sweet old lady full of wickedness and she feels that she has committed an unpardonable sin. She feels that she is going to die and will go to hell. There is another kind of loquacity belonging to Lachesis—patient is compelled to hurry in everything she does and wants everyone else to *hurry*. With that state of hurry is brought on a state of loquacity. The patient rapidly changes from one subject to another. Sentences are sometimes only half finished. She takes it for granted that you understand the balance and she will hurry on. Mental symptoms are closely connected to heart symptoms. Prolonged melancholy, *mental depression* with pain, gone sensation and weakness in the heart with difficult breathing. Person may quit a job because he or she is restricted. If asked to do something immediately by his wife he will feel the pressure.

Excess/overstimulation on the *sexual plane.* Lachesis is one of the remedies for masturbation. Sex suppression may bring on mental and physical symptoms.

HEADACHE

Cause—Stopping of a natural discharge—menses, coryza, perspiration, nose bleed etc. entering a warm room, sun headache (Glon. Bell). Headache in drunkards with high blood pressure Headache in hay fever with frequent and violent paroxysms of sneezing.

Location – pain comes surging in waves from back of neck, head and then over the head. Left sided headaches going on right side.

Sensation – Weight and pressure on the vertex. Pressing and bursting headache, oversensitive to touch but hard pressure often gives relief. Sensation as if head is hammered. Rush of blood to head.

Modalities – < Warmth, motion, after sleep, on waking in morning, noise and conversation.

> Flow of discharge.

Concomitants – Coldness of extremities with purple and mottled face, puffy eyes.

- Vertigo with nausea and vomiting.
- Pulsation all over the body.

EYE

- Inflammation in eyes worse after sleep.
- Eyes are oversensitive to touch and light.
- Eye symptoms with headache because of general disturbed circulation.
- Violent pains in the eyes from touching throat. In a sore throat when a tongue depressor touches the walls of the throat, there is violent pain in the eyes.
- Fistula lachrymalis with long standing eruptions on face.

EAR

Oversensitiveness of internal auditory meatus. Anything introduced in the canal will cause a violent spasmodic coughing and tickling in the throat.

FACE

Purple and mottled face with puffy eyelids – non pitting upon pressure. Face looks swollen and inflamed due to venous stasis, so it is purple and mottled. At times the face becomes pale and cold and the skin is covered with scaly eruptions which bleed easily. Jaundiced and sallow face. Livid, puffed and bloated face of the drunkards with a besotted look.

RESPIRATORY SYSTEM

Nose :

Person takes cold easily with frequent stuffing of nose and oversensitiveness to smell. Frequent bleeding of nose with watery discharge. In chronic form – congestive headache with coryza. Frequent bleeding from nose. Nose swells up and becomes purple, strawberry nose – red knob on the end of the nose. Lachesis is important and useful in drunkards who have a red nose with heart affections.

Throat (Tonsillitis, Diptheria) :

Location – Pain begins on the left side and goes to right side.

Symptoms :

- Throat and neck sensitive to external pressures and touch; everything about the throat distresses, even the weight of the bed covers. Person is obliged to loosen clothing. Sensation as if they hindered circulation with a kind of suffocative feeling.
- Empty swallowing or swallowing of saliva or liquids aggravates much more than solids.
- Pains in the throat run up to the ears.
- Much mucus in the fauces with painful hawking.
- Dark purple appearance of throat.
- Sensation of fullness in the neck with difficult breathing, pallor or plethoric face, choking when going to sleep.
- Elongation of uvula.
- Sensation of lump in the throat which decends on swallowing but soon returns. Patient is obliged to continuously keep hawking.
- Extreme dryness in the throat without thirst.
- *Modalities* – < after sleep, hot drinks, touch (Warm drinks cause suffocation).

Diptheria :

Swelling of throat – internal and external with unbearable odour, besotted appearance, rapid pulse and a high temperature, muttering delirium, purplish appearance of the membrane, lips, buccal cavity, throat and submaxillary gland. Lachesis is also helpful in syphilitic phagadaena of soft palate, fauces and gangrenous sore throat.

Glottis :

Spasm of the glottis with sensation as if something running from the neck to larynx, stopping the breath. Shortness of breath when walking. Least thing coming near the mouth or nose interferes with breathing. Tears off the collar or everything about the neck, throat or chest because it suffocates.

Asthma :

- Sudden flushes of heat or orgasm of blood.
- Must loosen clothing to prevent suffocation.
- Threatened paralysis of the heart and lungs.
- Dry hacking cough aggravated by touching throat or larynx.
- Cough during sleep.

Cough :

Dry hacking cough aggravated after sleep and is associated with a sensation as if the fluid has gone into the wrong passage. Cough is mostly dry and is raised with great difficulty. It is sympathetic with cardiac affections.

GIT

Mouth :

Gums are soft swollen and spongy with easy bleeding. Gums turn purple.

Tongue :

Tongue trembles and is protruded with great difficulty, dry tongue, trembles and catches under the lower teeth; bluish black appearance of tongue.

Stomach :

Pit of stomach is sore to touch or even to pressure of bed clothes. Cannot bear any pressure about the hypochondria. Warm drinks are hurtful and cause nausea and suffocation and increase palpitation and fullness in head. Cold drinks cause nausea with a tendency to vomit.

Abdomen :

Painful distension in the abdomen which is very annoying and can bear no pressure. Patient is obliged to loosen clothing and pull up the night dress to avoid pressure; surface nerves are sensitive. Cannot lay the arm across the abdomen on account of pressure.

Liver :

Jaundice, congestion, inflammation with nausea and vomiting of bile; white stool. Cannot endure any pressure about the hypochondria. Worse after sleep, heat

Stools :

Lachesis has peculiar stools. There is urging or rather a pressing down in the rectum which is worse when he attempts at stool. Painful constriction which prevents stool or is followed after an incomplete and unsatisfactory one. Stools are offensive. Heamorrhage from bowels of decomposed blood during the course of exhausting diseases like typhoid. Guerrecy says "Flakes of decomposed blood having form and appearance of perfectly charred wheat, straw in larger or shorter flat pieces, portions more or less grouped up."

Piles :

Blind or bleeding piles with a constricted feeling. Sensation as if *'little hammers'* beating in the rectum.

FEMALE

Menses at regular time.

Duration – short

Quantity – scanty

Character of blood – Dark watery and non coagulable.

Modalities – All troubles are relieved by menstrual flow. Menstrual sufferings before and after flow.

Concomitants – Headache during menses. Nausea and vomiting during menses.

Climacteric Ailments/menopause :

- Great circulatory disturbance with flushes of heat and surgings in the head.
- Headache with boring pain in the vertex.
- Pale face with faintings.
- Uterus does not bear contact, has to be relieved of all pressures; frequently lifts clothes as they cause an uneasiness in the abdomen without tenderness.

Ovary :

Affects the left ovary mostly (actual tumors, Cancer of ovary, suppuration, induration). Troubles begin in the left and go to the right. Engorgement of veins showing purple or mottled appearance.

Uterine Displacements :

Womb prolapse with congested and persistently obstinate heamorrhages. Hot flushes, hot vertex, pale face and fainting. Uterus is extremely sensitive to touch of even bed clothes.

Cancer of Breast/uterus :

Bluish and purplish appearance and if open or fungoid, bleeds easily a dark decomposed blood.

SKIN

Lachesis is useful in ulcers, carbuncles, abscesses, malignant pustules, black measles, erysipelas, small pox, boils, furuncles, bed sores, fungus heamatodes.

- Affected parts are very sensitive to touch and look bluish.
- Discharges are ichorous and offensive with intense burning. They must rise at night and bathe in water to relieve the burning.
- Tardy suppuration.
- Blood decomposes "breaks down" and becomes non coagulable. Bleeding is easily started and very persistent.

- Ulcers and wounds bleed profusely with a tendency to become gangrenous.

Cancers turn bluish or black; bleed much and often and burn; blood appears in the urine in many affections indicating a broken down constitution.

NERVOUS SYSTEM

- Trembling from extreme weakness.
- Person feels faint as if she must sink down. Great prostration both mental and physical on going to sleep.
- Prostration is accompanied by weak heart, nausea, pale face and vertigo.
- Left sided paralysis with apoplexy and cerebral exhaustion. Lesions are too extensive in apolexy with bluish black extravasation of blood.
- Weariness and prostration from hot weather.

General Modalities :

Aggravation – AFTER SLEEP, WARM DRINKS
SPRING, SUMMER
SUPPRESSION OF DISCHARGES
EXTREMES OF TEMPERATURE
ACIDS, ALCOHOL
PRESSURE OR CONSTRICTION
SUNS RAYS.

Amelioration – FLOW OF DISCHARGES.

Relation :

Complementry – Hep, Lyc, Nit Ac.

Incompatible – Acet. acid, Carbolic Acid.

Intermittent fever – Nat mur follows Lachesis well when type changes.

Important Questions ?

Q.1. Give indication of Lachesis in following :

1) Mind [1973, 74, 77, 79]
2) Diptheria [1979, 86, 88, 89]
3) Heart [1983, 87, 91]
4) Skin [1977, 81, 91]
5) Female [1972, 73, 75, 77, 95]
6) Tonsillitis [1975, 76, 76 S, 79]
7) Menopause [1966]
8) Drug Picture [1971, 77, 81, 93, 95]

52. LEDUM PALUSTRE

Hahnemann

Common Name – Marsh Tea.

Constitution – Adapted to full blooded and plethoric people who are robust. Such plethoric patients bleed easily, have red faces, they are fleshy, strong and of a robust constitution. Puffy bloated and besotted faces of the drunkards.

Remedy for Surgeon – Ledum pal is a great remedy for surgeons use during injury.

Diathesis – Rheumatic and gouty diathesis.

Relation with heat and cold – Chilly patient with desire for cold.

KEYNOTES

1) ***Chilly patient with lack of animal heat.*** Used for complaints of people who are cold all the time in bed, in the house, always feel cold and chilly.
2) Despite the chilly state all complaints of the people are ***relieved by cold application.***
3) Sufferings are *worse in warmth of bed.* Must get out of the bed which affords relief. *They always feel cold and chilly but still desire cold things.*
4) ***Punctured wounds*** – by sharp pointed instruments, also in rat bites, stings of insects, especially mosquitoes.
5) Injury followed by pain, puffiness and coldness (Lachesis : pain, puffiness and heat).
6) Swellings are pale, sometimes oedematous and aggravated at night in the heat of the bed, uncovering; cold water relieves.
7) *Emaciation of suffering parts.*
8) Ecchymosis ***"Black eye"*** from a blow or contusion.
9) Long remaining *discolouration* after injuries; ***black and blue places become green.***
10) ***Ascending rheumatism,*** begins in feet and ***travels upwards*** (Arnica). Affects principally left shoulder and right hip joint (Cactus and Kalmia have decending rheumatism).
11) Rheumatism and gout; joints become the seat of nodosities and *"gout stones"* which are painful.
12) Pains are worse from motion especially the joints, while walking, getting warm in bed and evening.

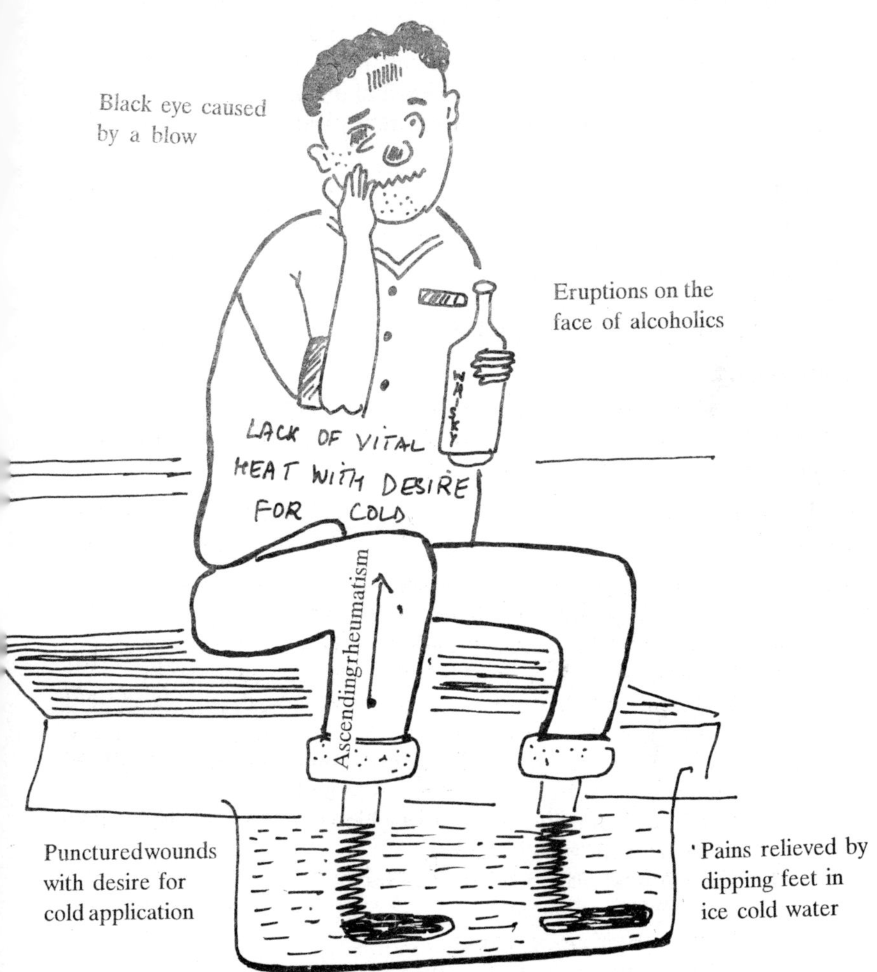
Black eye caused by a blow
Eruptions on the face of alcoholics
WHISKY
LACK OF VITAL HEAT WITH DESIRE FOR COLD
Ascending rheumatism
Puncturedwounds with desire for cold application
Pains relieved by dipping feet in ice cold water

LEDUM PAL

13) Pains are *better by holding feet in ice water.*
14) Stiffness of joints – can only move them after applying cold water.
15) Ledum is to whisky what Caladium is to smoking habit (Ledum helps the patient to break the habit of drinking).
16) Red pimples or tubercles on forehead and cheeks of brandy drinkers.

Particulars :

1) HEADACHE
2) INJURY
3) SKIN
4) RHEUMATISM and GOUT

HEADACHE

Pain in the head with cold body and extremities and hot head. Wants to bathe the head in cold water. Wants the head out in cold air, wants to put it out of the window.

INJURY

EYES

- Heamorrhage in the anterior chamber after iridectomy.
- Ledum is specific for a *'black eye'* from blow of a fist.
- Contusions of the eyes and lids especially if much extravasation of blood takes place. Ecchymosis of lids and conjunctiva.
- Ledum is excellent for *punctured wounds* such as sticking of a nail into the foot or an awl into the hand, for stings of insects, rat bites, mosquito bites. It makes no difference so as what kind of tissue is involved by this kind of wound.
- For black and blue spots from blows or bruises there is no better remedy than Ledum.
- *Open lacerations and cuts – Calendula.*
  Nerve injury – Hypericum
  Injury to Periosteum – Ruta
  Injury to Bone – Calcearea Phos, Symphytum
  Sore bruised injuries both acute and chronic – Arnica.
- Long remaining *discolouration after injuries;* black and blue places become green.
- Punctured wounds that bleed scantily but are followed by *pain, puffiness and coldness* (Pain, puffiness and heat – Lachesis).
- Ledum helps to finish up an Arnica case and removes the *discolouration* and ecchymosis more perfectly.
- Punctured wounds or wounds of septic nature, abscesses etc very sensitive to touch and *relieved by cold application*.
- Whitlows and felons caused by needle pricks.

- Ledum should be given when tetanus follows punctured wounds (Hypericum).
- *Emaciation of suffering parts* – A nerve that is injured by a puncture takes on infection and becomes inflamed, congested and oedematous. The part becomes cold to touch. The nerve that supplies the part takes on ascending neuritis; pains shoot along the nerves and the muscles that are supplied by the nerve dwindle and the part whithers (Puls).

SKIN

- Intense itching of feet and ankles, aggravated from scratching and warmth of bed (Puls, Rhus).
- Red pimples or tubercles on forehead and cheeks as in brandy drinkers, stinging when touched.
- Easy spraining of ankles and feet (Carbon An).
- Dropsical condition – Purple, mottled and bloated condition of the hands and feet with relief from putting the feet in ice water.

RHEUMATISM and GOUT

Cause – Altered secretion and deposit of solid substances like uric acid, sodium and other crystals.

Location – Rheumatism begins in the feet and ascends upwards. Throbbing pain in the left shoulder and right hip. Ledum especially affects the knee joint.

Sensation – Parts feel cold to touch and are better by dipping in cold water. Patients sit with joints exposed to cold, fanning it or putting on evaporating lotions.

Character of pain :

Acute rheumatism – Joints are swollen and hot but not red. The swellings are pale and the pains are worse at night and from heat of the bed; wants them uncovered.

Chronic rheumatism – Joints swollen and painful especially in the heat of the bed with painful hard nodes and concretions first in the joints of the feet, then hands. Periosteum of phalanges painful on pressure. Ankles swollen and soles painful and sensitive; can hardly step on them; (Ant crud, Lyco, Silicea).

Relief from cold is so prominent that the only relief is from dipping the feet in water, copious pale urine. Pains are *worse* from motion, warmth, covering.

Gout – Chalk stone deposits in the wrists, fingers and toes. Deposits affect the *great toe* and follow upwards. Gouty joints become suddenly inflamed and are *relieved by cold and copious urination. Aggravation by warmth and motion.* Urine in gouty states becomes diminished or increased and light in specific gravity, stream often stops during the flow. When there is clear and copious urine with little deposit, the gouty deposits in the joints become marked and the patient has marked aggravation. The patient feels better when there are great quantities of sandy deposits passing away.

General Modalities

Worse – WARMTH,
COVERING
MOTION.

Better – COLD WATER AND HOLDING FEET IN ICE COLD WATER. COPIOUS URINATION IN CASE OF RHEUMATISM.

Relations :

Remedies that follow well – Sulphuric acid, Acon, Bell, Bry, Chel, Nux, Puls, Rhus, Sulph.

Inimicals – China.

Antidotes – Camphor.

Important Questions ?

Q.1. Give indication of Ledum in the following :
1) Arthritis [1973, 79, 82, 93]
2) Gout [1973]
3) Injury [1977]

Q.2. Compare :
Ledum and Calendula in injury [1996]
Ledum and Staphysagria in injury [1987]
Ledum and Hypericum in injury [1977]

CALENDULA	STAPHYSAGRIA	HYPERICUM	LEDUM
Lacerated or *ragged* wounds with or without loss of substance accompanied with soreness and pain. It reduces inflammation and promotes granulation. Dr. Ludlam "*No suppuration* seems to be able to live in its presence."	*Incised wounds;* suitable in clean cut wounds especially after *surgical operations* where pains are excruciating, tearing causing great agony.	*Lacerated wounds*. Injuries to *nerves* or parts rich in nerves that are exceedingly painful. Nails or splinters in feet crushing of toes, smashing fingers with *ascending neuritis*.	*Punctured wounds* from nails and awls, mosquito bites, insect and rat bites. Coldness of wounded parts relieved by cold application. Long remaining discolouration after injury. *'Black eye'* from blow of fits.

53. LYCOPODIUM CLAVATUM

Hahnemann

Common Name – Wolfs foot : Club Moss.

Lycopodium is a constitutional *deep acting remedy for deep seated progressive diseases*. It is nicknamed as "Vegetable Sulphur'. It is rarely advisable to begin treatment of chronic diseases with Lycopodium unless clearly indicated. It is better to give another antipsoric first. Lyco being a *deep seated and long acting remedy* should rarely be repeated once improvement begins.

Constitution – *Intellectually keen but physically weak* people. Lean people tending towards lung and liver troubles. Subject is sallow and sunken with premature lines on face; looks older than he is. Emaciation of the upper part of body and dropsy of lower part.

CHILD – Weak with well developed heads but puny sickly bodies. Emaciation of the upper part of the body. Face has creases and wrinkles. Irritable child when sick, awakes out of sleep ugly and sick, scream and push away the nurse or parents.

Relation with heat and cold – *Chilly* patient and is sensitive to cold drinks and cold air. Head and spine symptoms aggravated by warmth.

Miasm – Trimiasmatic remedy. Lyco is antipsoric, antisycotic and antisyphilitic remedy.

Diathesis – *Lithic and uric acid diathesis Predisposed to lung and liver affections.*

Temperament – Irritable temperament.

KEYNOTES

1) ***Right sided remedy*** – Symptoms go from right to left. (Lachesis – left to right).
2) Dark complexioned people emaciated about the face and neck, bloated and swollen in lower parts. ***Intellectually keen but feeble muscular development.***
3) Dread of men and solitude, weeping tendency. Confused state of mind with great anticipation.
4) ***Aggravation*** of all complaints from ***4-8 P.M.***
5) ***Canine hunger but anxiety after a few mouthfuls.***
6) Patient ***desires warm things*** and warm drinks and is better by them. Skin, spine and head symptoms are aggravated by warm application.
7) *Craving* for *sweet things*.

8) Excessive accumulation of *flatulence* and he feels bloated after a few mouthfuls. Fermentation in the lower abdomen with loud grumbling and croaking.
9) *Fan like motion of alae nasi* occuring in cerebral, abdominal and respiratory complaints.
10) ***Red sand in urine.*** Child cries before urinating.
11) *Hungry* when waking at *night*. (Cina, Psor.)
12) *Impotence of old* and *young men* from sexual excess. Old men with strong desire but imperfect erections.
13) *Dryness of vagina* – burning before and after coition.
14) *One foot hot and the other cold.*
15) Right sided hernia.
16) Constipation due to constriction of anus (Nux vom : due to deficient peristalsis; Bryonia : dryness of rectum).
17) Rheumatic pains are better from warmth of bed and motion. Extreme restlessness and must keep turning.
18) Severe *backache better by passing urine*. Back burning as from glowing coals between the scapulae.
19) Eruptions of Lycopodium – ulcers, abscesses are better by cool application and aggravation by warm poultices.

Particulars :

1) MIND
2) HEADACHE
3) FACE
4) CHILD
5) RESPIRATORY SYSTEM
6) GIT
7) URINARY SYSTEM
8) MALE SEXUAL SYMPTOMS
9) FEMALE SEXUAL SYMPTOMS
10) SKIN
11) FEVER

MIND

Intellectually keen but *physically weak people*. Person generally tries to *avoid responsibilities*. They feel they are weak and unable to cooperate with responsibilities. They put up to the world an image of capability, extroverted friendliness and courage. The patient seeks a situation in which desire for sexual gratification can be satisfied without having to face personal resposibilities. Because Lycopodium fits *intelligent people* it is found frequently in professors requiring public performance, priests lawyers, school teachers and even politicians. A priest may feel perfectly well before giving a sermon but upon reaching the dias he realises that so

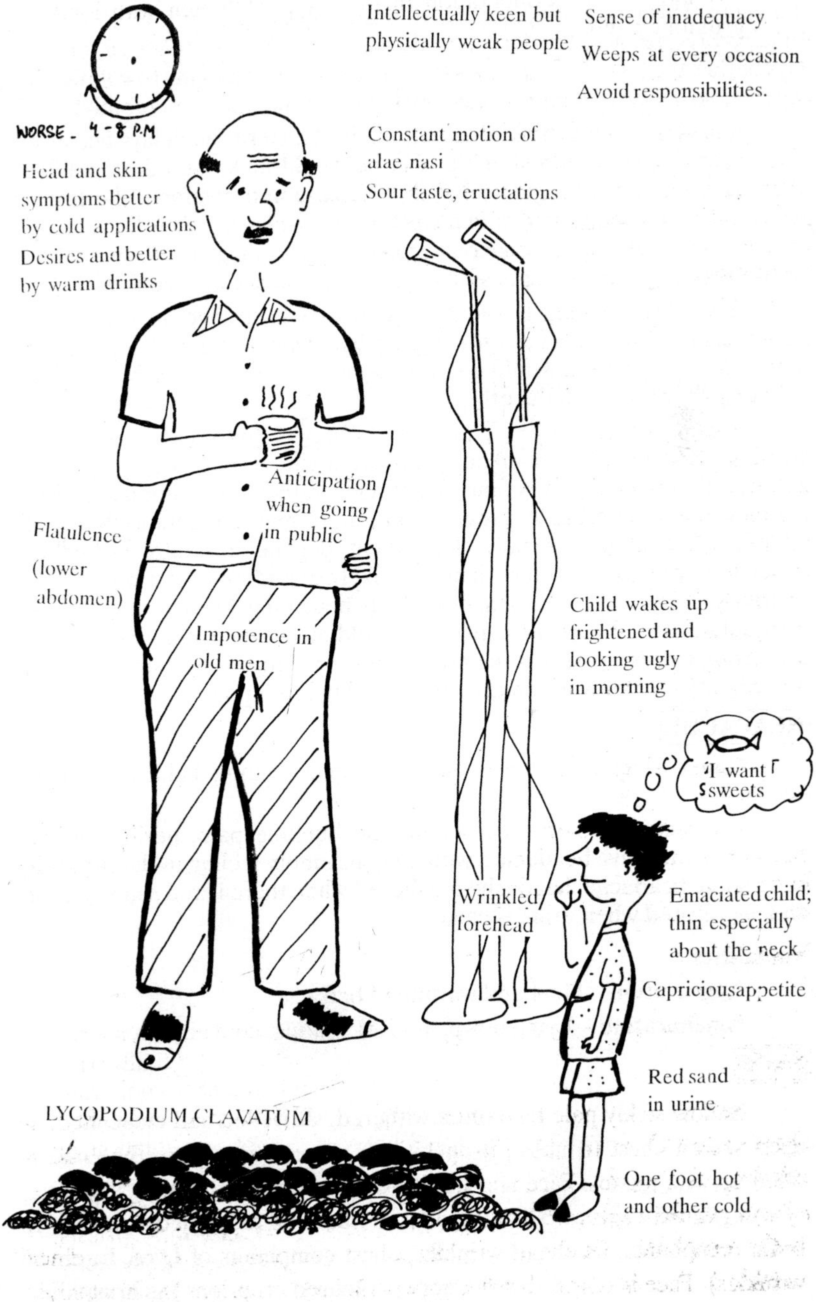

Intellectually keen but physically weak people

Sense of inadequacy

Weeps at every occasion

Avoid responsibilities.

WORSE - 4 - 8 P.M

Constant motion of alae nasi

Sour taste, eructations

Head and skin symptoms better by cold applications

Desires and better by warm drinks

Anticipation when going in public

Flatulence (lower abdomen)

Child wakes up frightened and looking ugly in morning

Impotence in old men

'I want sweets'

Wrinkled forehead

Emaciated child; thin especially about the neck

Capriciousappetite

Red sand in urine

LYCOPODIUM CLAVATUM

One foot hot and other cold

many people are waiting for him, he develops gastritis due to apprehension or anxiety. This is again an example of anxiety in the face of responsibility. *Anticipatory anxiety* in Lyco. is more during the actual task (*Gels* : hours or days before the task; *Silicea* – lack of self confidence, inability to coop with any responsibility; *Nat mur* – emotional and sentimental vulnerability).

A lawyer cannot think of appearing in the court; he delays because of the fear that he would stumble, that he would make mistakes and yet when he undertakes he goes through with ease and comfort. The Lyco. person suffers from a *sense of inadequacy and weakness* – thus he actually presents with a strong, courageous and competent image to the world but his bluff is called when responsibility and performance are required.

Fear – Lyco patient has fear of ghosts, dark, strange things, fear of facing responsibility. *They desire company but in next room*. If there are two rooms the Lyco patient would go into one and stay there though very glad to have someone else in the other.

Weak internally – Lyco. patient often breaks down and weeps when meeting a friend, when thanked, receiving a gift. In later stages there is deterioration of mental functions. They begin initially with poor memory in the morning and gradually progress to a more marked memory loss and intellectual weakness. Finally the patient degenerates into a state of imbecility or senility. Such patients are likely to end up in rest homes at a relatively early stage. They may end up becoming loners, spinsters or spiritual seekers. *Failure of sensorium* of old men – the memory fails, they use wrong words to express themselves, mix up things in writing, unable to do ordinary mental work on account of failing brain power.

HEADACHE

Cause – Heat, gastric trouble, irregular eating habits, Ureamic headaches.

Character of pain – Throbbing and bursting pain, periodical and bursting, congestive headaches with all gone empty feeling in the stomach. In ureamic headache, headache is relieved when there is red sand in urine and aggravated when urine is clear.

Modalities :

Aggravation – Heat and warmth of bed.

Amelioration – Lying down, 4-5 P.M., eating, cold air, open air.

FACE

Sallow sickly pale face often withered, shrivelled and emaciated. In deep seated chest troubles, bronchitis or pneumonia where the chest is filled up with mucus. Face and forehead are *wrinkled* from pain and *wings of nose flap with efforts to breathe*. This occurs in all forms of dyspnoea. (In brain complaints, forehead wrinkles; chest complaints of Lyco. forehead wrinkles). Face is covered with copper coloured eruptions (as in syphilis).

Oversensitive patient and with every slamming of the door, ringing of the bell the face wrinkles. *Jaw drops* as a mark of great exhaustion.

CHILD

Lyco. is extremely useful in children who wither after pneumonia or bronchitis, emaciate about the face and neck, take cold on slightest provocation, suffer from headache from being overheated, nightly headaches with a state of congestion that affects the mind more or less in which they arouse out of sleep in *confusion*. Little one screams out in sleep, *awakes frightened, looks ugly* and cannot recognise his parents until a few moments pass when he is able to collect his senses after a few minutes. Child *wakes up in fright and looks strange and confused*. Throbbing and bursting headaches better from cold and worse from heat and 4-8 P.M.

Eczema of infants – Eczema in a lean hungry and withered child with more or less head trouble, moist oozing behing the ears, red sand in urine, wrinkled forehead, kicks off covers, a child whose left foot is cold and other hot, capricious appetite, great thirst and yet losing weight steadily will often be cured by Lycopodium. It will throw out a greater amount of eruption first but will subside finally and child would return to health. Child desires sweets.

RESPIRATORY SYSTEM

Coryza :

Cause – Exposure to cold.

Character of discharge – Violent coryza with acrid discharge from nose and profuse lachrymation. In chronic catarrah discharge of crusts and elastic plugs with great dryness and stopping of nose causing frequent starting and choking during sleep. Patient has to breathe through open mouth especially during sleep.

Modalities :

Aggravation – Cold air.

Amelioration – Warmth.

Tonsillitis :

Location – Complaints start from right side and go to the left side.

Symptoms – Swelling and suppuration of tonsils aggravated from cold things. Great dryness, even saliva dries on the palate and lips and becomes stiff. Gums and palate get a lardaceous coating and stick very badly.

Modalities :

Worse – Cold things.

Better – Warm drinks, tea etc.

Diptheria :

Dirty greyish membrane starts from right side and goes to left. Feeling of contraction in the throat which prevents food and water from going down. They regurgitate through nose and cause a sensation of choking. Constant desire to swallow but swallowing is accompanied by violent stinging pains – > Cold drinks
< Warm things.

Pneumonia :

Stage of Hepatisation

Site – Later stages of acute attack when generally the lower lobe of right lung is affected and especially if liver complaints arise (Chel., Bry, Merc sol, Kali carb).

Symptoms – There is neither free expectoration nor perfect absorption of the diseased product taking place. Extreme dyspnoea and the cough sounds as if the entire parenchyma of the lung were softened. Even raising whole *mouthfuls of mucus does not afford relief*. Short breath and wings of the nose expand to their utmost with *fan like motion of the alae nasi* – Lycopodium is indispensible in such cases.

Aggravation – 4-8 P.M.

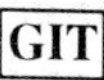

Mouth :

Sour taste in the mouth with a white coated tongue. Tongue is covered with numerous small blisters that burn and scald.

Dyspepsia :

- Atonic type of dyspepsia in persons of weak health.
- *Canine hunger but satiety after a few mouthfuls*.
- Complaints aggravate between *4-8 P.M.*
- Epigastric region is extremely sensitive to touch and tight clothing.
- One of the leading *trio of flatulent* remedies (Lyco, China, Carbo veg). Constant fermentation of gas going on in the abdomen which produces a loud croaking and rumbling. Rumbling of flatulence is found particularly in region of splenic flexure of colon or left hypochondria.

- Nausea and vomiting in gastric catarrah.

Sour stomach – sour vomiting, distension, flatus, pain after eating with a sense of fullness. Lyco. patients are always *belching*, they have eructations that are sour acrid like strong acid burning in the pharynx.

< Cold things, oyesters

> Warm drinks.

Liver :

Lyco. is indicated in chronic liver troubles of *atrophic* variety (China : liver troubles of hypertrophic variety).

Tenderness in the right hypochondrium. Due to atrophy of liver there is stagnation of circulation causing swelling and *enlargement of veins*. Big tortuous varices in the legs, genitilia etc that bring on fatigue and weariness after slight walking. Labia too are swollen with varices particulary during pregnancy.

Piles :

Bleeding piles which contain far great quantity of blood than the size of the vein involved. Piles which do not mature but from which partial absorption of their contents remain as hard bluish lumps.

Stools :

Constipation – Caused due to constriction of rectum. Rectum is full without urging. Nux vom – Constipation due to deficient peristalsis; Bry – Constipation due to dryness of rectum.)

Diarrhoea – Any kind of stool with chilliness in rectum before stools.

URINARY SYSTEM

Lithic and uric acid diathesis

Site – Lyco. is suitable in right sided renal colic, chronic cystitis, diabetes insipidus.

Character of urine – Red sand in urine. Inactivity of bladder and the patient has to wait a long time for the urine to pass. Feeble stream and is slow to flow. Child cries before urination.

Enuresis in children – Involuntary urination during sleep; *polyuria at night*. Patient has to get up many times at night to pass urine. Normal urine in daytime.

Concomitant – Backache is relieved after urination.

Aggravation – 4-8 P.M.

MALE SEXUAL SYMPTOMS

Strong desire without or with feeble erections. Persons of feeble vitality, overtired persons with feeble genital organs. A young man who has indulged in secret vices realises that he is sexually impotent after marriage.

The penis becomes small cold and relaxed with feeble erections; he falls asleep during an embrace.

FEMALE SEXUAL SYMPTOMS

Dryness of vagina due to which coition becomes painful. Burning in vagina before and after coition. Neuralgia of uterus especially the right ovary. Young girls who do not menstruate at puberty with underdeveloped breasts, Lyc. estabilishes a reaction, breasts begin to grow and child becomes a woman. (Calc. phos.)

Physometra – Discharge of flatus from vagina.

Pregnancy – Varices of genitilia .Lyco. is a medicine for morning sickness. Nausea, vomiting and anorexia in the first month of pregnancy. During pregnancy when the *movement of foetus in the womb* becomes a regular source of annoyance and distress to the mother Lyc. checks the excessive movement and also helps in ultimate expulsion of the child at proper time.

SKIN

Ulcers, abscesses, cellular troubles, eruptions with violent itching, vesicles and scaly eruptions, eruptions about the lips, behind the ears, fissures. Ulcers bleed and form great quantities of thick, yellow offensive and green pus. All complaints are *worse from warmth,* warm poultices and better by cool application.

Feeble state of arteries, veins with poor tone and circulation. Numbness in spots. Deadness of fingers and toes.

FEVER

- All types of fever which aggravate between 4-8 P.M. Dirty pale and sallow complexion.
- One foot hot and other cold.
- Sour vomiting between chill and heat.
- Great thirst with desire to uncover during heat stage.
- Great thirst after sweat.
- Perspiration immediately after chill.

Typhoid Fever :

Indicated between second and third week due to suppressed rash. Patient becomes stupid and lies with dropped jaws and half open eyes. Patient lies stupid and eyes do not react to light. Depression of sensorium with confused state of mind. Muttering delirium, picking at bed clothes, involuntary urine or retention of urine; blistered tongue with distension of abdomen.

General Modalities

Aggravation – 4-8 P.M.
COLD DRINKS AND FOOD
OYESTERS

(Head and skin symptoms are aggravated by warmth.)

Amelioration – WARM FOOD AND DRINK
UNCOVERING HEAD
LOOSENING GARMENTS

Relations :

Complementry – Iodine.

Bad affects of Onions, Breads, Wine, Oyesters, Spirituous liquors, tobacco smoking and chewing.

Follows well after – Calc., Carbo veg, Lach, Sulph.

Important Questions ?

Q.1. Give indication of Lycopodium in the following :

1) Diptheria [1989]
2) Female sexual symptoms [1987, 88, 89]
3) Male sexual symptoms [1990, 95]
4) GIT [1986, 88, 74, 87, 93]
5) Impotency [1993]
6) Drug picture [1970, 73, 74]
7) Marasmus [1976]
8) Urinary Disorders [1992]
9) Hepatitis [1987]
10) Desires and Aversions [1991]
11) Flatulence [1968]

Q.2. Compare :

1) Lycopodium and Silicea in Mental Generals. [1987 S]
2) Gastric complaints of Lycopodium, Raphanus, Carbo veg, China. [1993]
3) Liver complaints of Lycopodium and Chelidoneum. [1994 S]

I. MENTAL GENERALS :

LYCOPODIUM	SILICEA
• Sense of inadequacy. Avoids responsibilities. Tendency to weep. Desires company but in next room. • Anticipation on going in public gathering .	• Timid person – lack of self confidence and inability to coop with any responsibility; pin mania. There is want of grit both mental and physical. Lack of stamina and much afraid of failure.

II. GASTRIC COMPLAINTS :

LYCOPODIUM	CHINA	CARBO VEG	RAPHANUS
Flatulence in lower abdomen with sour stomach and canine hunger. No relief from passing flatus.	Flatulence in whole abdomen. No relief from passing flatus or belching.	Flatulence in upper abdomen. Patient is cold to touch, desires open air, fanning and loose clothing.	Tympanic abdomen which becomes full to a bursting state. No passage of gas whatsoever through eructations or through bowels.
< 4-8 P.M. cold food and drinks, oyesters.	< Fruits, fresh wine and slightest touch.	< Eating driking, Lying down.	
> Warm drinks and food.	> Hard pressure.	> Eructations and passing flatus.	

III. LIVER TROUBLES :

LYCOPODIUM	CHELIDONEUM
• Atrophic liver leading to pale face, varicosities in various places in body – legs, genitilia etc.	• Chelidoneum is indicated in liver diseases with constant pain under the lower and inner angle of scapula.
• Desire warm drinks and sweets.	• Desires hot drinks.
• Sour stomach with canine hunger but a few mouthfuls fill up the stomach.	• Yellow grey colour of whole skin.
• Aggravation – 4-8 P.M., cold food and drinks.	• Nausea and vomiting with bitter taste in mouth.

54. MAGNESIA PHOSPHORICA

T.A. Gann

Common Name – Phosphate of Magnesia.

"A NUTRITION AND FUNCTIONAL REMEDY FOR NERVE TISSUES." Magnesia phos acts best when given in hot water.

Constitution – Best adapted to thin emaciated persons of a highly nervous organisation, dark complexion.

Relation with heat and cold – Chilly patient : cold air is intolerable and cause of most complaints.

KEYNOTES

1) ***Right sided affections*** – head, ear, face, chest, ovary, sciatic nerve (Bell, Bry, Chel, Kali carb, Lyco., Podo.).
2) ***Neuralgia*** anywhere in the body with sharp *shooting lightning like pain coming and going.* Intermittent pain which *changes places* and drives the patient to frenzy (Lac. can, Puls).
3) *Cramping pain* in neuralgic affections of stomach, abdomen and pelvis. (Caul., Colo). Pains radiate from one part to another.
4) *Great dread of cold air* – uncovering, cold bathing, washing, touching the affected part.
5) ***Amelioration of complaints by heat and pressure.***
6) Colic flatulent, forcing the patient to bend double. Amelioration by heat, rubbing and hard pressure. (Colo., Plumb.)
7) *Dysmenorrhoea* with characteristic *cramping pains*, doubling up the patient and only relieved by heat.
8) *Cramps from prolonged exertion. "Writers cramp".* Cramps that come in the fingers from writing, piano playing, labourers, calves.
9) Cramps of stomach with clean tongue as if a band was drawn tightly around the body.
10) Mag. phos is a wonderful remedy for *spasmodic hiccoughing.*
11) *Violent toothache aggravated by cold things and better by warmth* (better by cold – Puls, Bry, Coff.).
12) *Facial neuralgia*, headache better by pressure and external heat and aggravated by cold air.
13) Ailments of *teething children with spasms* during dentition and no fever. (Bell – with fever, hot head and skin).

14) *Nocturnal enuresis*; from nervous irritation, after catheterisation.

Particulars :

1) HEADACHE
2) NEURALGIA
3) CRAMPS/CONVULSIONS
4) COLIC
5) DYSMENORRHOEA

HEADACHE

Cause – Cold air, cold place, headache of school girls from mental emotion and exertion of hard study (Calc. phos, Nat mur, Psor., Tuber.)

Location – Occiput and extends over to head;right sided headache (Sang, Sil.).

Sensation – Violent attacks of headache with throbbing pain. Chronic congestive headache with red face (Bell.).

Modalities :

< Cold air, mental exertion.

> Heat and tight bandaging.

NEURALGIA

Cause – Cold air, cold damp weather etc.

Location – Right sided neuralgia. Trigeminal neuralgia (Supra and Infra orbital neuralgia of face).

Character of pain :

- Lightning like pain coming and going; intermittent pains.
- Wandering pains with great periodicity.
- Sharp shooting unendurable pains which drive the patient frantic.

Modalities :

< Cold air and cold application.

> Heat, hot fomentation and hard pressure.

CRAMPS/CONVULSIONS

Cause – Prolonged exertion, cold air, uncovering.

Symptoms :

- *Writers cramp* – Useful in cramps that come in fingers from writing, playing piano, labourers, carpenters.
- Sudden stiffness of fingers and fingers cannot perform their use.
- Patient screams with violent cramps in dysentry and cholera morbus.

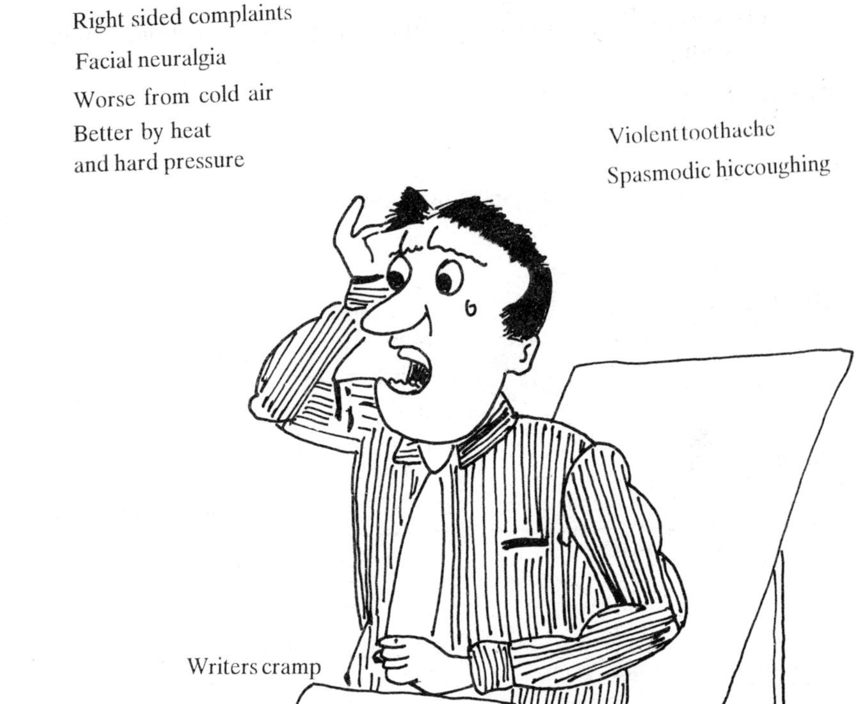

Right sided complaints
Facial neuralgia
Worse from cold air
Better by heat
and hard pressure

Violent toothache
Spasmodic hiccoughing

Writers cramp

Severe colic
Cramping and wandering
pains. Worse by
cold air. Better
by heat and
doubling up.

MAGNESIA PHOSPHORICA

- Convulsions in adults and children (dentition) followed by extreme sensitiveness to touch, wind, noise, excitement. Convulsions with stiffness of limbs and thumbs drawn in.
- Spasms of stomach with clean tongue.

Modalities :

< cold air, uncovering

> warmth, heat, hard pressure.

GIT

Colic (flatulent colic) :

- *Cramping pains* that *radiate* in the abdomen.
- Pains are unendurable and compel the patient to bend double.

< cold things and application, slightest touch.

> warmth and hard pressure, doubling up.

Mag. phos. is a wonderful remedy for spasmodic hiccoughing.

COLIC NEURALGIA :

MAG PHOS	COLOCYNTH
• Right sided	• Left sided
• **Cause** – Cold air, cold damp weather. Cramping pains better by hard pressure, heat and bending double.	• **Cause** – Anger, vexation cramping pains better by bending double.
• **Worse** – 4-9 P.M., Cold air.	• **Worse** – Anger, 4-9 P.M.

FEMALE SYMPTOMS

Membranous Dysmenorrhoea :

Menses :

Time – Early.

Quantity – Profuse.

Character of blood – Dark and stringy.

Concomitants – Sharp shooting pains like lightning more on right side. Better by bending double, hot application and warm drinks.

Pains < before menses

> when flow begins (Lach., Zinc. met.)

General Modalities :

Aggravation – A DRAFT OF COLD AIR
COLD WIND, COLD BATHING
WASHING, MOTION, TOUCH.

Amelioration – BENDING DOUBLE
HEAT, WARMTH
PRESSURE.

Important Questions ?

Q. 1. Give indications of Mag. phos in :
1) Abdominal Colic [1972, 73, 78]
2) Neuralgic pains [1976]

Q. 2. Compare :
Neuralgia – Ars alb/Mag phos [1988]
Toothache – Mag Phos/Chamomilla [1987 S]
Colic – Mag phos, Medorrhinum, Puls., Staph, Verat alb [1973]

NEURALGIA :

ARS. ALBUM	MAG. PHOS
• Burning pains relieved by heat.	• Shooting pains, wandering from one part to another < cold air > heat, hard pressure

TOOTHACHE :

CHAMOMILLA	MAG PHOS
• Violent toothache caused by anger or taking anything warm, coffee, during menses, pregnancy < heat > wet weather	• Violent toothache < cold air > warm food and drinks, hard pressure

COLIC :

VERATRUM ALBUM	PULSATILLA	STAPH.	MAG PHOS	MEDORRHINUM
• Colic with cramps commencing in hands and feet, spreading all over the body. Cold sweat on forehead. Profuseness of all discharges with great prostration.	• Paroxysmal pain : one sided neuralgia accompanied by great chilliness. More the pain greater the chilliness. Desires cold or open air.	• Neuralgia of shoulder joint and arm. Right sided affections. > cold air <warmth	• Right sided affections. Shooting pains wandering from one part to another <cold air > heat, hard pressure.	• Hot patient with coldness all over and burning of extremities. Despite the coldness the patient wants to be uncovered and fanned. Restless patient with trembling all over the body and soreness of all parts. < heat, uncovering, sunrise to sunset, thinking about complaints. > seashore, lying on stomach, damp weather.

55. MERCURIUS SOLUBILIS

Hahnemann

Common Name – Quick Silver (The element of mercury).

Mercurius is the *king of Antisyphilitic remedies*.

Constitution – Best adapted to light haired persons with a lax skin and lax muscles. In some cases jaundice and yellow colouration is marked.

Temperament – Easily frightened nature with rapid and hurried speech.

Relation with heat and cold – *Human Barometer* – Due to lack of defensive power Mercurius patient is sensitive to everything heat, cold, outdoor, wet weather, change of weather, warmth of bed, perspiration, exertion, various food.

Diathesis – Syphilitic/Rheumatic and gouty.

Miasm – Syphilis. King of anti-syphilitic remedies.

KEYNOTES

1) ***Lack of defensive power*** – Mercurius patient is aggravated by everything. Living thermometer affected by both heat and cold.
2) All complaints are ***worse at night.***
3) ***Glandular swellings*** with or without suppuration, but especially if suppuration is too profuse (Hep., Sil.).
4) *Lack of reactive power* is the underlying cause for Mercurius aggravation from suppression of discharges. When a suppuration or ulceration is established there is not enough power to heal them so a progressive decomposition results.
5) ***Profuse perspiration*** attends nearly all complaints. Sweating does not relieve the suffering. (Profuse perspiration relieves – Nat. mur, Psor, Verat.).
6) ***Offensiveness*** of discharges is marked (due to decomposition, breath and body smell foul.).
7) *Catarrah* – with much sneezing; fluent acrid corossive; nostrils raw, ulcerated; yellow green foetid pus like discharge, nasal bones swollen < night, damp weather.
8) ***Increased salivation*** – Foetid, coppery metallic tasting saliva.
9) *Tongue* – flabby, large and shows imprint of teeth. (Chel, Podo, Rhus).
10) *Intense thirst* although *tongue looks moist* and saliva is profuse (Puls, Nux mosch – dry mouth without thirst).

11) *Diptheria* – inflamed tonsils, swollen uvula, elongated with constant desire to swallow, profuse offensive saliva.
12) *Dysentry* – *Slimy, bloody stools* with colic and fainting. – Great tenesmus during and after stools. Tenesmus not relieved by stool. Tenesmus not relieved by stool and is followed by chilliness and "cannot finish" sensation. The 'more the blood' better is Merc sol. indicated.
13) Quantity of *urine voided* is *greater than the amount of water*; frequent urging to urinate.
14) *Leucorrhoea* – Acrid burning with itching and rawness; always worse at night, pruritis < contact of urine which must be washed off.
15) Painful mammae as if they would ulcerate at every menstrual period; milk in the breasts instead of menses.
16) *Trembling of extremities* especially hands, paralysis agitans (unable to hold a glass of water).
17) *Ulcers*; on gums, tongue, throat, inside cheeks with profuse salivation, *irregular and underfined – dirty and unhealthy look* (do not have the power to heal). Discharge of pus with blood. More the amount of blood more is Mercury indicated.

Particulars :

1) MIND
2) HEAD, SCALP
3) EYE
4) EAR
5) GIT
6) RESPIRATORY SYSTEM
7) RHEUMATISM
8) FEMALE SYMPTOMS
9) FEVER
10) SKIN
11) NERVOUS SYSTEM

MIND

Slowness of action – The patient is slow to comprehend and there is slowness of action. *Hurriedness with inefficiency of action* – hurry and restlessness in which the person does not accomplish anything.

Impulsivity – The Mercurius mind because of *vulnerability to stimuli* from without and from within is unable to keep his mind concentrated purely in a particular direction. There is inefficiency of mind with no strength for concentration and the patient becomes susceptible to every

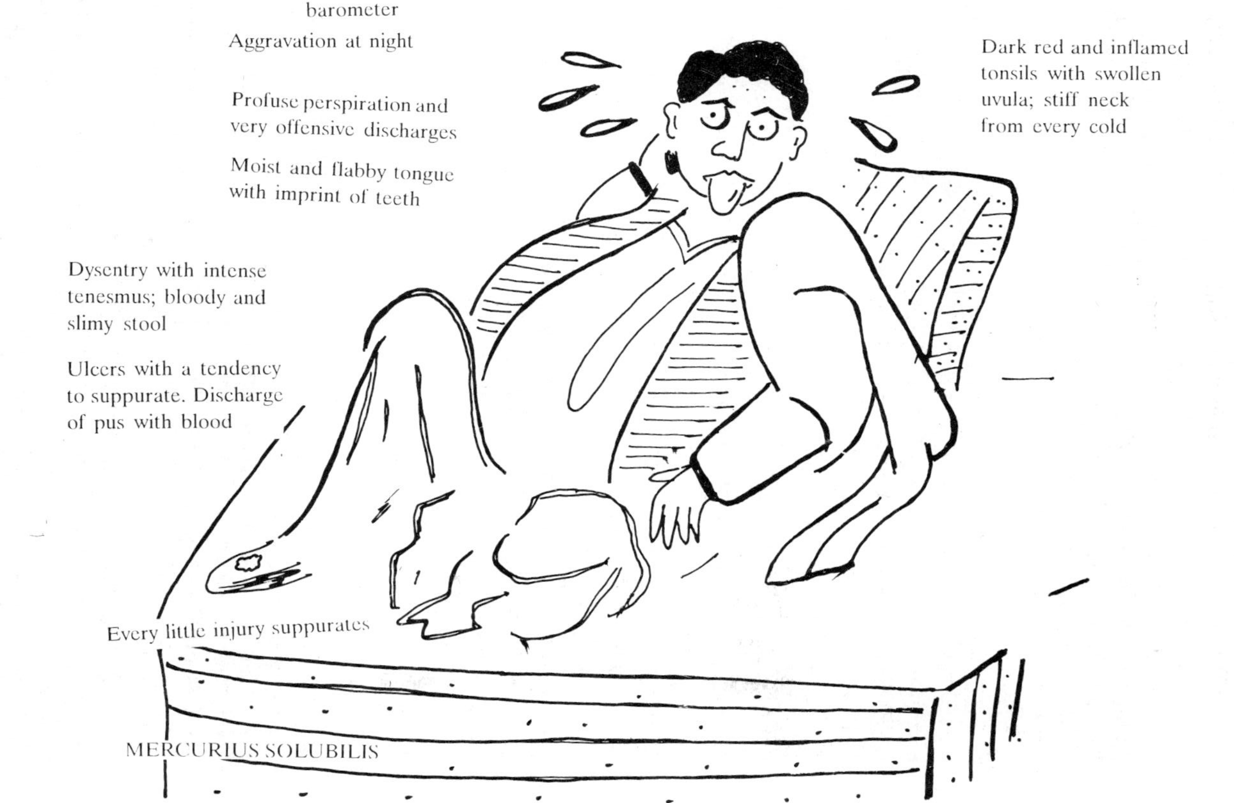
barometer
Aggravation at night
Profuse perspiration and very offensive discharges
Moist and flabby tongue with imprint of teeth
Dysentry with intense tenesmus; bloody and slimy stool
Ulcers with a tendency to suppurate. Discharge of pus with blood
Every little injury suppurates
Dark red and inflamed tonsils with swollen uvula; stiff neck from every cold
MERCURIUS SOLUBILIS

kind of impulse. The person may have an impulse to strike, to smash things, to kill someone over a merely slight offense (Nux vom, Platina).

Closed individual—Slow to answer, reluctant to reveal to others what he is feeling, recognising that his susceptibility can produce trouble for him, he simply holds them inside, not allowing them to be socially visible. This is a fragile strategy and the patient is still just as vulnerable and must expend considerable energy keeping himself under control.

HEAD

Head troubles caused by suppressed discharges (Merc—helps to establish the discharges and relieve the trouble). Rheumatic troubles of scalp/neuralgias/brain troubles with burning and stinging pains, sweating of head, dilated pupils, rolling of the head and aggravation at night with *suppressed discharges*.

HEADACHE

Cause—Suppressed discharges, catarrhal headaches, sudden changes in weather, heat, cold and damp weather.

Location—Pain in the temples, periosteum, above the bridge of the nose, around the eyes as if tied with a tape.

Sensation—Bursting headache with fullness of brain and constriction like a band. Much heat in the head.

Modalities— <Cold, damp weather, night, changes in weather, suppressed discharges, suppressed foot sweat.

> Flow of discharges.

EYE

Catarrah of the eye worse from *looking into the fire or sitting close to the fire*. Mist or fog before the eyes with eyelids forcefully drawn together as if long deprived of sleep.

Iritis of syphilitics—Teasing pains with burning around the eyes and in temples, ulceration and inflammation of cornea. There is copious lachrymation with all eye symptoms and the tears excoriate causing a red line down the cheeks. Lids spasmodically closed. Discharge of thin acrid mucopus.

Syphilitic condylomata—Purulent opthalmia—disturbed vision with great tumefaction and swollen lids—Merc. sol cures in a few days.

EAR

Otitis media with a ruptured drum, *purulent and offensive otorrhoea*. Horribly stinking greenish discharges with stinging pains. (Mercurius is indicated in later stages of inflammation when inflammation merges into suppuration).

GIT

Mouth :

Gums are spongy and swollen with tendency towards bleeding.

Tongue :

Broad, swollen and flabby almost filling up the buccal cavity. Its broad edge is invariably dented with imprints of teeth.

Odour of the mouth is very offensive and disgusting. Tumor of the tongue with difficulty in speech.

Salivation :

Constant overflow of saliva from the mouth. The saliva is tenacious, soapy, stringy and profuse; it gives him a peculiar coppery metallic taste; moist tongue with intense thirst.

Teeth :

Decaying of crowns of teeth, roots remaining black dirty and carious. Sometimes a bright red margin is noticed on the gums which have a tendency to recede, thus exposing the roots of the teeth and making them loose and painful.

Toothache :

Merc sol is the capital remedy for toothache. Tearing and lacerating pains < Damp weather, evening, warmth of bed, taking cold things.

Taste :

Sweetish and metallic taste in the mouth.

Ulcers/apthae – in the mouth with a characteristic offensive discharge. Ulcers have a tendency to extend to the depth.

Stomach :

Aversion – Meat, wine, brandy, coffee, greasy food, milk, sweets.

Gastritis (Acute/Chronic) :

Cause – Liquors, beers, wine, whisky, milk, sweets, change of weather.

Symptoms – Chronically disordered stomach with eructations, regurgitation and vomiting.

- Bad taste in the mouth with constant salivation.
- Half digested food is vomited.
- Fullness in the region of the stomach < Lying on right side, night.

Dysentry :

Cause – Fright, suppressed sweat.

Character of stool – Slimy, bloody, very offensive stool, excoriating the anus. (More the blood, better is Merc sol. indicated). Cannot finish sensation. Tenesmus not relieved after stool. (Nux vom – temporary relief after stool).

Modalities – Aggravated at night.

Concomitants – Colic and fainting with creeping chilliness and thirst. Great tenesmus during and after colic (Maximum tenesmus in Merc. cor after passing stools).

RESPIRATORY SYSTEM

Nose : – Coryza.

Cause – damp chilly weather, damp cool evening air.

Symptoms – Acrid nasal discharge, red and excoriating nose. Bridge of the nose may swell upon both sides. Afterward the discharges become thicker and more bland.

Aggravation – Night, damp weather.

Throat :

Inflammation of throat with spongy appearance, general tumefaction, swelling of the parotids, fullness and stiffness of neck. Great dryness in throat. Swelling impairs the motion of all the muscles that take part in swallowing. Difficulty, pain and paralytic weakness attends swallowing and effort to swallow forces the bolus of food up into the nose. *Dark red and inflamed tonsils* – quinsy after pus has formed with swollen uvula. *Offensive odour* from mouth with *profuse salivation*. *Stiff neck* with swollen glands and goitre. Stiffness from every cold.

Pneumonia :

Stage – Late in hepatisation and resolution stages.

Location – Affects the lower lobe of right lung (Bry, Chel, Kali carb, Lyco).

Character of cough – Dry fatiguing cough usually coming on in two paroxysms. Cough with yellow mucopurulent expectoration which may be mixed with blood, putrid or salty taste, offensive breath.

Modality – Cough aggravated at night and from warmth of bed, when lying on right side; in damp weather. Inability to lie on the right side (Bry, Nat mur, Phos.).

Concomitants – Fever with chilliness, offensive non relieving sweat, moist salivation, flabby tongue with intense thirst.

RHEUMATISM

Merc sol especially affects the joints, inflammatory rheumatism of the joints with much swelling < Night, sweat, warmth of bed and uncovering (it is difficult to get just the right weight of clothing.).

FEMALE

Leucorrhoea – Copious and excoriating leucorrhoea, parts feel raw, inflamed and itchy.

Menstrual flow :

Quantity – Profuse or scanty.

Character of blood – Pale, acrid and clotted.

Concomitants :

- Milk in the breast of the non pregnant women at the menstrual period.
- Chancres on the female genitals.
- Itching in the genitals from the contact of urine, it must be washed off. In children (boys/girls) – urine burns after urinating and they are always carrying their hands to the genitals.
- Boils and abscesses at the menstrual period, little elongated abscesses along the mucous membrane and the skin.

Pregnancy :

- Oedematous swelling of the genitals, diffused inflammation, soreness and fullness of the genitals and pelvis causing difficulty in walking.
- Merc. is an important remedy in pelvic cellulitis in the early months of pregnancy.
- Repeated miscarriages from sheer weakness. Merc sol is an excellent strengthener. Hepar sulph is an excellent palliative in Cancer of uterus and mammae.

FEVER

Type – Surgical, bilious, worm fever, remittent fever, low forms of continued fever.

Symptoms – Very chilly patient sensitive to moving air in a warm room. Cold hand and feet, profuse and offensive sweat.

In catarrhal fever when colds extend to the chest and there are copious discharges everywhere < sweating, night.

SKIN

Every little injury suppurates (Sil, Hep, Graph). Scurfy eruptions, vesicular eruptions, eruptions discharging pus. Violent itching of the skin especially in the warmth of bed at night. Ulcers on parts where skin and flesh are thin over the bone. Ulcers have a tendency to extend to the depth. Profuse offensive, non relieving sweat. *Boils and abscesses* when suppuration has set in with intense pain at night, not relieved by either heat/cold, with fever and chilliness, offensive non relieving sweat with intense thrist.

Ulcers – Irregular in shape, bleed easily, offensive and painful. Pains aggravated at night. More the bleeding more is Merc sol indicated.

- Rawness between thighs and between scrotum and thighs. Rawness and bleeding of the perineum rending walking difficult.
- *Fissures* at the commisures, at the corners of the mouth and eyes.

(In low potency Merc sol hastens suppuration and in high potency aborts suppuration. Persistent dryness of skin contraindicates Merc sol.)

NERVOUS SYSTEM

Trembling runs through the remedy with quivering all over. Tremors of the hands so that he cannot lift anything or eat or write. Merc sol is a great remedy in children with epiletiform fits, twitching and disorderly motion. Merc sol helps children to grow out of these incoordinate angular movements of hand and feet. *Extreme Restlessness* (Even speech is stammering and shows sign of great tremor).

General Modalities :

Aggravation – NIGHT, WARMTH OF BED
WHILE SWEATING
LYING ON RIGHT SIDE
DAMP WEATHER.

Important Questions ?

Q.1. Give indications of Merc sol in the following :

a) GIT [1995, 96]
b) Apthae [1987]
c) Otorrhoea [1987, 79]
d) Skin [1976, 77, 87, 91]
e) Keynotes [1987]
f) Drug picture [1976]
g) Modalities [1973, 77]
i) Generalities [1989]
j) Dysentry [1973, 75, 76, 79, 78, 82]
k) Urinary system [1981]

l) Surgical cases [1981]
m) Cough [1975, 81]
n) Tongue [1977, 82]
o) Tooth decay [1981]
p) Mumps [1981]
q) Breast [1982]
r) Jaundice [1975]
s) Glandular problems [1977]
t) Diptheria [1979]

Q.2. Compare Merc sol and Merc cynatus in diptheria.

DIPTHERIA :

MERC. SOL	MERC. CYN.
• Right sided diptheria.	• Adynamic and malignant diptheria.
• Thick grey membrane with adherent or free borders.	• Quick pulse (130-140 beats/mt).
• Constant desire to swallow although swallowing is painful.	• Membrane is white, covering the velum, palate and tonsils.
• Large flabby moist tongue with imprint of teeth.	• Glands soon begin to swell and the membrane becomes dark threatening to grow gangrenous.
• Intense thirst, moist, tongue, profuse salivation, fetid coppery metallic taste.	• Extreme weakness with fetid breath.
• Swollen and tender cervical glands.	• Necrotic destruction of soft palate with intense redness of fauces.
	• Nose bleed sets in later stages.

56. MERCURIUS CORROSIVUS

Buchner

Common Name – Corossive sublimate.

KEYNOTES

1) ***Dysentry and summer complaints of intestinal canal.***
2) ***Most persistent and terrible tenesmus before during and after stool;*** scanty stool, mucus tinged with blood.
3) *Tenesmus of bladder* with intense burning in urethra; urine hot and burning. Scanty or suppressed urine in drops with great pain.
4) *Throat intensely inflamed,* swollen, burning with swollen gums which bleed easily.
5) *Gonorrhoea* : *second stage*, greenish discharge worse at night with great burning and tenesmus.
6) *Deep ulcers that spread rapidly.*
7) *Corossive nature* of discharges that leave the parts raw and inflamed.
8) Ailments from syphilis, sun, summer weather.

Particulars :

1) EYE
2) THROAT
3) DYSENTRY
4) GONORRHOEA

EYE

Disorders of syphilitic origin, cystitis, choroiditis, iridocyclitis, episcleritis, retinitis heamorrhagica, kerato iritis.

Symptoms :

- Excessive photophobia and acrid lachrymation.
- Lids become red, inflamed and oedematous.
- Trouble starts with excessive photophobia and lachrymation.
- Patient sits in some dark corner to occlude any strong light.
- Gradually the inflammation becomes purulent. Pustules with ulceration on the cornea, phlyctenule discharging ichorous acrid matter. The corossive nature of the discharge from the inflamed area disfigures and excorites the surrounding parts.

THORAT

Sore throat with ulcers spreading rapidly with burning and smarting like coals of fire. Merc cor has *violence, intense burning and rapid spread.* Throat is enormously swollen with swollen glands and insatiable thirst, swollen uvula < external pressure.

DYSENTRY

Cause – Summer weather.

Character of stool – Copious bleeding, slimy, contains streaks of mucus, offensive and frequent evacuation. Sometimes the patient may be passing pure blood in large quantity.

Great urging and tenesmus before, during and after stool. Anus gets raw and inflamed after stool. *Tenesmus not relieved after passing stools.* Number of stools are generally many (constricting pain, prolapse of rectum, constant urging to stool and tenesmus of bladder with suppression of urine are some keynotes for giving Merc cor.)

CYSTITIS

Intense tenesmus of bladder, passing out of hot burning bloody urine in drops with great pain and presence of flesh like pieces of mucus and filaments in urine. *Albuminuria* especially during pregnancy.

MALE ORGANS

Merc cor is an efficient remedy in second stage of *gonorrhoea* when the greenish discharge has set in and burning with tenesmus continues < Night.

General Modalities :

Aggravation – Afternoon, at night during summer.

Amelioration – By rest.

Important Questions ?

Q.1. Give indications of Merc. cor. in the following :

a) Dysentry [1975, 76, 77, 79, 82, 87]
b) Rectal prolapse [1976, 83]
c) Urinary complaints [1981]
d) GIT [1987]

Q.2. Compare Nux vomica and Merc. cor in Dysentry.

MERC. COR	NUX VOMICA
• Dysentry with violent urging for stool.	• Violent urging for stool.
• Tenesmus before, during and after stool.	• Tenesmus before and during but better after stool.
• Passage of pure blood.	• Ineffectual urging for stool.

57. NATRUM MURIATICUM

Hahnemann

Common Name – Chloride of Sodium; Common Salt.

Constitution – Face is sickly looking, greasy, skin shiny, sallow, yellow and often chlorotic covered with vesicular eruptions around the edges of the hair, ears and back of the neck. Scaly and squamous eruptions with great itching, oozing a watery fluid or may be dry. An exfoliation takes place and a shiny surface is left. Watery vesicles form about the lips, wings of nose, genitals. Great itching of skin. Skin looks waxy and dropsical. Emaciation from above downward.

Miasm – All three miasms – Psora, Sycosis and Syphilis are present.

Diathesis – Scrofulous Diathesis.

Relation with heat and cold – Hot patient.

KEYNOTES

1) ***Great emaciation*** – Losing flesh while living well. Well marked emaciation in the neck with losing of flesh while living well. Infant looks like an old man. Collar bone becomes prominent and neck looks scrawny but hips and lower limbs remain plump and round.
2) Symptoms are *worse at sunrise* (10-11 A.M.). Better by perspiration.
3) ***Mapped tongue*** with red insular patches like ringworm on sides (Ars. alb. Kali carb, Rhus tox, Taraxacum).
4) ***Left sided headache*** in school girls which is relieved by perspiration.
5) *Involuntary urination* when walking, laughing and coughing. Cannot pass urine in presence of others (Caust, Puls, Arg. nit).
6) Great ***dryness of mucous membranes*** causes dryness of throat, constipation etc.
7) ***Intense craving for salt***, bitter things, fish, milk.
8) *Aversion* – Bread, coffee, tobacco.
9) *Fluttering of heart* – Hearts pulsations shake the whole body. On account of aneamia, circulation becomes readily excited so that every little exertion produces *throbbing* all over the body. Palpitation of heart is excited by every motion and noise.
10) *Hair fall* out when touched in nursing women.
11) *Hangnails* – Skin around the nails is dry and cracked.

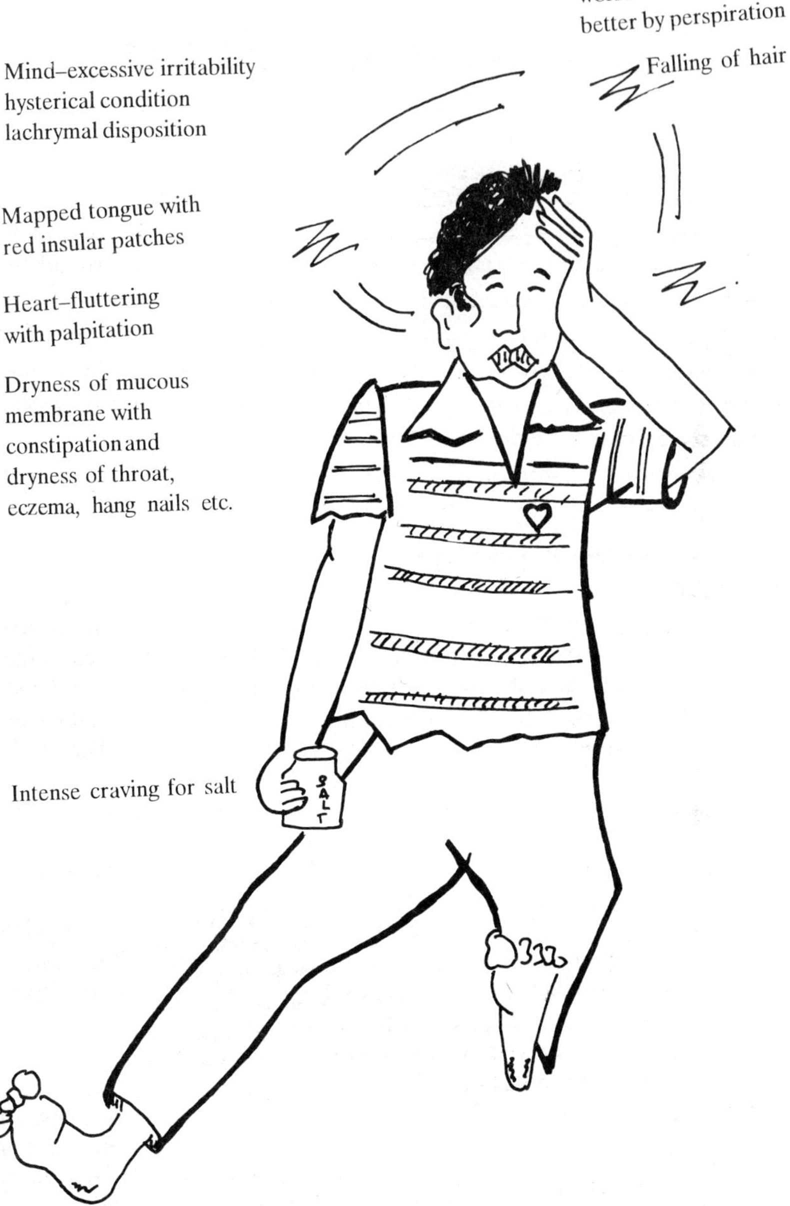
Left sided headache;
worse in sunlight;
better by perspiration
Falling of hair
Mind–excessive irritability
hysterical condition
lachrymal disposition
Mapped tongue with
red insular patches
Heart–fluttering
with palpitation
Dryness of mucous
membrane with
constipation and
dryness of throat,
eczema, hang nails etc.
Intense craving for salt
SALT

NATRUM MURIATICUM

Particulars :

1) MIND
2) ANEAMIA
3) HEAD
4) EYES
5) NERVES
6) NOSE
7) MUCOUS MEMBRANE
8) TONSILS
9) SKIN
10) GIT
11) FEMALE SYMPTOMS
12) MALE GENITAL ORGANS
13) URINARY SYMPTOMS
14) FEVER
15) CHILD

MIND

Depression – Patient is sad and tearful and is made worse by any attempt at condolence. Consolation aggravates her troubles. *Tearful condition* is accompanied with palpitation of heart and intermittent pulse

Hypochondriasis – This keeps up with the degree of indigestion and consolation. Patient keeps angry at trifles. Forgetful patient.

Unrequited affection brings her complaints. She is unable to control her affections and falls in love with a married man or a coachman. She knows she is unwise but cannot help it. In cases of this kind Natrum mur turns her mind into order and she looks back and wonders how silly she was.

ANEAMIA

Natrum mur is indicated when blood is impoverished. The nutrition of the whole system suffers. It is indicated in aneamia particularly in aneamia provoked by loss of animal fluids, in women who suffer from menstrual diseases, men who suffer from loss of semen. Nat mur can be used in scurvy as it is caused due to prolonged use of salted meat. Mapped tongue caused due to ulcers on tongue, gums with a foetid breath and odour. Due to impoverishment of blood the nervous system is secondarily affected.

HEADACHE

Cause – Individuals living in malarial districts, over use of mind, aneamic school girls.

Location – Left sided headache.

Sensation – Pain is so severe that it makes the patient frantic. Bruised feeling about the eyeballs.

Concomitant – *Heaviness of limbs* along with headache especially in aneamic girls whose faces are yellow. Skin is dry and shrivelled and menses are scanty. Periodical headaches associated with intermittent fever. *Dry tongue* that clings to the roof of the mouth. Insatiable thirst.

Aggravation – Sunlight, (10-11 A.M.), overuse of mind.

Amelioration – Sleep, sweating, patient being perfectly quiet.

EYES

Natrum mur produces weakness of muscles. This is especially manifest in muscles of eyes. Muscles of eyelids feel stiff when moving them. Nat. mur is especialy indicated when *internal recti* are affected. Letters blur and run together when looking steadily at them as they are reading. *Scrofulus opthalmia* (inflamed structure being subject to tuberculous and cheesy degeneration). There is smarting and burning pain and feeling of sand beneath the eyelids. Tears are acrid and there is very marked spasmodic closure of the eyelids. Eyelids cannot be forced apart. Ulcers form in the cornea. Eyelids are inflamed and agglutinated in the morning.

(In addition to the eye symptoms scabs form on the scalp and from there oozes a corossive matter. There are moist scabs in the angles of the lips and wings of nose along with emaciation.)

Ciliary neuralgia – especially when pains are periodical returning from sunrise to sunset – (Spigelia, Gels., Glonoine)

NERVES

Spinal irritation – Backache relieved by lying on something hard. Small of back pains as if broken. *Paralysed feeling* – in the lumbar region aggravated in the morning after rising. *Joints* feel weak especially the ankles that are worse in the morning. Coughing and walking aggravate spinal troubles. A general nervous trembling pervades the whole body.

RESPIRATORY SYSTEM

Nose :

Catarrah – Patient easily takes cold in the head and is constantly obliged to wrap it up. If he allows it to be uncovered during the day he has stoppage of nose at night. Inflammation and swelling of the left half of the nose with itching and pain when touched. *Hypersecretion of mucous is* accompanied by paroxysms of *sneezing*. Fluent coryza alternates with dry coryza. Every exposure to fresh air gives the patient cold. Wings of the nose are sore and sensitive. Loss of smell and loss of taste due to catarrah. Nat mur is best indicated in *"Hawking of mucous from throat in the morning."*

Tonsils :

Excess salt intake causes relaxation of muscles. This causes the uvula to be elongated. There is constant feeling of plug in the throat and the patient chokes easily when swallowing. Tongue is mapped and coated with insular patches. *Dryness of mucous membranes* causes the throat to be dry. *Fishbone sensation* in the throat. Inability to swallow without washing down the food with liquids sticking all the way down the oesophagus. Cough is caused due to tickling in the throat or pit of the stomach. It is accompanied with bursting headache.

[**Hepar-S** – Tonsils are swollen, full and purple. Pain in throat and patient is sensitive to slightest draught of cold air.

Nitric acid – Yellow patches in throat with jagged ulcers Urine smells like horses urine.

Arg. nit – Hoarseness. Vocal cords are disturbed . Patulous throat; patient wants cold things and cold water.]

SKIN

Harsh, dry and yellow skin. Patient feels greatly exhausted from little exertion of mind and body. *Dropsical and waxy skin* in old lingering cases of malaria. Urticaria when itching is very annoying. It occurs about the joint particularly about the ankles. Weals form on different parts of the body which itch, smart and burn. Nat mur is doubly indicated when symptoms follow intermittent fever or occur after exposure to damp cold air. Exercise makes this nettlerash intolerably worse. (Acute cases of urticarea – Apis. Chronic cases of urticaria – Nat mur, Sulphur, Sepia, Calc. carb.)

Herpes :

Nat mur is used for hydroa labialis. They are little blisters which form on the borders of the lips and which accompany every marked case of chills and fever.

Eczema :

Especially on margins of hair, scalp and behind the ears. Scabs may ooze pus and cause matting of hair. < Salt, seashore

> Open air.

Warts – On palms of hands.

GIT

Dyspepsia – Bread disagrees. Patient who was fond of bread at one time is totally averse to it. There is distressed and indescribable feeling in the pit of the stomach. This is relieved by tightening the clothing.

(Floric acid, opp – Lachesis, H. Sulph)

Constipation – Constipation causes hypochondriasis. Patient is low spirited and ill humoured during constipation. When bowels are removed the mind is relieved.

Rectum – There is slimy discharge as in chronic prostatitis. Prolapsus ani with a discharge of bloody mucus and water, burning that prevents sleep. Dryness and smarting of rectum and anus with a tendency to erosion of mucous membrane.

Stools – Hard, dry and crumbling.

[*Mag mur* – Crumbling stools.

Phos – Long hard, narrow, dog like stools.

Verat alb – Large stools with much straining until exhausted. Cold and clammy sweat on forehead.

Alumina – Smarting soreness.

Ratanhia – Feeling of splinters or glass and fissures in the rectum.]

FEMALE SYMPTOMS

Females requiring Nat mur are generally chlorotic.

Menses – First menses at puberty is delayed.

Time – Too early.

Duration – Irregular menses lasting for too long or too short duration.

Quantity – Scanty or profuse.

Concomitants – Bearing down pain which is worse in the morning. 'When she gets up in the morning she must sit down to prevent prolapse." Prolapse is due to muscles and ligaments which support the organ. Headache after menses. Uterine symptoms are accompanied with backache and decided spinal irritation which is greatly relieved by lying flat on the back or by pressing the pillow firmly against the back.

MALE GENITAL ORGANS

Great weakness of genital organs giving rise to seminal emissions during sleep. Genital organs are greatly relaxed. As a consequence there is entire emptying of seminal organs with some weakness remaining there. Due to excess seminal loss there is backache, night sweat and weakness in legs. Gonorrhoea is curable by Nat. mur in chronic form. Discharge is generally clear. Cutting in the urethra after urination.

URINARY SYMPTOMS

Slow action of bladder, due to weakness of abdominal muscles. As a result of this, urine slowly dribbles out of force. Involuntary urination while walking, coughing or laughing. Patient cannot pass urine in presence of others. Cutting pain in urethra after urination (Thuja, Sarsaparilla). Sensation as if more urine remained. Frequent urging for urination. Must pass urine very often.

INTERMITTENT FEVER

Nat. mur is used as frequently as China and Arsenic in intermittent fever.

Chill Stage :

Chill comes chacteristically between 10-11 A.M. Chill comes in the small of the back or in the feet. It is accompanied by thirst and aching pains all over the body. Sometimes urticaria may complicate this case. A person freezing to death may want warm clothing but a Nat mur patient wants cold drinks. There is a marked tendency to develop fever blisters.

Heat Stage :

Fever is very violent. Thirst increases with heat. Headache is throbbing and severe with cerebral congestion at times that the patient becomes delirious and unconscious.

Sweat stage

Sweat stage occurs after heat stage. Sweat breaks out copiously and relieves headache and other symptoms.

Apyrexia :

Marked cachexia, canine hunger, obstinate constipaton, enlargement and induration of both liver and spleen (chronic cases). Nat. mur is indicated in people who live in malarial swamps. The patient is aneamic and dropsical. Nat mur removes the tendency to intermittents and patients susceptibility to take cold.

CHILD

Nutrition is greatly impaired in the child. Used in children who suffer from marasmus from defective nourishment. *Look of the baby* – Pale, aneamic, weak and emaciated. Emaciation marked about the neck – (long neck).

Desires – Child craves cold water all the time. There is constant heat and dryness of the mouth all the time which is relieved by cold water. Intense craving for *salt*.

Hot baby with a tendency to catch cold easily.

Aversion to bread.

Tongue – Mapped tongue. Slow learning to talk.

Constipation – Dry and hard stool which is difficult to expel. Due to passage of hard stool there is fissuring of anus accompanied with bleeding during the stool.

Important Questions ?

Q. 1. Give indications of Natrum mur in following :

a) Malaria [1988, 89]
b) Constipation [1986, 89]
c) Headache [1966, 72, 73, 76, 82]

- d) Worm infestations [1994]
- e) Modalities [1973]
- f) Apthae [1987]
- g) Mind [1972, 73, 74, 78, 87, 97]
- h) Female [1976, 81, 82, 86]
- i) Fever [1975, 76, 79, 82, 88]
- j) Tongue [1976, 77]
- k) Heart [1982]
- l) Emaciation [1974, 75, 82]
- m) Drug picture [1972, 74, 76, 82]

Q.2. Compare :

Headache of Sanguinarea and Nat. mur [1982]
Marasmus of Sarsaparilla and Nat mur [1983, 87]
Coryza – Nat. mur/Euphrasia/Allium cepa [1986]
Mind – Sepia/Puls./Nat mur [1971, 72]
Marasmus – Nat mur/Abort/Lyc./Nit. acid [1987]

58. NATRUM PHOSPHORICUM

E. Farrington

Common Name – Sodium Posphate.

Diathesis – Acid Diathesis.

The fluids of the body contain both alkali and acid but a deficiency in acid never occurs because it is organic and like albumin it is always present in sufficient quantities. "An excess of acid" is a misnomer – there is a *deficiency in the phosphate of sodium an alkali* that helps to balance the acid production. A lack of proper balance of the alkali cell salt in gastric juice will allow ferments to arise and so retard digestion such that the lining quickly becomes involved. An inspissation of bile occurs and bilious diarrhoea and other bilious disorders follow.

KEYNOTES

1. ***Acidity* is** preeminently marked.
2) *Sour eructations*, vomit, stool and perspiration *smell acid*.
3) ***Yellow creamy coating at back part of the roof of tongue and mouth***.
4) *Intense acidity* of expectoration so as to cause *soreness* of mouth and *rawness of lips*.
5) *Inflammation of the eyes* – Eyes are glued together especially in the morning with a secretion of golden yellow creamy matter.
6) *Trembling of the heart worse after eating* (Irregular action of the heart caused by imperfect digestion.).
7) ***Worms*** of all kinds with accompanying symptoms of picking the nose, itching at the anus, pain in the abdomen, acidity of stomach, restless sleep.
8) *Rheumatic troubles* (acute or chronic) with *acid diathesis*.
9) *Acidity* also characterises the secretion from *uterus and vagina* (such extreme *acidity* is an important cause of *sterility*.)

Particulars :

1) HEADACHE
2) EYES
3) GIT
4) RESPIRATORY SYSTEM
5) CIRCULATORY SYSTEM
6) RHEUMATISM
7) URINARY SYSTEM
8) FEMALE SEXUAL ORGANS
9) SLEEP

HEADACHE

Cause – Gastric derangement.

Location – Top of the head.

Sensation – Intense pressure and heat in the head.

Concomitants – Yellow coated tongue, vomiting of sour fluids with giddiness and acid eructations.

EYES

Inflammation of the eyes when *secreting a golden yellow creamy matter*. Eyes glued together in the morning. Squinting of eyes when caused by irritation due to worms.

NOSE

Picking at the nose due to acid condition of the stomach. Cold in the head with creamy discharge from the nose and itching of the nose.

GIT

Mouth :

Creamy yellow coating at the back part of roof of mouth. Sour acid taste of the mouth accompanied with canker sores.

Teeth :

Gastric derangements during teething or due to worms.

Tongue :

Creamy yellow golden coating at the back part of the tongue.

Stomach :

All conditions of the stomach with *sour* eructations and sour vomiting. Acid risings with flatulence, headaches, giddiness and morning sickness with vomiting of sour fluid. Stomachache from presence of worms or acidity. *Ulceration* of the stomach where least amount of food causes pain and the tongue and palate have a characteristic creamy yellow coating. Ulceration with vomiting of sour acid fluids or substance like coffee grounds.

Diarrhoea :

Character of stool – Green sour smelling stools caused by acid condition. Much straining and constant urging to stool with passing of jelly like stools indicating acidity. *Worm* troubles with accompanying symptoms of picking at nose, itching at the anus, pain in the abdomen, acidity of the stomach, restlessness and sleep.

RESPIRATORY SYSTEM

Nose :

Picking at the nose due to acid condition of the stomach. Cold in the head with creamy discharge from the nose and itching of nose.

Throat :

Tonsils and throat inflamed with creamy, yellow moist coating of the tongue. False diptheria with creamy coating at the palate and back part of the tongue.

Constipation :

Expectoration causes soreness of the lips, rawness of the tongue and mouth.

CIRCULATORY SYSTEM

Palpitation and irregularity of action of heart from weak digestion. Trembling about the heart aggravated by eating.

RHEUMATISM

Acute and chronic articular rheumatism with an acid diathesis. Rheumatic pains in the joints, weak feeling in the leg. Metastasis of rheumatism to heart. Pains in base of heart relieving pains in limbs and toe.

URINARY SYSTEM

Frequent urination with inability to retain urine with corresponding symptoms of acidity.

FEMALE SEXUAL SYMPTOMS

All secretions from uterus and vagina which are acid, creamy, yellow and watery. Sterility caused by acid secretions from the vagina proving fatal to the spermatozoa. Irregularity of the monthly periods when accompanied with acid leucorrhoea and frontal headache, also vomiting of acid fluids.

SLEEP

Restless sleep from worm troubles gritting teeth and screaming in sleep with itching of anus and picking of nose.

Modalities – No characteristic modalities.

59. NATRUM SULPHURICUM

Glauber

Common Name – Sodium Sulphate.

Natrum sulph. keeps the blood, bile and pancreatic juice at normal consistency by eliminating excess of water in the system caused by malassimilation and want of harmony in the various influences of life and health. The deficiency of this salt prevents the elimination of such water from tissue as is produced by oxidation of the organic matter.

Constitution – *Hydrogenoid constitution*

These patients feel keenly every change of temperature. They cannot tolerate air or atmosphere surcharged with moisture, nor can they eat with impunity plants or vegetables that thrive in or near about water. They feel healthy and happy in dry weather.

Miasm – Deep seated anti sycotic remedy.

Relation with heat and cold – *Easily affected by dampness of weather, damp houses or cellars.*

KEYNOTES

1) ***Mental traumatism*** – Mental affects from injuries to head; chronic brain affects from blows, falls (physical affects from blow – Arnica).
2) ***Patient feels every change of weather from dry to wet;*** cannot tolerate sea air, cannot tolerate plants that thrive near water.
3) ***Skin affections reappear every spring (Psor).***
4) *Diarrhoea with sudden urging* on first rising and standing on feet with much flatulence and rumbling in the abdomen (Aloes, Calc phos).

   (*Bry, Nat sulph* – Diarrhoea occurs after rising.

   Sulph – Hurries the patient out of bed.

   Thuja – Gets an urgent call as soon as he takes his first cup of tea.)
5) *Sad, gloomy and irritable* – Worse in morning. Must use great self control to prevent from shouting himself. Lively music makes her sad and tearful.
6) *Granular lids* – like small blisters; green pus with terrible photophobia (Thuja) – gonorrhoeal or sycotic.
7) Gonorrhoea – Painless, greenish, yellow thick discharge (Puls). Chronic or suppressed gonorrhoea (Kali Iod).

8) *Humid asthma* – in children-with every change to wet weather, with every fresh cold, always worse in damp rainy weather, sputa is greenish and copious.
9) Dyspnoea – Great desire to take a deep breath during damp wet weather.
10) *Sycotic pneumonia* – Lower lobe of left lung, great soreness of chest during cough such that the patient has to sit up in bed and hold the chest with both hands.
11) *Spinal meningitis* – Violent crushing growing pains at base of brain, head drawn back with mental irritability and delirium, violent congestion of blood to head.
12) *Aggravation during damp weather,* touch, pressure and morning hours.

Particulars :

1) MIND
2) HEAD
3) EYES
4) GIT
5) RESPIRATORY SYSTEM
6) SKIN
7) FEVER
8) URINARY SYSTEM

MIND

- *Depressed and tearful patients* – Sadness is aggravated by music.
- Inclination to commit suicide and self destruction.
  (Aurum has a desire to commit suicide and no desire to live.)
- There is a struggle between the desire to die and desire to live.
- Smallest noises drive her cold – even music – music makes her weep.
- *Morning aggravation* of all mental symptoms.
- There is intense wildness and irritability and there is a wonderful restraint to prevent doing herself bodily harm. Patient has to greatly control herself from shouting.
- *Mental symptoms from injuries to head*, fall, blows – headache, loss of memory, twitchings, epileptiform convulsions.

HEADACHE

Location – Basal headache. Top of the head feels hot. Violent pains felt in great depth of brain.

Sensation – Brain feels loose when stooping as if it would fall forward. Great deal of congestion felt in the brain with heaviness of head.

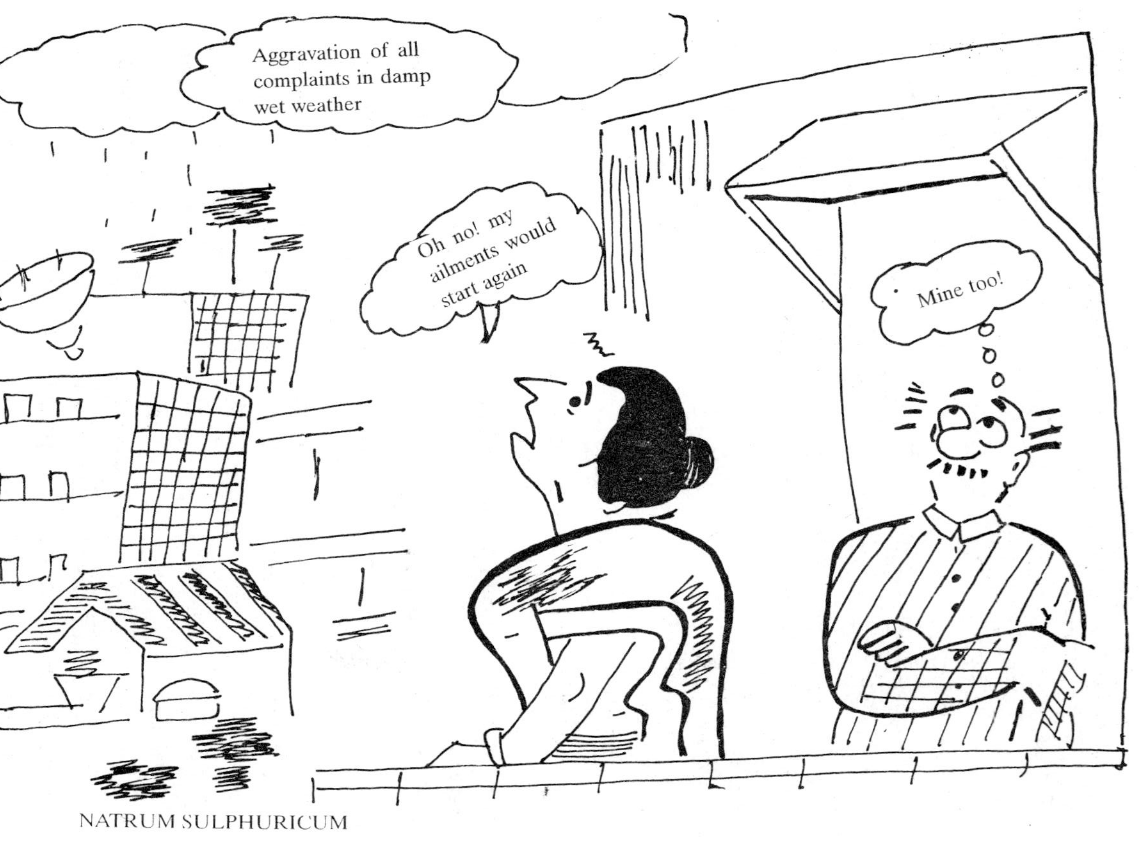
Aggravation of all complaints in damp wet weather
Oh no! my ailments would start again
Mine too!

NATRUM SULPHURICUM

Concomitants – Excess salivation with headache causing the patient to spit continuously.

- Greyish greenish coating of tongue.
- Giddiness with bilious taste in mouth, vomiting and bilious diarrhoea.
- *Spinal meningitis* with violent crushing pains at the base of the brain, mental irritablity and delirium, violent congestion of blood to head, delirium and opisthotonos.

EYES

Eye troubles with greenish thick catarrhal discharges, intense photophobia – patient can hardly open his eyes to light. Light from room brings on headache. Burning of edges of lids with lachrymation. Chronic conjunctivitis with large blister like granulations.

GIT

Tongue :

Dirty greenish grey or dirty brown coating at the back of tongue. Bitter taste in mouth.

Stomach :

Troubles with regurgitation of food. Food always welling up. Bitter taste, distension, weight with almost constant nausea. Cannot digest starchy foods, milk and potatoes disagree.

Liver :

Bilious disturbance is a grand feature of Natrum sulph. Engorgement of liver with great pain and soreness in the right hypochondrium. Stitching pains while walking and taking a deep breath. Vomiting of bitter fluids, greenish brown and greenish grey tongue. Constant taste of bile in mouth with a yellow complexion, loss of appetite, rising of sour water in mouth, disgust for bread and great desire for ice cold water. Torpidity of liver is the root cause of diarrhoea.

Diarrhoea :

Nat sulph is a great remedy for both acute and chronic diarrhoea.

Cause – Liver troubles, damp wet weather.

Time – Morning. Patient starts getting stools after he gets up and moves about.

Character of stools – Sudden urging and gushing stool is accompanied with flatulence. There is a great deal of rumbling, gurgling in bowels, then sudden gushing, noisy spluttering stools after rising in morning.

- Rumbling in the abdomen especially the right ileo ceacal region.
- Soreness in the right hypochondrium.

Aggravation – Morning, damp weather.

Amelioration – After stools – immediate relief of colic and patient feels cheerful after passage of stools.

RESPIRATORY SYSTEM

Cough :

Cause – Damp weather.

Character of cough – Mucopus is expectorated with thick ropy and yellowish green looking like pus.

Sensation – Cough with all gone sensation in chest. Great soreness and rawness felt in the chest and patient holds the chest while coughing (Bry – Dry cough; Nat sulph – Loose cough).

Humid Asthma (acute and chronic)

- Aggravated during damp wet weather.
- Violent spasmodic asthma with copious greenish purulent sputa, loose evacuation immediately on rising.
- Short breath with piercing pain in left chest – lower lobe of left lung involved.
- Great dyspnoea with a desire to take a deep breath during damp and cloudy weather.
- Looseness of bowels with each attack of asthma.
- Soreness of chest on coughing relieved by pressure.
- Loud rales with empty all gone feeling in chest.

(Kent – Asthma when hereditary is one of the sycotic complaints of Hahnemann. Asthma is a sycotic disease and hence it should be cured by Anti-Sycotic remedies. (Nat sulph being a deep seated antisycotic remedy has given great results in curing asthma).

SKIN

Skin affections reappear every spring, damp wet weather. Itch, scabies and vesicular eruptions, vesicular eczema with a thin watery discharge. Fingers are swollen, stiff and stand out stiffened by swelling. Skin affections are accompanied with bilious symptoms. Palms of hands are raw and sore and exude a watery fluid.

- *Vesicular eruptions* around the mouth, chin and various parts of the body; little fine water blisters.
- Barbers itch – sycotic disease of hair follicles.
- *Wart like eruptions* on the arms, thighs, anus betray the sycotic taint.

- Condylomata and soft fleshy excrecences on the male genital organs also belie some of the constitutional taint.

FEVER

Types – Remittent, bilious, malarial and intermittent fevers.

Symptoms – Icy coldness of limbs. Absence of thirst in all stages. Bilious vomiting. Itching anywhere during fever is an invaluable symptom.

Modalities – Aggravation – Damp wet weather.

Concomitants – Greyish, green or brown coating of tongue.

URINARY SYMPTOMS

Diabetes – Nat sulph is a chief remedy for sugar and general wastes from kidneys. Lithic deposits in urine looks like brick dust and clings to the sides of the vessel. Excessive secretion of urine in diabetes.

General Modalities :

Aggravation – DAMP BASEMENTS, WET WEATHER
(Aran, Ars iod, Dulc.)
REST, LYING DOWN.

Amelioration – DRY WEATHER
PRESSURE, SITTING UP
CHANGING POSITION
OPEN AIR.

Relations :

Complements – Ars, Thuja.

Remedies that follow well – Bell, Thuja.

Important Quesions ?

Q.1. Give indications of Nat. sulph in the following :

1) Diarrhoea [1972, 74, 75, 77, 84]
2) GIT [1973]
3) Asthma [1976, 77, 79]
4) Bronchitis [1987]
5) Mental symptoms [1982]
6) Skin symptoms [1979]
7) Head injury [1981]
8) Drug picture [1988, 89, 90]

COMPARE :

1) Respiratory symptoms of Rumex/Nat sulph [1977,82]
2) Bowel symptoms – Nat sulph./Thuja/Verat. alb [1973]
3) Asthma – Nat sulph/Bromium [1991]

RESPIRATORY SYMPTOMS :

RUMEX	NAT. SULPH
• < Cold dry weather, open air, slightest inhalation of cold air.	• < Damp wet weather, morning. > Open air.
• Dry teasing cough in the first stage. Later the cough becomes yellowish, thick, tenacious, ropy and stringy that the patient is exhausted from his efforts to expectorate.	• Loose cough and the patient holds the chest while coughing. Expectoration – copious greenish purulent sputa expectorated immediately after rising.

BOWEL SYMPTOMS :

NAT. SULPH	THUJA	VERAT. ALB.
• Patient starts getting stools after he gets up in the morning and moves about.	• Diarrhoea especially after having tea or morning breakfast.	• Diarrhoea from fright, eating, drinking and taking fruits.
• Acute and chronic diarrhoea with rumbling and gurgling in bowels, then sudden gushing, noisy spluttering stools after rising in the morning.	• Stool is forcibly discharged as if water is passing through a bunghole with rumbling and colicky pains in the abdomen.	• Profuse watery stools with cramps and cold sweat on the forehead. Desire for cold drinks.
• Feels better and cheerful after stool.	• Great debility after stool.	• Great prostration after stools.

ASTHMA

BROMIUM	NAT. SULPH
• < Hot weather, dust.	• < Damp wet weather.
• Sensation as if air tubes were full of smoke.	• Dyspnoea with desire to take a deep breath.
• Asthma of sailors as soon as they go ashore; relieved as soon as they are at sea.	• Violent spasmodic attack with copious greenish purulent sputa and loose evacuations immediately on rising.
• Little expectoration with stony hardness of glands.	• Looseness of bowels with each attack of asthma.

60. NITRIC ACID

Hahnemann

Constitution – Nitric acid is especially suited to thin weak and debilitated persons with rigid musculature, dark complexion, black eyes and hair. Ugly looking appearance with broken down cachetic constitution, aneamic and emaciated people with morning diarrhoea (Phos.).

Temperament – Nervous and Irritable.

Relation with heat and cold – Chilly patient.

Miasm – Covers all there miasms – Psora, Sycosis and Syphilis.

Diathesis – Heamorrhagic diathesis.

KEYNOTES

1) ***Affects the mucous outlets of the body at the junction of skin and mucous membranes*** – mouth, nose, rectum, anus, urethra – cracks, rhagades, fissures etc.
2) ***Bright red heamorrhage*** from all outlets of the body.
3) Great general weakness, feeble, extreme sensitivity and nervous trembling with marked ***aneamia and emaciation***.
4) Nit. acid is suited to persons suffering from chronic diseases, who take cold easily and easily disposed to diarrhoea.
5) Old people who suffer from great weakness and diarrhoea.
6) ***Excessive physical irritability*** – Sensitive to least noise, touch, pain and jar.
7) Sticking and pricking pains as from *splinters* suddenly appearing and disappearing on change of temperature, weather, during sleep.
8) *Sensation of band around head, bones* (Carb Ac., Sulph.); of a *splinter* in affected parts. Ulcers, piles, ingrowing toe nails < least contact.
9) ***Thin, offensive acrid discharges*** of a dirty brown yellowish colour. *Corossiveness* of discharges is marked.
10) *Urine* is scanty, dark brown, strong smelling like *horses urine*; cold when it passes, turbid, looks like remains of sides of barrel (Benz Ac, Sepia).
11) *Ulcers* – *easily bleeding* in corners of mouth; splinter like pain especially on contact, zig zag irregular edges, base looks like raw flesh.
12) *Cracking* in ears on masticating joints (Coc., Graph.).

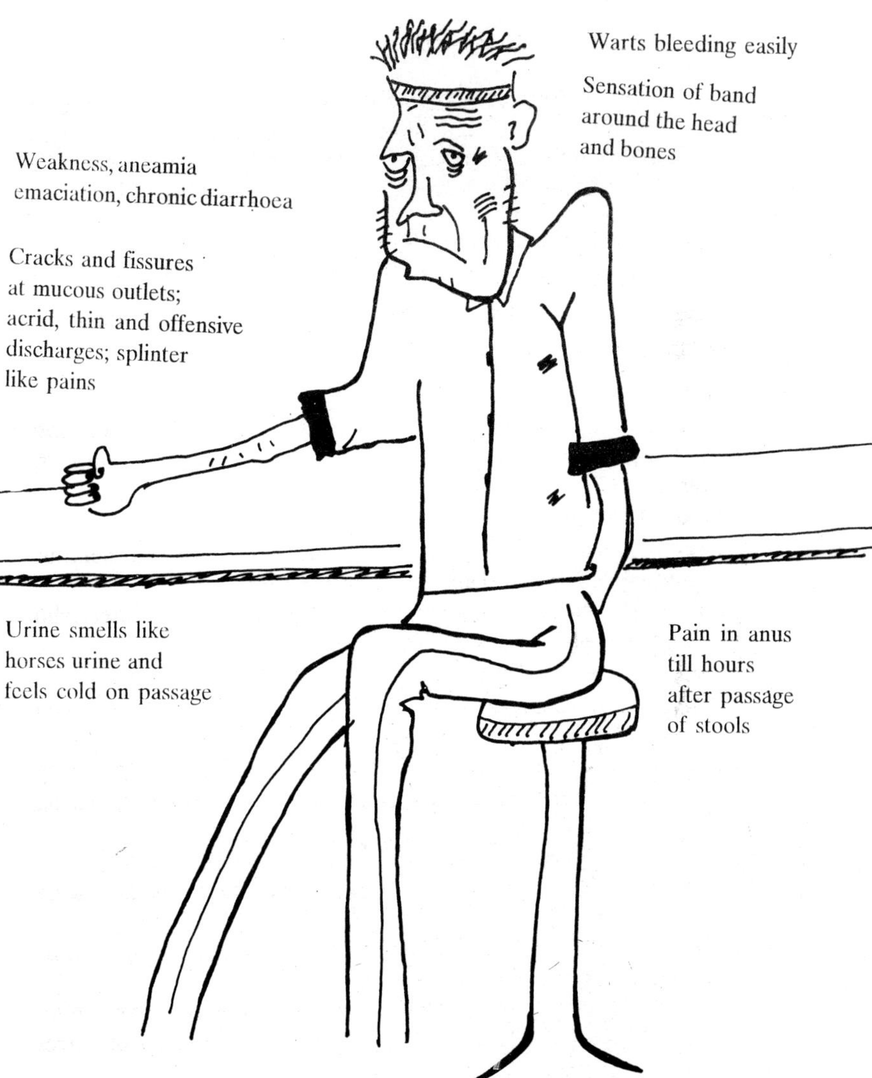
Mental and physical irritability
Warts bleeding easily
Sensation of band around the head and bones
Weakness, aneamia emaciation, chronic diarrhoea
Cracks and fissures at mucous outlets; acrid, thin and offensive discharges; splinter like pains
Urine smells like horses urine and feels cold on passage
Pain in anus till hours after passage of stools

NITRIC ACID

13) *Warts* – large, jagged and pedunculated that bleed easily on washing; moist oozing with sticking pains (Staph, Thuja).
14) *Fissures in rectum* – tearing spasmodic pains during stools and remains for hours after passage of stools (ever after soft stools). (Alum, Nat mur, Rat).
    (*Merc sol* – Tenesmus before and after stools.
    Nux vom – better after stools.)
15) Irritable, head strong and vindictive persons unmoved by apologies.
16) *Syphilitic bone pains* as if flesh were torn from bones with a splinter felt in inflamed parts.
17) ***Desire for salt, fat, chilliness and indifference*** are a symptom complex that puts on to Nit acid.
18) Mucous membranes – ulcerations, fissures, stitching, splinter pains, bleeding and offensiveness.

Particulars :

1) MIND
2) HEADACHE
3) FACE
4) RESPIRATORY SYSTEM
5) GIT
6) URINARY SYSTEM
7) SKIN
8) FEMALE SYMPTOMS
9) FEVER

HEADACHE

Cause – Loss of sleep, overexertion, virulent poisoning, chronic headaches of syphilitic origin.

Sensation – Band around the head. Hammering pains in the head with extreme sensitivity of scalp.

Aggravation – least motion, jar, noise, morning on waking.

Amelioration – wrapping up, rising, riding in a carraige.

MIND

General *indifference* to all matters *hopelessness, despair and sadness with indifference and mental irritability.*

Self willed, headstrong and obstinate person – entreaty, apology, love are equally incapable of moving him.

Anxious state of mind – Anxious about his health, future and things that don't concern him. This state of mind is due to continued loss of sleep or from loss of a dear friend. *Marked fear of cholera* (Ars.). Patient is *very weak and exhausted* that he is obliged to lie down. Every now and then slightest exertion causes him loss of breath. He trembles in all his limbs and complains of great debility and heaviness particulary in the morning hours. Constitution is tainted by poisons of syphilis, mercury and scrofula.

FACE

Deep lines of suffering characterise the face. Pale yellow sallow and sunken face with sunken eyes. Lids are tumid in morning. Skin feels drawn over the face with pigmented warty spots on the forehead. Cracking in the jaw when chewing. Corners of the mouth cracked, ulcerated and scabby. Raw sore and bleeding lips.

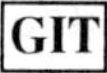

GIT

Teeth :

Tearing pains in the teeth aggravated from cold or warmth. Easy bleeding of gums.

Tongue :

Ulcerated, raw, sore and fissured tongue.

Mouth :

Ulcers or apthae in the mouth with burning pains. Foul cadaveric odour from the mouth. Acrid saliva from the mouth excoriates the lips.

Stomach :

- Longing for fat, salt, lime, chalk etc.
- Bread and meat cause strong aversion to food; milk disagrees.
- Generally thirstless.
- Bitter vomiting of sour contents with pain in the cardiac opening. Food sours and causes sour eructations. Nausea after eating, better by riding in a carraige. Liver is enormously affected as a result of which there is jaundice.

Abdomen :

Distended and tender abdomen with great pain in ileo ceacal region aggravated from motion. Relaxed condition in weakly infant boys that disposes to inguinal hernia.

Diarrhoea :

Cause – cold changes in weather, broken down subjects who are disposed to frequent attacks of diarrhoea.

Character of stool – putrid undigested, green slimy, excoriated and sour stools.

Before stools – Great desire for stool but passes little at a time.

During stool – Ineffectual urging for stool. Feel that a large amount of stool remains in the rectum but is unable to expel.

After stool – great pain in rectum hours after stool. The person walks about the floor with this intense burning, tearing, splinter like pain in the anus, still urging with exhaustion and soreness of anus.

Sensation – as if rectum was full but cannot expel.

(**Keynotes** – Sero croupous discharge, ineffectual urging for stool with sharp splinter like cutting pains. Excoriated fissured anus with warts. Rectal complaints with ulceration, fissures, stitching and splinter pains with bleeding and offensiveness.)

PILES

External and internal piles that are extremely painful with burning and sticking during stools. Piles that ulcerate and discharge copiously of blood and pus. *Foetid moisture at anus.* Piles are so painful that the person breaks out in sweat and pulsates all over on slightest touch or at stool (Peonia, Staph.). Constant urging and tenesmus are very exhausting.

RESPIRATORY SYSTEM

Nose :

Ozeana – Ozeana of syphilitic origin. He expels yellow plugs and green crusts from the nose. Frequent epistaxis and disagreeable odour from the nose. Excoriating discharge from the nose makes the lips sour; corners of the mouth crack so that the child cannot open its mouth on account of soreness.

Nasal diptheria – with offensiveness and excoriating discharge, frequent epistaxis with well developed white deposit in the nose. As the membrane decends to the throat there is a sensation of fish bone, splinter or a piece of glass in the affected part.

Pthisis – Sudden rush of blood to the chest and decided hectic fever which indicates ulceration of lungs from breaking down of tubercles. Person suffers from frequent heamorrhages from the lungs with bright red and profuse blood. Great dyspnoea so that the patient cannot talk without getting out of bed. Tickling cough with offensive and bloody expectoration. Morning hoarseness with exhausting physical diarrhoea. Intermittent pulse. Least exertion causes palpitaton of heart and dyspnoea.

URINARY SYSTEM

Nitric acid is extremely useful in albuminous urine of syphilitic patients. Excessive prostration, nausea, sour taste, bilious diarrhoea, fetid, turbid urine and oedema of feet are strong indications. Dark brown and strong smelling urine. *Urine smells like horses urine* and feels *cold when passing.*

Difficult micturition – Patient has to press a long while before urine appears but once the stream starts it continues uninterruptedly.

SKIN

Ulcers – Irregular in outline tending to spread towards periphery but more deeply than that arising from action of mercury. Ulcers are filled with profuse exuberant granulations which bleed readily from slightest touch. Pains are sticking in character as if splinter were sticking into the affected parts. Splinter like burning pains in the ulcers < cold water. Thin offensive and acrid discharge of a brown or dirty yellowish green colour comes out. Dry scaly and yellow skin with deep cracks and fissures.

- Junction of skin and mucous membranes are most affected – *cracks and fissures* with lancinating and sticking, *splinter like pains*.
- There is profuse bright red bleeding from these cracks, fissures and ulcers.
- Warts and condylomata of syphilitic origin in various parts of the body. Warts may be large peduculated and bleed easily on slightest touch. There may be moist oozing, offensive and acrid discharges with typical pricking and splinter like pains.
- Tendency to *fungal growth* – pains are sore and splinter like; they burn and smart and are worse from application of cold water.
- *Chilblains* on hands and feet.
- Yellow curved nails with splinter sensation under the nails.
- *Primary and secondary syphilis* with nocturnal bone pains, particularly on head of long bones. Development of warts and copper coloured spots associated with pronounced debility and exhaustion. Buboes and syphilitic chancres with splinter like pains. (Nitric acid is most useful after abuse of mercury.)

FEMALE

- Bleeding excrecences in the vagina and on the mouth of uterus. Menses are too early and profuse, dark red blood with muddy water. During menses the patient complains of pains in the thighs, labor like pains in the abdomen and back, palpitation, anxiety, trembling and tiredness.

Leucorrhoea – Greenish, yellow acrid and offensive discharge.

FEVER

- Thirstless in all stages.
- Cold hands and feet.
- Chronic intermittent and cachetic constitutions, copious night sweats, extreme weakness and characteristic odour of urine, bleeding of dark blood from some part. Intermittent pulse. In

ulcerative stage of typhoid fever there may be profuse bright red heamorrhage from the bowels with fainting on slightest motion. In pneumonic complications there is threatening paralysis of lungs with loud rattling of mucus.

General Modalities :

Aggravation – EVENING, NIGHT, AFTER MIDNIGHT CONTACT, CHANGE OF WEATHER AND TEMPERATURE, DURING SWEAT ON WAKING, WHILE WALKING.

Amelioration – While riding in a carriage (opp of Cocc.).

Relations :

Complementry – Ars, Calad.

Inimical to – Lach.

Resembles – Ars – morbid fear of cholera relieves ailments resulting from abuse of mercury especially if there is erethism, bad effects of repeated doses of Digitalis.

Follows well – Calc, Hep, Merc, Nat. carb, Puls, Thuja, but most affective after Kali carb.

Important Questions ?

Q.1. Compare Piles of Nitric acid/Aesc. hipp – [1988]

NITRIC ACID	AESC. HIPP.
• Extremely painful heamorrhoids that bleed easily during stool.	• Blind and painful heamorrhoids.
• Sticking and pricking pain as from splinters. Pain is so severe that the patient may break in sweat and becomes anxious.	• Fullness of rectum with intense pain in back and anus. Sensation as if rectum is full of sticks. Fullness in parts due to undue amount of blood.
• Blood from piles is profuse, dark and offensive.	
• Heamorrhoids discharge thin acrid offensive yellow green pus.	• Constipation with hard dry stools that are difficult to pass.
• Piles associated with diarrhoea. Rectum feels full but nothing comes out as expulsion is difficult < cold application.	• Dryness and heat of the rectum.

Q.2. Give indications of Nit acid in the following :

1) Apthae	[1987]
2) Marasmus	[1987]
3) GIT	[1993]
4) Keynotes	[1978 S, 87, 91]
5) Eczema	[1984]
6) Urinary symptoms	[1973, 79, 81, 95]
7) Heamorrhage	[1972, 73, 75]
8) Mind	[1982]
9) Ear discharge	[1976]
10) Uterine cancer	[1979]
11) Skin	[1975, 76, 82]
12) Rectal troubles	[1973, 74, 79]

61. NUX VOMICA

Hahnemann

Common Name – Poison Nut.

- Nux is the *king of polychrest remedies*.
- Suitable for all age, sex and temperament.
- It is *an antidote* to post drugging affects of ***allopathic** medicines*.
- It is a remedy for the present day attitude *'modern trend of life'*.
- Nux is the male counterpart of Ignatia and Pulsatilla.
- It is a remedy which is capable of working wonders with people from all walks of life.
- Nux should be given on retiring or what is better *several hours before going to bed as* it acts best during repose of mind (Sulphur should be given in the morning).

Constitution – Adapted to thin irritable nervous, zealous persons with dark hair and bilious or sanguine temperament. Nux is chiefly successful with persons of an ardent character, of an irritable, impatient temperament, disposed to anger, spite and deception. Persons who are very particular, careful but inclined to become easily excited or angered. Hypochondriac, literary studious persons who are too much at home, suffer from want of exercise, with gastric abdominal complaints and costiveness especially in drunkards.

Temperament – Nervous and irritable, bilious and sanguine temperament.

Relation with heat and cold – Very chilly person.

Miasm – Psora in the background.

KEYNOTES

1) ***Oversensitive person*** – sensitive to noise, light, least current of air, to his surroundings, extremely touchy in regard to his food, trifling ailments are unbearable.
2) Nux is an *antidote* to bad affects of allopathic medicines.
3) ***Aggravation*** of complaints mostly in the ***morning*** after waking.
4) ***Very chilly person*** – oversensitive to open air, to draft of air, always taking cold and it settles in the nose and goes to the chest. Least uncovering brings on chilliness.
5) Actions are turned in the *opposite direction*.

Keeps doors and windows closed
Headache with gastric symptoms
Morning aggravation
Sensitive, nervous and chilly person
Oversensitive, angry and irritable person
NEWS +
Symptoms turn in opposite directions
Constant nausea and retching with a sensation as if only he could vomit he would feel much better
Pressure in stomach an hour or two after eating
Unfinished sensation in rectum, passage or small quantities of stool at a time
WHISKY
NUX VOMICA

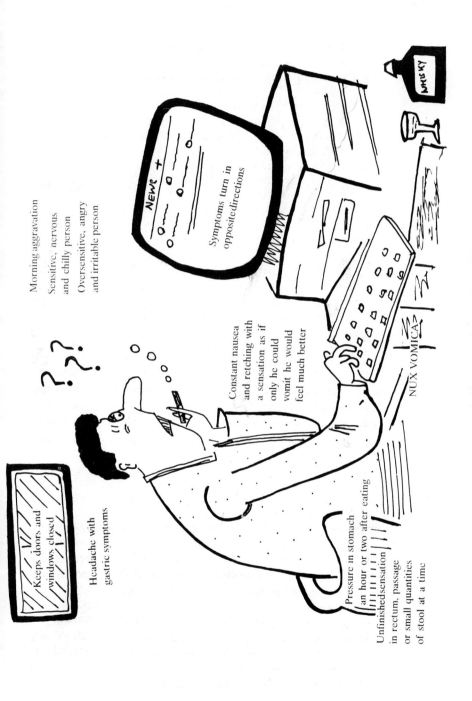

- When the stomach is sick it does not empty its contents but there is a lot of retching, gagging and straining and after a prolonged effort the stomach empties its contents.
- In constipation the more he strains the harder it is to pass stools.
- When the bladder is full, the urine dribbles away and as soon as the person strains, it ceases to urinate.
- Diarrhoea – little squirting of stool when the person sits on the commode and then comes on the tenesmus so that he cannot stop straining and when he does strain there comes a sensation of forcing back, the stool seems to go back, a kind of *anti-peristalsis*.

6) Bad affects of coffee, tobacco, alcoholic stimulants, highly spiced or seasoned food, overeating, long continued mental overexertion, sedentry habits, loss of sleep, aromatic or patent medicines.
7) Persons who are very particular, careful but inclined to become easily exited or angered, irrascible and tenacious.
8) ***Hypochondria*** – literary studious persons who are too much at home, suffer from want of exercise, with gastric abdominal complaints and costiveness.
9) Cannot keep from falling asleep in the evening while sitting or reading hours before bedtime and awakes at 3-4 A.M., then wants to sleep late in the morning.
10) *Awakes tired* and weak generaly worse with many complaints < morning on waking.
11) Stomach – pressure an hour or two after eating as from a stone (immediately after – Kali bi, Nux. mosh.)
12) *Constant nausea* after eating in morning "If I could only vomit I would feel much better."
13) ***Constipation*** with frequent unsuccessful desire, passing small quantities of feaces; ***sensation as if not finished*** after passage of stools. Alternate constipation and diarrhoea.
14) Spasms (from simple twitchings to clonic form) sensitiveness, nervousness and chilliness are the general characteristic of Nux vom.
15) Twitchings, spasms, convulsions slightest touch.
16) *Convulsions with conciousness* < anger, emotion, touch, moving.
17) ***Backache***; must sit up to turn in bed, lumbago, from sexual weakness, from masturbation.
18) *Menses* are too early, profuse and lasting too long, with aggravation of all other complaints during their countenance.
19) *Fever* with great heat of the whole body, burning hot body with a red face, patient cannot move or uncover without being chilly.

Particulars :

1) MIND
2) HEADACHE
3) GIT
4) RESPIRATORY SYSTEM
5) URINARY SYSTEM
6) FEMALE SEXUAL SYSTEM
7) EXTREMITIES
8) FEVER

MIND

Mental symptoms are consequent upon *modern civilised life and high living.* Nux persons are *ambitious, intelligent,* quick, capable and competent. They are self reliant rather than dependent. Their intelligence is pragmatic and efficient rather than philosophical or intellectual. Nux persons in their non pathological states make excellent employees and their talents lead them to occupations like supervisors, businessmen, accountants, salesman. Nux person becomes *ruled by his ambition*. He lays overemphasis on achievement and competition – *workaholic* dominated by work. He accepts promotions and responsibilities. Person is *fastidious* and wants all work to be done efficiently. He firmly believes that any challenge, any problem can be overcome by sheer effort and ability. One of the most difficult things for a Nux person is to accept limitation and to resign himself to the inevitable. To keep up with the work pressure he *comes to use various artificial means* to keep himself stimulated, coffee, cigarettes, drugs, alcohol, sex and continued loss of sleep. Despite abuse of these stimulants the Nux persons are unusually sensitive to many of these substances and consequently suffer consequence of their over indulgence. As overstimulation and toxicity take their toll – that leads to gastric and nervous disorders. The patient becomes irritable to slight stresses such as noise, light etc. Finally the pressure becomes so much that the patient becomes *impatient and irritable*. Nux person is intolerable to contradiction, not out of arrogance but because he knows he is right and he usually is.

Patient may even become very cruel and *impulsive* in the later stages. Anxiety and irritability with inclination to commit suicide prevail though the patient is afraid to die. Nux is *self reliant, independent, compulsively hard working, overly efficient, irritable and impulsive.*

HEADACHE

Cause – sweating, wine drinkers, night watching, unrefreshed sleep, abuse of coffee, alcohol, light, noise, high living, highly seasoned food, drugging.

Time – Aggravation in the morning hours after waking.

Location – Vertex, occiput.

Sensation – Head has been beaten with an axe. **As if head would** split. Heat and redness of face.

Aggravation – Eating, open air, mental **exertion, anger,** alcohol, masturbation, constipation, debauchery.

Amelioration – Warm room, wrapping up.

GIT

Mouth :

Putrid and bitter taste in the morning.

Tongue :

Anterior half of the tongue clean and posterior **coated white**, furred cracked on edges.

Stomach :

Gastric upsets caused by coffee, alcoholic drinks, debauchery, abuse of drugs, business, anxiety, sedentry habits, broken rest from long night watching, too high living etc.

Sour taste, heartburn, ***pressure in the stomach an hour or two after eating.*** Stomach symptoms are worse in morning.

Craving for fats, alcohol, beer. Person *loathes* beer, coffee, food etc. Actions are turned in opposite direction – constant retching and straining as if actions were going the wrong way. Hypochondriacal mood, pyrosis, tightness about waist, must loosen clothing, confused, cannot use mind two or three hours after meal, epigastrium bloated with pressure as from a stone in the stomach. Patient feels *"only if I could vomit I'd feel much better."* Constant ***scraped*** sensation in the throat, chest and stomach.

Nux is a *routine remedy for loss of appetite*. Nux is an old dyspeptic – **lean, hungry,** whithered and bent forward, premature age always **selecting his food and digesting** almost none. Patient craves **pungent bitter things and tonics.** Aversion to meat as it makes him sick.

Liver :

Induration and swelling of liver caused by high living, debauchery and **drunkeness. The region** of the liver is so sore that the patient **constantly looses his clothings** to release the oppression.

Abdomen :

Great accumulation of wind which presses on the heart, causing **palpitation, uneasiness and difficulty** in breathing; pressing downwards on **the intestines and bladder** it causes frequent desire for stool and urine. **Frequent colic with** periodical belching, tearing in the abdomen, jaundice, **aversion to food,** constipation, bilious attack, loss of appetite, yellow skin, **high coloured** urine, backache are violent and characteristic symptoms.

Constipation :

Alternate constipation and diarrhoea. Constipation in people who lead a sedentry life. *Anti-peristaltic* action of bowels. *Frequent ineffectual desire* for stools but passes little at a time (caused due to irregular peristalsis). Character of stools *large and hard stools.*

Diarrhoea :

Diarrhoea alternates with constipation in persons who have taken laxatives, aromatic medicines throughout their lives. *Frequent desire for stool*; stool is offensive and watery, passes a little quantity at a time with temporary satisfaction. Urge for stools comes in the morning after rising from the bed or immediately after eating some food.

Dysentry :

- Stools consist of slimy mucus and blood but are *small in quantity and unsatisfactory*. The tenesmus is greatly relieved for a short time after every stool. Constant sensation **"As if not finished"**. As a result of ineffectual urging heamorrhoids become plentiful in a Nux vom patient. Prolapsus recti due to severe pressing, tearing, itching, painful spasmodic closing.

Hernia :

Pressure and weakness in the left inguinal ring and hence cures hernia in babies (Lyc. – R.H.S.).

RESPIRATORY SYSTEM

Cold :

Cause – disordered stomach, least draft of cold air. Patient takes cold from least provocation; perspires easily, least current of air causes headache with coryza.

Character of discharge – Completely filled up and stuffed nose out doors but fluent in doors. Thin watery discharge during the day.

Concomitant – catarrah with headache, heat in face, chilliness, much mucus in throat.

Cough :

Burning and scraped feeling in the air passages. Dry teasing cough with great soreness in chest.

Asthma :

Asthma from *every disordered stomach*. The patient may eat something that disagrees and they sit up all night with asthma (It is due to upward pressure of gas on diaphragm). Asthma associated with cough and rattling in the chest; retching and gagging cough, as if chest is filled with mucus < heavy meal, cold air, exercise.

URINARY SYMPTOMS

"Ineffectual urging to urination" is a keynote that would lead to prescription of Nux vom in diabetes, renal colic, heamaturia and cystitis.

FEMALE SEXUAL SYMPTOMS

Menses –

Time – too early.

Quantity – too profuse.

Duration – Menses occur too soon and last too long.

Concomitants – A great tendency to fainting and oversensitiveness to nervous impressions, constant chilliness frequent palpitation and great irritabitity of temperament.

Pregnancy :

Nux vom is a remedy for morning sickness with constant nausea and a sensation of "only if I could vomit I'd feel much better." There is a strong predominance of retching over vomiting. Inefficient labor pains extending to the rectum with desire for stool or frequent urination are quickly relieved by Nux vom. *Prolapse of uterus* with great excitement of sexual organs leading on to sexual dreams and orgasms in sexual and irritable women. They lead an idle life, partake of rich and highly seasoned food and drink large quantities of stimulating liquors which stimulate excessive venery and exaggerated passion.

EXTREMITIES

Convulsions with conciousness – spasm, sensitiveness and chilliness are three characteristics of Nux vomica. Convulsions of all muscles of the body with pimple face and loss of breath from movements < slightest draught of air.

Paralysis :

Paralysis of the bowels with no passage of stools; paralysis of bladder with difficulty in vioding urine; paralysis of extremities of the face, hands or single muscles. Sticking pains are important. *Neuralgia* about the face, head with a sensation of tension in the muscles.

Backache :

Backache worse on lying down. Must sit up to turn over as turning and twisting the body aggravates. Drawing pains in the sacrum and hips.

FEVER

Nux vom. is very useful in *intermittent* fevers with constant chilliness. The patient is chilly in all stages and all time. Cannot move or uncover without being chilly.

< even lifting the covers, least draft of air.

> keeping warmth, covering up.

Typhoid :

Gastric symptoms predominate over cerebral symptoms. Vertigo with bitter taste in mouth, pressure in epigastrium, constipation, restless and disturbed sleep, chilliness on slightest movement, constant headache generally located in occiput.

General Modalities :

Aggravation – MORNING, WAKING AT 4 A.M.
MENTAL EXERTION, AFTER EATING
OR OVEREATING, TOUCH, NOISE
ANGER, SPICES, NARCOTICS
DRY WEATHER, COLD AIR.

Amelioration – EVENING, WHILE AT REST
LYING DOWN, DAMP WET WEATHER.

Relations :

Complementry – Sulphur in all diseases.

Inimical – Zincum (must not be used before or after).

Follows well – after – Ars., Ipec, Phos, Sep., Sulph.

Is followed well by – Bry, Puls, Sulph.

Important Questions ?

Q.1. Give the indications of Nux vom in the following :

1) Rectal symptoms [1991]
2) Intermittent fever [1990, 91, 94]
3) Convulsions [1976, 86, 88, 89]
4) Modalities [1986 C, 69, 72, 87]
5) Constipation [1981]
6) Epilepsy [1988]
7) Stoppage of nose [1982]
8) Asthma [1987]
9) Mind [1968, 72, 73, 79, 81]
10) Keynotes [1970, 72, 73, 79, 81]
11) Toothache [1996]
12) Dysentry [1991]
13) Headache [1974, 76]
14) Backache [1974]
15) Piles [1976]
16) Labor [1977, 82]
17) Drug picture [1973, 74, 78]

GIT SYMPTOMS [1994]

NUX VOMICA	BISMUTH
• *Pure gastralgia without catarrah.*	
• Irritable and nervous persons with sedentry habits.	• Cannot bear solitude, always desires company, restless person.
• Constant sensation of retching and feels only if he could vomit he would feel much better.	• Vomiting of water as soon as it reaches the stomach; solid food is vomited out later in decomposed form.
• Intolerance of tight clothing	• Headache alternates with gastralgia.
• < Coffee, drugs, night watching, high living, sedentry habits, cold air, uncovering.	• < heat
• > Warmth.	• > cold application

CONSTIPATION – [1966)

ALUMINA	NUX VOM	BRYONIA
• Deficient peristalsis with inactivity of rectum. Even soft stool requires great straining.	• Constipation due to irregular peristalsis causing frequent desires and an unfinished sensation. Passage of small quantities of stool at a time.	• Constipation due to lack of secretion in the intestines. Dry and hard stools.

III. RENAL COLIC – [1967]

LYCOPODIUM	NUX VOM.	BERB. VULG.
• Right sided renal colic.	• "Ineffectual urging" to urinate.	• *Left sided kidney* troubles with numbness, bubbling sensation, stiffness, burning and soreness in the kidney region.

• Red sand in the urine with scanty urine during day and copious, frequent at night. • < 4-8 P.M. Backache is better by urination.	• Urine passes in drops with tearing and burning pains in the urethra.	• *Acute condition :* Bloody greenish and thick slimy mucus and jelly like sediment. • *Chronic condition :* dark and turbid urine with copious sedimentation.

RECTAL SYMPTOMS – [1993]

NUX VOMICA	AESCULUS HIPP.
• *Blind, bleeding piles* which burn and itch violently at night. Compelled to sit in a tub of cold water for relief.	• *Dryness* and heat in the rectum; it feels full of sticks with knife like pains shooting up in the rectum.
• *Unfinished sensation* in the rectum; passage of small quantity of feaces at a time.	
• *Backache* in the bed and must sit up to turn over. < Morning, after mental exertion, after eating, cool air.	• *Blind and painful* heamorrhoids. Backache worse on walking or stooping.

62. PODOPHYLLUM

Jeanes

Common Name – May Apple.

Podophyllum is a *long and deep acting drug.*

Constitution – Adapted to persons who suffer from gastro intestinal derangements, especially after abuse of mercury. Children who suffer from diarrhoea during the time of dentition.

Temperament – Bilious temperament.

Relations with heat and cold – Affected by extremes of both heat and cold.

Miasm – Psora is in the background.

KEYNOTES

1) ***Diarrhoea—stools are profuse, painless, putrid, polychromatic with prolapse of rectum and prostration***.
   Aggravation – Morning, dentition, hot summer weather, taking fruits. Diarrhoea is accompanied by a sensation of weakness or *sinking in abdomen* or rectum.
2) *Right sided remedy.* Affects right throat, right ovary, right hypochondrium.
3) *Difficult dentition*. Grinding the teeth at night, *intense desire to press the gums together* (Phyto), hot head-rolling the head from side the side.
4) ***Thirst for large quantities of cold water*** (Bry).
5) *Alternating condition* – alternating diarrhoea and constipation, headache alternates with diarrhoea – headache in winters and diarrhoea in summers.
6) Painless cholera morbus, cholera infantum (Phyto.)
7) *Tongue* yellow or white coated with imprint of teeth (Merc. sol, Rhus tox, Stram.).
8) Patient is constantly *rubbing and shaking the liver region* with his hand.
9) *"**Bile**"is a constant feature of Podophyllum. Liver is out of order with bitter taste in mouth, spitting up of bile with yellow colour; in diarrhoea it is a green substance.*
10) Constant *nausea* and *gagging* without vomiting .
11) *Fever* paroxysm at *7. A.M.* with great *loquacity* during chill and heat.

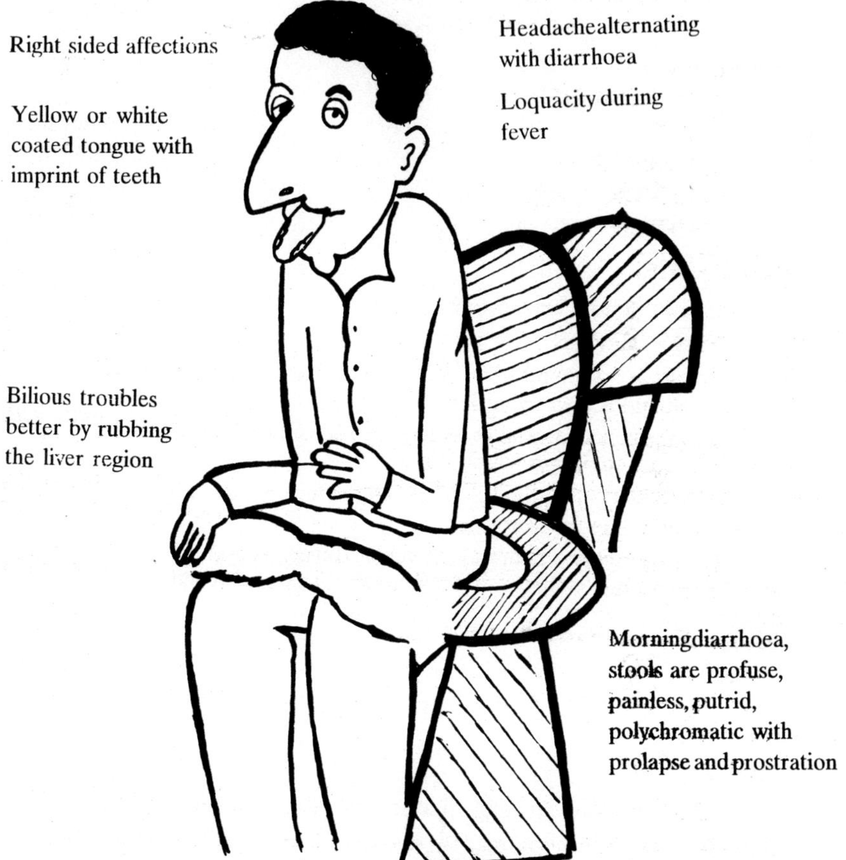
Right sided affections
Yellow or white coated tongue with imprint of teeth
Headachealternating with diarrhoea
Loquacity during fever
Bilious troubles better by rubbing the liver region
Morningdiarrhoea, stools are profuse, painless, putrid, polychromatic with prolapse andprostration

PODOPHYLLUM

12) *Prolapse of uterus* from over lifting or straining from constipation, after parturition with subinvolution (Nux vom, Rhus tox.).
13) Can *lie comfortably on stomach* in the early months of pregnancy.
14) ***Pain in the right ovary*** – running down the thigh of that side (great keynote of Podo.).

Particulars :

1) HEADACHE
2) GIT
3) FEMALE
4) FEVER
5) CHILD

HEADACHE

Bilious headache, winters.

Time – Morning.

Location – Occipital protruberance. Pain extends from the occiput down to the neck and shoulder.

Sensation – Congestive headache : sensation as if the head is full of blood and that the head would burst.

Modalities – Headache alternates with diarrhoea. As diarrhoea slackens up headache increases.

Concomitants – Blurring of vision during headache and the objects look hazy and misty. There is disgusting nausea and vomiting.

GIT

Tongue :

Yellow or white coated tongue with imprint of teeth. Bitter taste in the mouth.

Liver :

'Bile' is the striking feature of Podophyllum. Liver troubles (jaundice, chronic hepatitis, hyperemia of liver, gall stones) with great fullness, soreness and pain in the liver region. Stitches in the epigastrium from coughing, sour regurgitation of food, acute pain in the region of pyloric orifice, jaundice, bilious nausea, giddiness, dark urine, bitter taste, clayed stools, alternate constipation and diarrhoea, sensation of weight in the hypogastric region and piles with prolapsus ani.

- Uneasiness and *distress 2-3 hrs after eating.*
- *Green profuse vomiting* – vomits everything.
- Deathly overpowering nausea and prostration.
- *Prolapse of anus and rectum* during vomiting and stools. Hunger after vomiting.
- Clay coloured stools.

Relief is oblained by constantly rubbing the hypochondriac region.

Abdomen :

Podophyllum acts profoundly upon the the abdominal viscera causing rumbling and gurgling. The glands of the stomach are as if paralysed thus there is no digestion; this goes on until there is vomiting and diarrhoea. Abdomen is so sensitive that the person can hardly endure pressure. The soreness extends to the stomach, intestines and finally to the liver. After this comes a gurgling watery stool pouring out of the anus.

Diarrhoea :

Cause – Liver disturbance, hot weather, dentition, eating fruits.

Time – Morning. *"All gone sensation in stomach."*

Sensation – Weakness and sinking in the abdomen or rectum. The patient feels as if everything would drop through the pelvis. Diarrhoea alternates with constipation.

Character of stools – Painless, profuse, putrid, polychromatic with prostration and prolapse of rectum. Sometimes they are yellow coloured with meat like sediment in it and sometimes greenish yellow, slimy or bloody. Profuseness of stools is a mystry – every time the patient seems to be drained dry but he fills up again.

(*Sulph, Rumex* – Urging is felt before rising.

Bry; Nat. sulph – Urging comes on after rising in the morning and moving about.

Aloes – Want of confidence in sphincter ani.

Podo – Patient goes to the closet on the trot.)

Before stools – Loud gurgling in the abdomen with a gripping colic. Great weakness in the abdomen.

During stools – Patient experiences great heat and pain in the anus. Sensation as if the genital organs would come out during stools.

After stools – Patient experiences great weakness and exhaustion. Patient feels better after stools.

Concomitant – Prolapsus ani – sleep with eyes half closed and rolling the head from side to side, frequent gagging or empty retching. (Podo. is hardly indicated when the stool is not offensive). Complaints are worse in morning.

FEMALE SYMPTOMS

Podo. is useful in ovarian tumors, leucorrhoea, prolapsus uteri and other kind of uterine troubles.

- *Prolapse of uterus* caused by indiscriminate straining and lifting.

- *"Amelioration of pains is by lying on the stomach."* – it relieves morning sickness and excessive vomiting in pregnancy caused by congestion of pelvic viscera.

Menses :

Suppressed in young females with bearing down sensation felt mostly in hypogastric and sacral regions.

Concomitants – Chronic prolapse of anus, thick transparent leucorrhoea, pain in ovary, nausea, heamorrhoids and relief of pain from lying down.

Ovaries :

"Pain in the right ovary, running down the thigh of that side." (Lil. tig.) (Dr. Nash says ovarian tumors have disappeared under Podo. with the above symptoms.)

FEVER

Intermittent and Remittent fever.

Paroxysm – 7 A.M. morning.

Symptoms – Patient wakes up in the morning with a dull throbbing headache.

- Dry mouth with a bad taste.
- Yellow or white coated tongue with imprint of teeth.
- 'Nausea' is a prominent symptom and the patient vomits bilious substance, it is accompanied by a yellow and greenish diarrhoea.
- *'Loquacity'* is a grand feature of Podo which continues all through the chill and partly through the stage of heat.
- Person is sleepy.
- During chill the patient has pain in the hypochondria, knees, elbows and wrists.

CHILD

Dentition :

- Pressing of gums during dentition (Phytolacca).
- Podo. causes reflex cerebral irritation whether from abdominal symptoms or from the teeth. The child grates its teeth – the head is thrown back and rolled from side to side.
- Diarrhoea during dentition and hot weather with profuse, offensive and coloured stools.

General Modalities :

Aggravation – EARLY IN MORNING
(Aloes, Nux vom, Sulph.)
SUMMER, HOT WEATHER
DURING DENTITION.

Relations :

Compare – Aloe, Chel, Collin, Lil,Merc, Nux, Sulph.

It ***antidotes*** bad affects of mercury. After Ipec. and Nux in gastric affections and after Calc. and Sulph in liver diseases.

Important Questions ?

Q.1. Give indications of Podophyllum in the following conditions :

1) Intermittent fever [1990, 91]
2) Keynotes [1987]
3) Diarrhoea [1972, 73, 74, 75, 76, 77, 78, 84]
4) Drug picture [1986]
5) Liver disorder [1986]

63. PULSATILLA NIGRICANS
'Female Remedy'

Hahnemann

Common name – Wild flower 'Anemone'.

The following lines potray a Pulsatilla patient :

"Passive patients come for consultation.
Unlike Ignatia craves consolation.
Like April day has changeable mood
Stomach cannot hold rich and fatty food.
All complaints accompany thirstlessness and dry tongue.
Thick green yellowish discharges make her funk.
Irregular and painful menses – suppressed delayed and scanty.
Leucorrhoea is also acrid burning and creamy.
In labor pains wants doors and windows open.
And cannot lie on the back for desire to urine sharpens."

Silicea is chronic of Pulsatilla.

Constitution – Sandy hair, blue eyes, pale face easily moved to laughter or tears, affectionate, mild, timid, gentle, yielding disposition, inclined to be fleshy. *Tendency to weep* is a very important feature. *Changeability with softness.*

Relation with heat and cold – Worse in a warm room relieved by gentle motion in open air.

Miasm – Psora and Sycosis are in the background.

KEYNOTES

1) ***Mild, gentle and yielding disposition,*** sad and despondent, weeps easily, pale and aneamic.
2) ***Weeps easily*** – almost impossible to detail her complaints without weeping.
3) ***Ailments during and after puberty/menarche*** – Have never been well since that time – aneamia, chlorosis, bronchitis, pthisis.
4) ***Changeability of symptoms*** – pains travel from one joint to another; heamorrhages flow, stop and flow again; no stools are alike; no two chills are alike; no head or tail to the case – *mixed case'.*
5) *Pains* are accompanied with *constant chilliness (more severe the pain more the chill)* –

    With profuse sweating – *Cham.*

    With fainting – *Hepar sulph.*

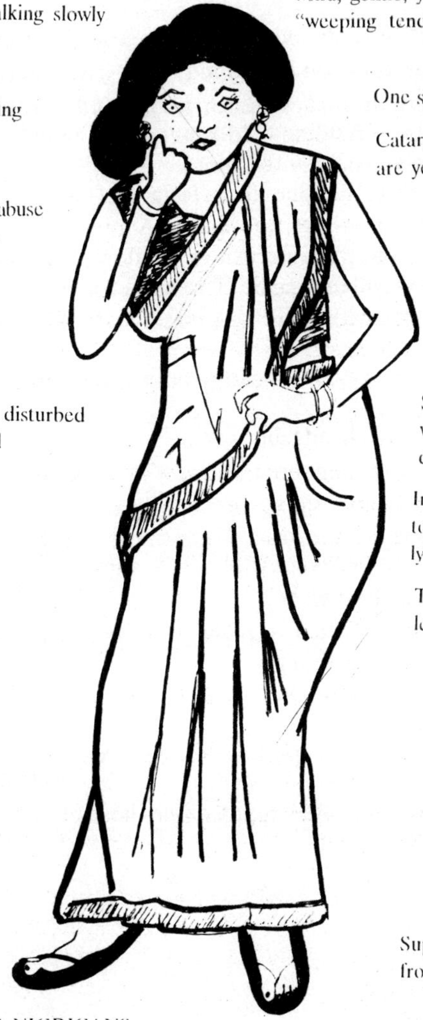

Aggravation–warmth, fatty food

Amelioration–coldair, cold things, walking slowly in open air

Bad taste in mouth in morning

Ailments from abuse of iron, quinine

Stomach easily disturbed from fatty food

Thirstlessness

Ailments from puberty or menarche–"have never been well since that time".

Mild, gentle, yielding, disposition "weeping tendency".

One sided symptoms

Catarrhaldischarges are yellowish green

Scanty menses with venous congestion and dysmenorrhoea

Increasedinclination to urinate on lying down

Thick milky white leucorrhoea

Suppresseddischarges from getting feet wet

PULSATILLA NIGRICANS

Frequent micturiton – *Thuja.*

Delirium – *Verat album.*

- *Shifting pains* from one joint to another.
- Pains come suddenly and disappear gradually and vice versa – "lets up with a snap."

6) Bad taste in the mouth aggravated in morning with great dryness but no thirst.

7) ***Thirstlessness with a dry mouth*** – with nearly all complaints.

8) ***Stomach easily disturbed by rich fatty food,*** cakes and pastry.

9) ***Thick bland, greenish yellow discharges from all mucous membranes.***

10) Toothache from holding cold water in the mouth – worse from warm things and heat of the room.

11) *Menses – Suppressed* due to getting feet wet, irregular since puberty. Flow is *scanty*, too late or suppressed by wetting the feet. Changeable characteristic in the flow of menses – they stop and flow, stop and flow again. Threatened abortion – flow ceases and then starts with increased force; suffocation with fainting, must have fresh air.

12) *Styes on upper eyelid* from eating fatty, greasy, rich food or pork (Lyc, Staph.).

13) *One sided sweats*, headache.

14) Affections consequent upon *abuse of iron, quinine.*

15) Increased inclination to *micturate*, aggravated *when lying down.* As soon as she lies she has a desire to pass urine.

16) *Metastasis of mumps to mammae* or testicles.

17) *Diarrhoea* usually at *night.*

18) *Sleep* – sleepless in first of night from ideas crowding in mind. Sleeps late in the morning.

19) Pulsatilla is one of the best remedies to start the treatment in a *chronic case.*

20) *Better* – Cold air, cold applications, while walking slowly in open air.

Worse – Warm room, warm applications, heat of bed, cold drinks retained – warm vomited.

Particulars :

1) MIND
2) HEADACHE
3) FACE
4) TOOTHACHE
5) EYES
6) EARS
7) RESPIRATORY SYMPTOMS

8) GIT
9) FEMALE SYMPTOMS
10) MALE SYMPTOMS
11) URINARY SYMPTOMS
12) FEVER
13) RHEUMATISM

MIND

Mild, gentle and tearful disposition – She is so gentle that she can hardly say a cruel word to anybody. People very often take advantage of her sweet disposition. A Puls. wife never quarrels with her husband. Puls person moulds herself to what others want.

Weeping tendency – She cries even when nothing has happened. Relieved by weeping and consolation.

Aversion to marriage – She imagines that the company of opposite sex is dangerous. Relationships are very important *Needs a steadying anchoring force.*

High sexual desire – Sexual physically and emotionally. May become an extreme fanatic, apathy in the end stage.

HEADACHE

Headache in school girls who are about to menstruate, uterine/neuralgic origin.

Cause – Menstrual disorders, gastric disturbances due to overeating, fatty food, warm room.

Location – One sided headaches. Pains through the temples and side of the head. Frontal and supraorbital headache.

Sensation – Throbbing congestive headache, wandering pains from one part of head to another.

Better – Cold application, open air, walking slowly in open air, flow of menses.

Worse – Warm room, evening, stooping, mental exertion.

Concomitants – Perspiration on one side of head.

FACE

Pulsatilla person has a venous constitution. The veins are engorged and in a state of stasis and hence overheat of skin. False plethora – unusual fullness, redness and purple aspect of the face. This leads to puffiness and swelling especially at menstrual periods. Considerable bloating of the face and eyes, bloating of abdomen, feet puffed so that she cannot wear shoes, feet red and swollen at menstrual periods > menstrual flow, slow motion, in open air.

TOOTHACHE

- Severe tense tearing and throbbing pain shooting into the gum every now and then that makes the eyes water.
  < evening, warm things, heat of room.
  > holding cold water in mouth.

EYES

Catarrhal condition of the eyes – lids become swollen and itchy – the conjunctiva becomes full of minute pustules and keeps on discharging a bland thick yellow or yellowish green secretion. *Styes* (Puls. has great predilection) especially on the upper lids, from eating fat greasy rich food or pork.

EAR

Puls is commonly indicated in children when the child is gentle, fat plump. Vascular red faced child always pitifully crying. Catarrhal affections of the ear with thick yellow offensive, purulent bland discharge, very fetid sometimes bloody.

Otitis media – Ear troubles with ruptured ear drum and no healing, abscess with inflammation in the middle ear – copious thick bloody and yellow green discharge.

RESPIRATORY SYSTEM

Catarrah :

Wherever there is mucous membrane there is catarrah. Mucous membrane is covered with purple spots, dry spots, tumid puffed looks. *Bland thick green yellowish discharges are characteristic.*

Nose :

Coryza (chronic character) – Puls is suitable for chronic catarrah with yellowish green discharges. Bland discharges with offensiveness (Puls. is not indicated in an acute stage with watery discharge). Large bloody thick yellow crusts accumulate in the nose, harden up and are blown out in the morning accompanied by thick yellow pus. Relief from the horrible stench by blowing out crusts > Open air:<Warm room (Nose stuffs up in a warm room, he feels more stuffy in a warm room).

Epistaxis – 'passive character'– The flow comes steadily but is not bright red. Vicarious menses – epistaxis instead of menses.

Mumps – *Metastasis* of mumps to breasts in females or testicles in males. Puls is one of the most important remedies.

Chest – Feeling of *soreness* referred to either the right or left sub clavicular region or to the apex of one or the other lung. This soreness is felt when the patient lies on the affected side or presses against the chest. It seems to involve the muscular structure about the shoulder and even the arm of the affected side – this symptom indicates venous congestion or sluggish circulation in upper part of the lung. (Valuable symptoms in incipiency of T.B.).

Heart :

Puls. affects the right heart – the vascular system especially upon the veins and capillaries.

A warm room provokes symptoms as the temperature is too high and the veins will become tortuous and there will be some oppression about the chest and hearts action. Open air despite chilliness caused due to aneamia stimulates the venous circulation and that improves the symptoms caused due to sluggish flow of blood.

Larynx :

Bronchitis with thick yellow expectoration or dry tickling cough from irritation in the trachea < evening, lying down. Dry air passages with a raw and scraped feeling. Dyspnoea < walking fast, becoming overheated after eating, stopping of nose, emotions, suppressed asthma, suppressed menses, chronic loose cough, after measles; > open air, slow motion. Wandering tearing pains in the chest with dryness and rawness. Puls. is useful in catarrhal pthisis in chlorotic girls.

GIT

Bitter taste in the mouth in the morning. Dry mouth without thirst. Saliva gives sweetish taste. Constant spitting of frothy cotton like mucus.

Dyspepsia :

[Mouth, throat and stomach symptoms < night. Mind symptoms < evening]

Cause – Rich fatty food, little exercise, sedentry life.

Sensation – Pressure in the pit of the stomach as from a stone. This is accompanied with gnawing distress as from ulceration in the stomach.

Symptoms – *Slow digestion* – as a consequence the smell and taste of food remains in the mouth for long. Frequent attacks of vomiting in which all foods taken for days are brought out. Due to bad assimilation eating does not satisfy, due to slow digestion the patient goes to the next meal hungry. Scraping sensation in the stomach and oesophagus with heartburn. Bloating, gas and sour stomach are characteristic. Epigastric pain of changeable character, shifting pains that go from one part to the other >pressure, cold applications.

< hot applications, lying on painless side.

Desires things he cannot digest—lemonade, cheese, pungent things, juicy things.

Craves—Ice cream, pastries, highly spiced food.

Aversion to—meat, butter, fat food, pork, bread, milk.

Modalities < Warm room.

> Open air, cold air, slow motion.

Flatulence :

Caused by free indulgence in ice creams, fruits and pastries. Flatulence gives rise to colic which makes her bend double and unlace her clothes <Evening, warm room,before menses.

Concomitants—Coated tongue, dry mouth with thirstlessness.

Diarrhoea :

Cause—Fatty food, fruits, cold drinks, ice creams.

Time—Night.

character of stool—No two stools are alike. Loose watery yellow green slimy stools constantly changing character.

Constipation :

Ineffectual urging to stool with backache or they are insufficient and finally consist of nothing but yellow mucus.

Piles :

Extremely painful, protruding, blind with itching and stitches in the anus.

<lying down, warmth of bed.

>gentle motion in open air.

FEMALE

Complaints generally start at *'puberty'* or *'menarche'*—patient says "I've never been will since that time".

Premenstrual Syndrome :

Bloating of abdomen with a stuffed feeling, has to throw off her clothes, wants to get into a loose dress or go to the bed. Bloating of face, lips, feet are puffed so she cannot wear shoes. Funnelling or dragging down sensation in the uterus as if the parts would come out.

Dysmenorrhoea :

Violent menstrual colic with soreness in the region of uterus, wants windows open, tearful and weeps without cause (menses with absence of thirst and pains of shifting nature). In girls of mild disposition, when puberty is unduly delayed or menstrual function is defectively or irregularly performed, they are pale and languid, complain of headache and chilliness and lassitude. Another striking feature which may be present during menses is when the menstrual flow is present, there is milk in the breasts.

Menses :

Suppression or scanty menstrual flow from getting feet wet.

Time – Too late.
Duration – Short.
Quantity – Scanty discharge.
Character of blood – Thick black clotted blood or thin and watery. Changeability is marked.

Leucorrhoea :

Thick and milky white and appears in young girls during puberty.

Amenorrhoea :

Occurs during ordinary period of menses or as a result of cold feet; when nose bleed acts vicariously for the menses. Amenorrhoea may be accompanied with headache, anorexia, dysuria, opthalmia, nausea etc.

Labor :

During labor – pains are slow, weak and ineffectual – spasmodic and irregular and may excite fainting. Intermittent pains – sharp and crampy and appear in bladder, groins, lower extremities, shifting in character. Desire for open air, wants doors and windows open, feels suffocated in a stuffed room.

After Labor :

When the placenta remains adherent Puls brings out the release of the placenta and also tones up the uterus as to avoid post partum heamorrhage. Pulsatilla corrects *malpositions of foetus in utero* (it does not make the foetus turn around but acts on the muscular walls of the uterus and stimulate their growth and thus permits the foetus to assume its proper position).

Abortion :

Threatened abortion. Flow ceases and starts again with double force and ceases again. Puls promotes expulsion of moles.

Mammary glands are affected before during and after pregnancy. It is indicated when mechanical irritation excites the flow of milk for instance carrying school books excite the flow of the milk. Agalactica (absence or failure of secretion of milk). After labor the breast is swollen and painful, flow of milk is scanty or absent, patient is gloomy and tearful.

MALES

Having a very strong sexual desire. Long lasting morning erections, sexual desire leads to headache, backache, heavy limbs. Burning or aching in testicles.

Suppressed gonorrhoea that gives rise to complications like orchitis, epididimitis, prostatitis. Great tenesmus and stinging in the neck of the bladder. Gonorrhoeal discharge is thick yellowish green and patient is sensitive to heat and is better by walking in open air.

URINE

Trouble caused by taking chill, getting feet wet. It spurts out on least movement or strain. She is afraid therefore to go out into company. She soils her clothes even while moving or walking. Coughing, sneezing or laughing also causes involuntary spurting of urine.

She cannot lie on the back without the desire to urinate.

Nocturnal enuresis in little mild gentle yielding girls of florid complexion who kick off their covers at night.

(Loss of urine during first part of sleep – Caust, Sep.)

FEVER

Puls. is an invaluable remedy in all fevers that are suppressed (Remittent and Intermittent).

- Morning and evening paroxysms – evening one being more pronounced (4 P.M.).
- Fever is preceded by gastric disturbances such as diarrhoea, nausea and vomiting. The broad and large tongue is coated white and yellow and is covered with tenacious mucus.
- Changeability of symptoms – no two paroxysms are alike.
- Patient keeps constantly licking his lips to moisten them and yet does not wish to drink.

Chill Stage :

Starts at 4 P.M. with vomiting of mucus and dyspepsia. Chilliness is flitting in nature but after a while the parts feel hot and he feels chilly in a different place.

Heat Stage :

Whole body burns like fire and external warmth is intolerable, the patient complains of the room being too stuffy and wants doors and windows open. Veins are distended and his face is red.

Sweat Stage :

One sided sweat < night, during sleep. *Thirstlessness* is a marked feature of Puls. though morning paroxysms are marked by thirst and evening paroxysms are free from thirst.

Measles :

Catarrah is prominent and there is profuse lachrymation. Cough is dry at night and loose in the daytime. Child sits up in bed to cough. Puls. is indicated in chronic affects of badly managed measles.

RHEUMATISM

Pains of shifting character attended with chilliness

< warmth, evening.

> cold air, cold applications, walking slowly in open air.

General Modalities :

Aggravation – WARM CLOSED ROOM
EVENING
BEGINNING TO MOVE
LYING ON LEFT OR PAINLESS SIDE
RICH FAT INDIGESTIBLE FOOD
WARM APPLICATIONS, HEAT.

Amelioration – OPEN AIR, LYING ON PAINFUL SIDE
COOL AIR, COOL ROOM, EATING
OR DRINKING COLD THINGS,
COLD APPLICATIONS.

Relations :

Complementry – Kali mur, Lyc, Silicea, Sulph. Acid.

Follows well and is followed by Kali mur. Puls is one of the best remedies to begin the treatment of a chronic case (Calc., Sulph.).

- Aneamic or chlorotic patients who have taken much iron, quinine and tonics even years before.
- **Follows well** – after – Kali bi, Lyc, Sep, Sil, Sulph.

Important Questions ?

Q.1. Give indications of Pulsatilla in the following :

1) Gastric Disorders [1973, 74, 75, 77, 78, 82, 86, 93]
2) Hysteria [1986]
3) Drug picture [1967, 69, 74, 77, 79, 82]
4) Diarrhoea [1977]
5) Leucorrhoea [1986]
6) Mental generals [1971, 72, 72 S, 73, 74, 79, 87, 91]

7) Toothache [1985]

8) Female disorders [1967, 72, 75, 76, 77, 78, 82, 93]

9) Constipation [1984]

10) Urinary disorders [1984]

11) Headache [1974, 76]

12) Cough [1975]

13) Eruptive fever/measles [1973, 77]

14) Mumps [1979, 81]

15) Orchitis [1977]

16) Eye troubles [1982]

Q.2. Silicea is the chronic of Pulsatilla. Justify. [1997]

Q. 3. Why is Nux vomica a remedy for Males and Pulsatilla a remedy for females.

[1976, 87]

Q. 4. Compare :

1) Female – Kali carb/Puls [1994]

2) Female – Kreos/Puls [1994]

3) Mental generals – Nat mur/Puls/Sepia/Platina [1971, 73]

4) Catarrhal symptoms – Kali bi/Puls [1991]

6) Menstrual disorders – Actea spicata/Puls [1990]

7) Prostatic affections – Sabal.S/Puls [1987]

8) Female – Puls/Murex [1983]

64. RHUS TOXICODENDRON

Hahnemann

Common Name – Poison Oak.

Constitution – Chilly patient – easily susceptible to cold and aggravated by cold. Acute remedy so no specific constitution is marked.

Relation with heat and cold – Very chilly patient.

Miasm – Psora is in the background of all troubles.

Diathesis – Rheumatic and Gouty diathesis. Adapted to persons of rheumatic diathesis, bad affects of getting wet, especially after being overheated.

KEYNOTES

1) ***Ailments from spraining or straining*** **a** single part, muscle or tendon (Calc, Nux.), Overlifting particularly from stretching high up to reach things, lying on damp ground, too much summer bathing in lake or river.

2) *Pains as if sprained* – as if a muscle or tendon was torn from its attachment, as if bones were scraped with knife, worse after midnight and in wet rainy weather.

3) ***Lameness, stiffness and pain on first motion***, after rest or on getting up in morning walking or continued motion.

4) ***Great restlessness*** – anxiety and apprehension (Acon., Ars.). Cannot remain in bed, must change position often to obtain relief from pain.

   Restlessness from mental anxiety – Ars alb.

   Restlessness from physical anxiety – Acon.

5) *Back* pain between the shoulders on swallowing; pain and stiffness in small of back.

   < sitting or lying.

   > motion, lying on something hard.

7) Muscular rheumatism, sciatica (left sided) – aching in the left arm with heart disease.

8) Great *sensitiveness to open air* – putting the hand from under the bed cover brings on cough (Bar., Hep.). Dry teasing cough before and during chill. In intermittent fever cough with taste of blood.

9) Headache – brain feels loose when stepping or shaking the head, sensation of swashing in the brain, stupefying as if torn.

10) Vertigo when standing or walking

< when lying down, rising from lying or stooping (Bry).
(better lying down – Apis).

11) Corners of mouth ulcerated with fever blisters around the mouth and on chin (Nat. mur).
12) ***Paralysis with numbness*** of affected parts from getting wet or lying on damp ground, after exertion, parturition, sexual excesses, paresis of limbs, ptosis.
13) *Erisipelas* extending from left to right. ***Vesicular eruptions*** with swelling, inflammation, burning, itching and stinging.
14) Aggravation – Cold, wet rainy weather, getting wet while perspiring, during rest.

Particulars :

1) HEADACHE
2) FACE
3) GIT
4) RESPIRATORY SYSTEM
5) FEVER
6) HEART
7) RHEUMATISM
8) MALE SEXUAL SYMPTOMS
9) FEMALE SYMPTOMS
10) SKIN

HEADACHE

Cause – Exposure to cold, damp weather, suppressing sweat on head, rheumatic headache.

Location – Whole head.

Sensation – Brain feels loose or there is undulating feeling in the head. Pain in the head as if the brain were torn. Rush of blood to head with humming in the ears. Sensation as if bones of skull were scraped together.

Modalities < wetting the hair, motion.
> holding head backward.

Concomitants – Great restlessness. Keeps the head in constant motion. Vertigo when standing or walking, motion, rising from bed.

Eruptions on the scalp are very sensitive to touch. Vesicular eruptions upon the scalp, erisipelas of scalp with large blisters, eruptions on scalp that suppurate, eczema of scalp in infants.

EYES

Inflammation of the eyes, pustules on the cornea, iritis, acute conjunctivitis, chemosis.

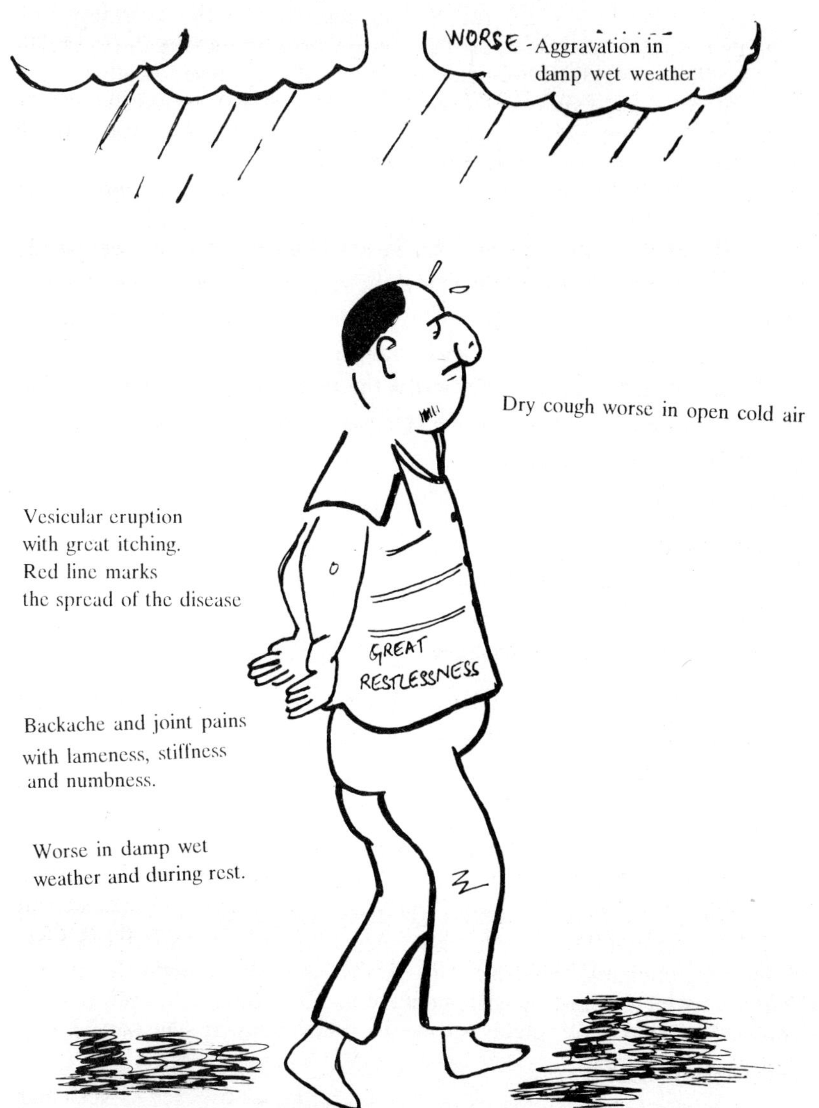
WORSE - Aggravation in
damp wet weather
Dry cough worse in open cold air
Vesicular eruption
with great itching.
Red line marks
the spread of the disease
GREAT
RESTLESSNESS
Backache and joint pains
with lameness, stiffness
and numbness.
Worse in damp wet
weather and during rest.

RHUS TOXICODENDRON

Cause – Rheumatic subjects from exposure to damp weather, suppressing perspiration.

Symptoms – Eyes are red and agglutinated in the morning with copious purulent mucous discharge. Pains worse on moving the eyeballs. Intense photophobia. Eyelids that are inflamed are spasmodically closed. If the lids are forced apart there is a gush. In iritis pains shoot through eyes to the back of the head. Ptosis in rheumatic patients after exposure to dampness. Styes on lower lids (Puls – upper lids).

FACE

Rheumatic patients with pain in maxillary joints as if joint would break. Every time the patient makes a chewing motion with mouth the jaw cracks. Erisipelas of the face with burning large blisters and rapidly extending inflammation which pits upon pressure. Erisipelas of the face often extends from left to right across the face. Eczema of the face with chronic suppurating eruptions on the face, stiffness of jaws, rheumatic conditions of jaws and joint.

GIT

Tongue :

Triangular red tipped tongue with imprint of teeth and bitter taste in mouth.

Mouth :

Dry mouth with accumulation of saliva and sometimes bloody saliva in the mouth which runs from mouth during sleep. Violent thirst, difficulty in swallowing solids from constriction of throat.

Stomach :

Desires – Oysters, cold milk, sweets.

Aversion – Meat.

Hunger without appetite. Hungry sensation or sensation of emptiness without desire for food. Dryness of mouth and throat with great thirst, unquenchable thirst for cold drinks especially at night. Desire for *cold milk* which relieves gastric complaints (In Iodum cold milk relieves constipation and in Graphites warm milk relieves gastric symptoms.)

Diarrhoea/Dysentry :

Cause – Damp wet weather, summer bathing.

character of stools – Blood and slime mixed with reddish yellow mucus.

Concomitants – Tearing pains in thighs during defeacation. Great thirst with dry tongue, mouth and throat.

RESPIRATORY SYSTEM

Bronchitis :

Cause – Exposure to cold or open air, damp wet weather, summer bathing, putting hands outside from under the bed cover brings on cough.

character of cough – Hoarseness and scraping rawness in larynx with roughness and soreness in chest. Short dry respiration very much oppressed and anxious. Cough before and during chill. Patient knows that chill is coming because of dry teasing cough.

Modalities – < before storm, after midnight, bathing, exposure to cold, inspiration and rest.

> Wrapping up in a warm application, dry clear weather.

Inflammation of lungs – pleura with stitching pains, much fever, progressing towards typhoid state with aching in bones and restlessness. Intense fever, marked thirst, great prostration with typhoid symptoms. Heamorrhage from chest due to overexertion.

FEVER

Rhus tox is an excellent remedy both for remittent and intermittent fever.

Cause – Drenching in rain, bathing in pond or streams, living in damp room, rheumatic fever, suppressed foot sweat.

Symtoms – Yawning and stretching are first symptoms noticed. Patient feels weary and languid with regular aching of limbs. A dry teasing and fatiguing cough soon makes its appearance. Hydroa, cold sores on the lips may be found (Nat mur).

INTERMITTENT FEVER

Chill Stage :

Chill starts in one leg, usually thigh, between the shoulders or over one scapula. Chill starts at around 7 P.M. Patient shivers with great chilliness and feels as though dashed with ice water. Least movement like eating and drinking aggravate his chill but still he moves about for movement eases his pain.

Heat Stage :

The blood that was so long running like ice water feels like boiling hot. Headache not attended by teasing cough. Urticarea breaks out instead of cough with violent itching and great thirst. Intense restlessness and the patient continuously changes his position but finds rest nowhere.

Sweat :

After the heat stage the patient breaks out into profuse odourless perspiration. Urticarea passes off with advent of sweat.

Ign. – Urticarea during heat stage.

Apis – Urticarea as soon as stage of chill is over.

Typhoid :

Intense weakness and exhaustion with mild delirium. Patient constantly wants to jump out of the bed and escape. Patient slowly passes into stage of delirium and later to a stage of apathy and indifference. This is followed by involuntary stool, urination and great thirst. The typhoid may affect the lungs producing pneumonia with usual cough, difficult breathing, rust coloured sputum.

Tongue :

Rhus tox has a characteristic broad and flabby tongue with imprint of teeth. It is covered with brownish tenacious mucus. At other times it is dry, cracked with red edges and triangular red tip.

Scarlatina :

Rhus tox child becomes drowsy and restless, fauces look dark red and oedematous. Cervical glands too are swollen. Swelling may even extend to the parotid glands. Glands of axilla are especially affected by Rhus tox.

HEART

Weak heart, tremulous with palpitation. Violent palpitation when sitting still. Hypertrophy of heart that comes from overexertion, violent exercise, hypertrophy that comes on in atheletes, runners. Organic diseases of heart with sticking pains. Numbness and lameness of the left arm that comes on with heart diseases.

RHEUMATISM

Backache/Lumbago/Rheumatism

Cause – Getting wet, overlifting, taking cold, suppressing the sweat.

Symptoms – Lameness and stiffness in the back. Pains between the shoulders on swallowing food, rheumatic stiffness, pain between the shoulder blades, small of the back aches while sitting in a draught, attempting to rise. Least exposure to draft of cold air brings on a general aggravation of all symptoms.

< First motion, beginning to move, sitting, damp weather, dwelling in damp place.

> When moving about, lying on something hard.

Paralysis :

Cause – Overexertion, getting wet, lying on damp ground, summer bathing. Paralytic weakness either of the lower limbs or one part of the body. Stiffness and lameness in the sacrum aggravated on resting after exercise. Numbness in the limbs with pain. Paralysis of the arms, erisipelas with much swelling in limbs, swelling of the hands and arms, lower limbs. Tingling and pricking sensation is felt in hands and fingers when grasping something, crawling and numbness in the finger tips and fingers, swelling of the fingers, eruptions upon the hands and fingers. *Rhus tox patient is very restless – never at ease. Desires to change position every little while followed by relief for a short time. After resting when first moving, a painful stiffness is felt which wears off from continued motion.* Tearing and drawing pain in the lower limbs. < rest, first motion.

> continued motion.

- *Pains and weakness in joints*, muscles and tendons following sprains.
- Projections of bones are sore to touch as for eg. cheekbones.
- *Infantile paralysis* (Rhus is a common remedy). The nurse takes the infants to the park, takes him out of carriage and pulls him down upon the cold damp ground and in a few days the child comes down with infantile paralysis.

MALE

Eczema of genitals with infammation of erisipelas character. Scrotum becomes thick and hard with intolerable itching, oedematous swelling of genitals, erisipelas of genitals, humid eruptions of genitals.

FEMALE

Erisipelas swelling of the genitals with some eruptions.

Menses :

Time – Too soon.

Quantity – Too profuse.

Duration – Lasts too long.

Character of blood – Acrid blood causing excoriation of parts. Membranous tissue in menstrual flow. Suppression of menses from becoming wet and getting feet wet or becoming chilled. Prolapse of uterus from straining, lifting, weakness of pelvic muscles, labor like pains in abdomen from straining.

SKIN

Vesicular eruptions are a characteristic of Rhus tox and so it becomes a remedy in herpes, eczema etc. Skin is covered with numerous vesicles and there is great itching and tingling. Skin is often swollen and oedematous. These vesicles have a red areola around them. Symptoms are worse at night, damp weather, winter.

Rhus tox is useful in *acute suppuration,* especially it has been useful in suppurative condition about the eye. It has proved curative in abscesses about the parotid and axillary glands, pus is bloody and serous, pain is intense with dark red swelling. Rhus corresponds very closely to septicemia. Cutaneous surface about the eruption is red and angry looking. Eruptions extend from left to right. (Apis – Right to left. Apis is inimical to Rhus tox and should never be used before or after Rhus tox.)

Eczema – If the face is attacked there is oedema of loose cellular tissue about the eyelids which we may denominate as burning, itching and tingling. The eruption is moist, offensive and suppurating, at times impetiginous. A red line marks the spread of disease.

Right sided herpes zoster with extensive vesications and is generally accompanied with rheumatic pains. Vesicles have red areola around them.

General Modalities :

Aggravation – BEFORE STORM, COLD WET RAINY WEATHER, AT NIGHT, ESPECIALLY AFTER MIDNIGHT, GETTING WET WHILE PERSPIRING, DURING REST.

Amelioration – WARM DRY WEATHER, WRAPPING UP, WARM OR HOT THINGS, MOTION, CHANGE OF POSITION, MOVING AFFECTED PARTS.

Relations :

- Rhus tox is complemetry to Bryonia.
- Rhus tox is Inimical to Apis – Apis must not be used before or after Rhus tox. (Can cause severe aggravation.)

Compare – Acon, Bry, Rhod, Nat. sulph, Sulph.

Important Questions ?

Q.1. Give indications of Rhus tox in following :

1) Fever [1986, 96]
2) Skin [1972, 73, 74, 76, 77, 79, 86, 8, 90, 96]
3) Typhoid [1972, 73, 74, 78, 79, 91]
4) Modalities [1968, 72, 75, 77, 79]
5) Injuries [1972]
6) Sprain [1977]
7) Paralysis [1976]
8) Herpes zoster [1977]
9) Eczema [1982]
10) Rheumatism [1975, 77, 79, 81]
11) Tongue [1977]
12) Hoarseness of voice [1977]
13) Restlessness [1976]
14) Cardiac troubles [1977]
15) Acute epidemic parotitis [1979]
16) Acute bacillary dysentry [1979]

Q.2. Compare :

I. Restlessness of Acon, Ars. alb, Rhus tox. [1993, 97]

ACONITE	ARS. ALBUM	RHUS TOX
• Aconite patient moves about quite frequently; he is physically strong.	• Intense prostration with mental restlessness. Person wants to keep moving but is very weak and prostrated to move about.	• Patient is very restless. Cannot stay in one place. Must change position frequently to obtain relief from pain.

II. Pain – Rhus tox and Bryonia – [1969]

BRYONIA	RHUS TOX
• Patient desires and remains perfectly still to relieve his pain.	• Pains are better by slow motion and aggravated by rest. Extreme restlessness and patient desires constant change of position.
• Pains < slightest motion. > rest and hard pressure.	
• Complaints are aggravated in heat and summer weather.	• Great sensitiveness to open air and damp weather.

III. Malarial Fever – China/Rhus tox – [1994]

CHINA	RHUS TOX
• Periodicity is well marked.	• Great restlessness is well marked.
• Pumped out, broken down constitution.	• All pains < rest > slow motion
• *Chill stage* – Chill is of short duration. Thirst before and after but not during chill.	• *Chill stage* – Chill starts in one leg usually thigh, between the shoulders or over one scapula. Patient is very restless. Least movement like eating or drinking aggravates chill, still the patient wants to keep moving. Dry cough during chill stage.
• *Heat stage* – Long lasting heat and patient wants to uncover. Even though the patient is very thirsty. He just wants to uncover the mouth.	• *Heat stage* – Urticarea breaks out instead of cough with violent itching and great thirst. Intense restlessness.
• *Sweat* – Profuse debilitating sweat with great thirst.	• *Sweat* – Profuse sweat after heat stage. Urticarea passes off with advent of sweat.

IV. Rheumatism – Ranunculus bulbosus and Rhus tox – [1972, 73, 83]

RHEUMATISM

RANUNCULUS	RHUS TOX
• Rheumatism of *chest wall :* sharp shooting neuralgic and myalgic pain that are aggravated by touch, motion or turning the body; during inspiration wet and stormy weather. Great sensitiveness to cold air and wet stormy weather.	• Rheumatism caused by lying on damp ground, summer bathing, working in a damp place. Pains as if sprained, as if muscles and tendons are scraped with knife. Parts are sore to touch. Great restlessness – patient wants to keep moving constantly.

65. SECALE CORNUTUM

Common Name – Spurred Rye (Ergot). A fungus – A nosode.

(Used in olden days as an abortificant.)

Constitution – Adapted to women of thin scrawny, feeble, cachetic appearance, irritable, nervous temperament with pale sunken countenance.

Look of the face – Emaciated, withered, wrinkled, unhealthy appearance of the skin, purplish bluish skin in general or in spots. Feeble circulation on back of hands, feet and on the tibia. These parts become numb, tingle and wither. Eyes are sunken with blue rings around them. Dim vision with a hoarse croacky voice. The extremities prickle burn and tingle with creeping and crawling as of insects under the skin. Toes become black and gangrenous.

Senile withering – Such as found in feeble old people, the blood vessels close up, no blood goes to the toes and they become numb and black devoid of sensation. Hence Secale improves the circulation of aged and postpones senile gangrene.

(*Looseness everywhere* – Uterus, blood vessels, skin, rectum.)

Relation with heat and cold – Hot patient though the skin feels cold to touch, the patient cannot tolerate covering.

Miasm – Psora is in the back ground.

Diathesis – Heamorrhagic diathesis. – The slightest wound causes bleeding for weeks (Phos, Lachesis) discharge of sanious fluid; blood with a strong tendency to putrescence, tingling in the limbs with great debility especially when weakness is not caused by previous loss of fluids.

KEYNOTES

1) ***Skin feels cold to touch and yet the patient cannot tolerate coverings, icy coldness of extremities internal burning with external coldness.***
2) *Pale pinched ashy skin* with *lax muscular* fiber, everything seems loose and open with *no action*, flabby muscles with passive heamorrhages, copious flow of thin black watery blood, the corpuscles are destroyed.
3) *Formication* – Tingling sensation all over the body especially after abortion or blood loss. The patient requests the attendant to rub her limbs.
4) *Burning* in all parts of the body as if sparks of fire were falling on the patient (Ars.).
5) *Boils* – small painful with green contents, mature very slowly and heal in the same manner, very debilitating.

6) *Unnatural ravenous appetitie* even with exhausting diarrhoea – craves acids and lemonades.
7) *Diarrhoea* – profuse watery putrid brown; discharged with great force (Gamb., Crot) very exhausting, painless, involuntary with a wide open anus (Apis, Phos).
8) *Collapse in cholera disease*, skin cold and yet cannot bear to be covered.
9) *Large ecchymosis* – blood blisters form at commencement of gangrene.
10) *Menses* – irregular copious dark fluid with pressing labor like pains in the abdomen, continuous ***discharge of watery blood until next period***.
11) ***Threatened abortion*** especially at *third month* (Sabina). Prolonged bearing down with forcing pains.
12) *During labor* – pains are irregular, too weak, feeble or ceasing. Everything seems loose and open with no expulsive action. After pains are too long and too painful.
13) *Suppression of milk* in scrawny exhausted women, the breasts do not fill up.
14) *Small* rapid contracted and *intermittent pulse*.

Particulars :

1) HEAMORRHAGE
2) GIT
3) FEMALE SEXUAL SYMPTOMS
4) NERVOUS SYSTEM

HEAMORRHAGE

Ergot affects the blood itself. It seems to lessen the coagulating function of the blood – *hence it causes and cures heamorrhages that are dark, thin and persistent* – heamorrhages from uterus or from any of the cavities of the body. It may be given in uterine heamorrhages when the flow is passive, dark in colour and it may be offensive. The women is reduced to such an extent that she is exsanguinated and lies unconcious and cold. Before losing her conciousness she complains of tingling all over the body.

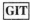

Cholera Infantum :

Character of stools – Profuse, undigested stools which are watery, thin and offensive and are discharged by fits and starts and followed by intense prostration. Stools are ejected with great violence.

Concomitants :

- *Cold and almost pulseless* with spasmodic twitching of muscles in various parts of the body. Despite the superficial coldness the *patient complains of great heat inside*. Heat makes him worse. Patient desires cold refreshing drinks such as lemonade and ice water.
- Unquenchable thirst.
- *Eyes are sunken with pinched* features.
- Great deal of spasmodic retching without much vomiting. Surface of the body is harsh, shrivelled and dry as though there were no moisture left in the system.
- Suppressed urine.

FEMALE SEXUAL SYMPTOMS

Abortion :

There are certain predisposing causes or exciting causes for abortions.

Predisposing causes – Syphilis in the parents is the most potent cause of abortions. Others are abnormalities of placenta, infectious diseases, malnutrition on the part of the mother, abnormalities in the generative tract such as displacement of uterus, retroflexion, prolapse etc.

Exciting causes – Injury, overexertion, intense mental emotions such as anger, fright and grief. In some women the uterus is in such a state that the slightest violence as caused by an act of coitus, a mis-step, tripping over a carpet or a ride over a rough road will bring on an abortion. In Secale cor – the abortion is caused generally by lifting, straining, hard labour. The miscarraige takes place around the *third* month with copious flow of black, bad smelling liquid blood. She gets cramps in the fingers with a tingling sensation. (*Ergot in crude state* acts more on pregnant than non pregnant uterus and more on multiparous than nulliparous uterus. It produces marked contraction and hence hastens expulsion of foetus when abortion is inevitable. It produces ineffectual uterine pains. In case of retained placenta there is hour glass contraction of uterus. This peculiar contraction prevents the expulsion of placenta.)

Retained Placenta :

Secale can be given in retained placenta especially that occuring in the early months of pregnancy. Discharge corresponding to lochia is offensive. Patient is almost cold and pulseless from loss of blood. The uterine contractions are very imperfect or else there are prolonged tonic contractions.

Labor :

During labor – Irregular pain which is too weak and ceasing occasionally.

After pains – Too long and painful with hour glass contraction.

Breast – Suppression of milk in thin,lean, and exhausted women. Breast is small and does not fill up properly.

Menses :

Time – Irregularly regular.

Duration – Long lasting.

Quantity – Copious.

Character of blood – Dark blood, continuous oozing of watery blood until next period.

Concomitants – Menstrual colic – labor like pains with coldness and intolerance of heat in scrawny feeble and cachetic women.

GANGRENE

Dry senile gangrene following injury with burning as if sparks of fire were falling on affected parts. Despite *coldness of parts* there is aggravation from external heat and relief from cold.

Convulsions :

Convulsions of *single parts* of whole muscular system, opisthotonos, cramps in calves, soles of feet and hands. Convulsions begin in face. Active manias with great excitement, exposes her body and tears at the genitals, puts her fingers in the vagina and scatches until the lips bleed, all idea of modesty lost. Extensor type of cramps in fingers and toes.

General Modalities :

Aggravation – HEAT, WARMTH
FROM COVERING.

Amelioration – COLD AIR, GETTING COLD
COVERING PARTS, RUBBING.

Relations :

Similar to – Arsenic album but cold and heat are opposite.

Resembles Colchicum in cholera morbus.

Compare – Cinnamon in post partum heamorrhage; it increases labor pains. Controls profuse or dangerous flooding. It is always safe. Ergot is dangerous.

Important Questions ?

Q.1. Give indications of Secale cor in following :

1) Menstrual symptoms [1986]

2) Female Genital symptoms [1967, 88, 89, 90, 91]

3) Diarrhoea [1973, 76]

4) Collapse [1981]
5) Labor [1972, 81, 82]
6) Heamorrhage [1972]
7) Mental Symptoms [1974]

Q.2. Compare :

I. Dysmenorrhoea of Secale cor and Sabina.

SECALE COR	SABINA
• Menstrual colic with labor like pain, coldness and intolerance of heat in scrawny feeble and cachetic women. Irregular, long lasting menses with copious blood. Dark blood with continuous oozing of watery blood until next period.	• Dysmenorrhoea with labor like pain which is drawing in character in small of the back especially from sacrum to pubes. Too early and profuse menses that are long lasting. Flow in paroxysms which is too protracted. Bright red liquid blood intermingled with clots i.e. partly fluid and partly clotted especially in those ladies who have menarche very early.

II. CHOLERA – Secale cor/Veratrum album

SECALE COR	VERATRUM ALBUM
• 1. Indicated in collapse stage of cholera.	• 1. Indicated in early stage of cholera, it is preventive against cholera.
• 2. Body cold to touch, extremities icy cold, cold sweat, sunken eyes but cannot tolerate covering.	• 2. Great internal chilliness, icy coldness of face, nose, tongue, vertex, extremities etc. Cold feeling in abdomen < drinking cold water > covering.
• 3. Unquenchable thirst for cold water, craving for cold refreshing things, acids and lemonades.	• 3. Unquenchable thirst for large quantities of icy cold water. Craving for acids, refreshing things and ice cubes.
• 4. Coldness and collapse is main indication.	• 4. Violent vomiting with profuse diarrhoea and collapse.

66. SILICEA

Hahnemann

Common Name – Pure Silicea.

It is a *long and deep acting remedy that is slow in action*. It is known as *'Surgeons knife'* it is capable of reaching and curing the derangement in the most vital process of life, in the internal sphere of man where the surgeons knife can never reach.

Silicea is complementry and chronic of Pulsatilla.

Constitution – Adapted to nervous, irritable people of sanguine temperament. Persons of light complexion, fine dry skin, weakly with lax muscles. Constitutions which suffer from deficient nutrition not because food is lacking in quantity but from imperfect assimilation (Bar carb, Calc. carb) Oversensitive physically and mentally.

Temperament – Sanguine temperament.

Relation with heat and cold – Chilly patient.

Miasm – Psora is in the background.

KEYNOTES

1) ***Silicea is chilly, easily perspiring with want of self confidence*** and grit.
2) *Scrofulous rachitic children* – with large heads, *open fontenelles* and sutures; much sweating about the head which must be kept warm by external covering (Sanic), distended abdomen, weak ankles and slow in learning to walk.
3) ***Great weakness and debility*** – Nervous debility; mental labour is very very difficult.
4) Ailments caused by :
    a) *Suppressed foot sweat* (Cup, Graph, Psor).
    b) Exposing the head or back to slightest draft of air.
    c) Bad affects of vaccination especially abscesses and convulsions.
    d) Chest complaints of stone cutters and total loss of strength.
5) ***Want of vital heat*** – always chilly even when taking active exercise (Led; Sep.).
6) ***Desires—Cold food, cold drinks and ice creams.***
7) *Has a wonderful control over suppurative process* of soft tissue, periosteum of bone, maturing abscesses when desired or reduces excessive suppuration (affects chiefly soft tissues) – (Camph, Hep.)

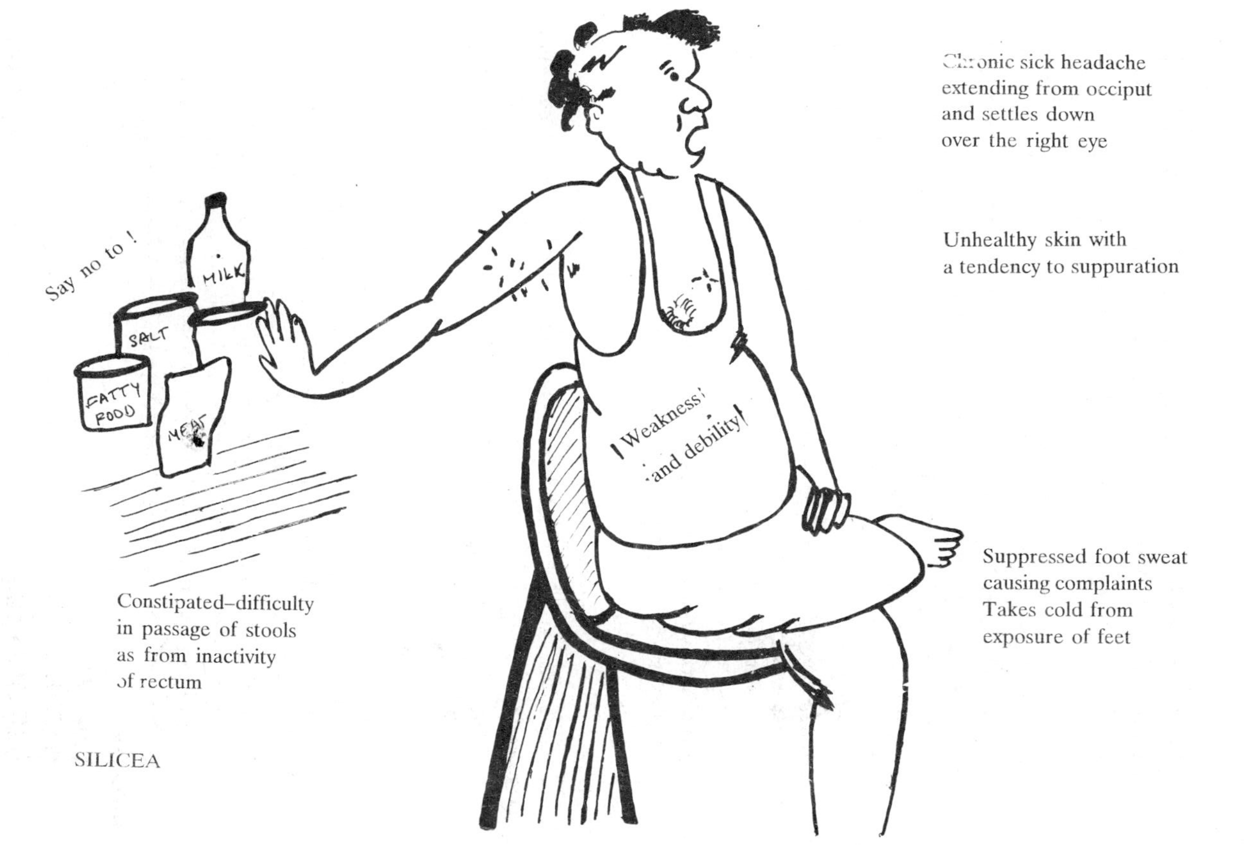
Chronic sick headache
extending from occiput
and settles down
over the right eye
Unhealthy skin with
a tendency to suppuration
Say no to !
MILK
SALT
FATTY FOOD
MEAT
Weakness!
and debility!
Suppressed foot sweat
causing complaints
Takes cold from
exposure of feet
Constipated–difficulty
in passage of stools
as from inactivity
of rectum

SILICEA

8) *Vertigo* – spinal, ascending from back of neck to head; as if one would fall forward from looking up (Puls; looking down – Kalmia, Spig.).

9) ***Chronic sick headache*** ascending from nape of the neck to vertex as if coming from spine and locating in one eye; especially the right (left – Spig). < draft of air or uncovering the head.
> pressure and wrapping up warmly, profuse urination.

10) Constipation – before and during menses; difficult as from inactivity of rectum with great straining as if rectum is paralysed; when partly expelled, the stools recede again (Thuja). Feaces remain for a long time in the rectum (diarrhoea before and during menses – Amm carb, Borax).

11) Fistula in ano alternates with chest complaints (Berb., Calc. phos.)

12) Discharge of blood from vagina every time the child takes to the breast (Crot)

13) ***Unhealthy skin*** – *Every little injury suppurates* (Graph., Hep, Petr., Merc sol.)

14) *Crippled nails* on fingers and toes (Ant. crud).

15) Takes *cold from exposure of feet* (Con., Cup.)

16) *Sweat of hands*, toes, feet and axillae – offensive.

17) Intolerable *carrion like odour* of feet without perspiration.

18) *Ingrowing toe nails*, fistula lachrymalis; blood boils, carbuncles, ulcers of all kinds, with painful offensive and highly spongy edges, proud flesh in them, fistula ani with great pain after stool.

19) ***Promotes expulsion of foreign bodies from the tissues;*** fish bones, needles, bone splinters. It will throw out abscesses in old cicatrices and opens them out.

(Silicea should not be used when the whole lung is tubercular since Silicea opens out old abscesses, establishes inflammation about tubercles as other foreign bodies and throws them out and in such a case it may lead to a general septic pneumonia.)

20) Silicea has *aggravation from milk* (Nat. carb, Aeth.). Mothers milk causes diarrhoea and vomiting. Silicea is one of the polycrests – *chilly, easily perspiring with want of self confidence of grit – to build up and give backbone to the weaklings.*

Particulars :

1) MIND
2) CHILD
3) HEADACHE
4) EYES
5) EAR

6) NOSE
7) FACE
8) RESPIRATORY SYSTEM
9) GIT
10) RHEUMATISM
11) SKIN
12) NERVOUS SYSTEM
13) FEMALE SYMPTOMS
14) FEVER

MIND

Silicea patient is very *yielding*–submissiveness that arises out of a lack of energy to insist upon her point of view. They are quite agreeable, mild and easy to get along with. Silicea patients are intellectuals but not aggressive or critical.

Mild and reserved–They are capable of freely talking about themselves when circumstances permit and they make friends easily. The Silicea patient will never challenge or become impatient. Silicea patients are tired, they lack stamina therefore they learn to conserve their energies. They are thin, pale, delicate and highly refined and aesthetic. The overstimulation of mind followed by lack of stamina is the basis for the descriptions in the books of professionals who develop an aversion to their work.

Pin mania–The patient always tries to collect pins. The child is afraid of pointed objects. Sometimes these patients develop fixed ideas and develop absolute prejudices. Its as if a small portion of brain has become sclerosed causing a loss of flexibility in thinking in regard to specific concepts. Silicea child is elite and delicate. They are delicate and easily develop curvatures of spine. Their intelligence is so great that it has pathological consequences. State of weakness with dread of failure–A lawyer dreads to appear in public but when he forces himself into work he goes on with ease and his usual self command returns.

CHILD

Silicea is used in marasmus of children (Abrot., Nat mur, Sulphur, Calcarea and Iodine); child has a pale sickly and suffering face. He is irritable and grumpy, scrofulous and rachitic children with large and open fontanelles and sutures. Much sweating about the head with distended abdomen. Head is disproportionately large for the body. *Sweat* on hands, toes, feet, axillae is very *offensive*. Suppression of sweat causes some pathological problems. Desire for cold drinks, cold foodand ice cream. Head is disproportionately large in comparison to the body. Head perspires profusely and is worse from getting wet. *Bad affects of vaccination.* Aggravation from milk and the infant is unable to take any kind of milk. Mothers milk causes diarrhoea and vomiting. Child suffers from damp changes in the weather and both are sensitive to cold about the head.

SILICEA	*BARYTA CARB*
• a)Profuse sweat on the head.	• a) Not present.
• b) Child is self willed and intelligent.	• b) Weakness of mind.

HEADACHE

Cause – chronic sick headache caused since some severe diseases of youth, suppressed foot sweat, mental exertion which causes congestion and heat of head.

Location – Headache goes up through the back of neck especially to the right side of the head and settles down over the right eye. Supra orbital neuralgia.

Sensation – Sharp tearing pains and at the height of paroxysm there is nausea and vomiting from sympathetic involvement of stomach.

Modalities – < Mental exertion, excess study, noise, motion, jarring foot steps, light, stooping, pressing at stool, touch.

> Warmth, wrapping up the head to avoid cold air, passage of profuse urine.

Concomitants – Sweat about the upper part of the body and the head, cold and clammy offensive sweat on the head. Vertigo which like the pains must rise from the spine into the head. There is a difficulty in balancing and the patient has a fear of falling to the left.

EYES

Many inflammatory conditions of eyes - - ulcers on cornea, pustules on the lids, falling of the lashes, suppuration of the margins of the lids with burning, stinging and redness. Intense photophobia with sore eyes. Spots and cicatrices on the cornea. Eyes inflamed from traumatic causes, foreign particles have lodged in the eyes with abscesses, boils, styes and tarsal tumors. [Where an indurated cicatrix forms around a lodged particle, Silicea throws out abscesses in these cicatrices and opens them out. It opens up old ulcers and heals them with a normal cicatrix.]

Tracoma with great hyperemia, swelling of conjunctiva, copious secretion of tears, mucus, violent supraorbital pain and intense photophobia.

EAR

Otorrhoea – Discharge from the ear being offensive watery and curdy. Perforation of membrana tympani with purulent discharge thence containing little pieces of bone, the result of involvement of mastoid process of the ossicles of middle ear by disease. Silicea is useful in beginning of dry catarrah of the middle ear and eustachian tube and the deafness goes on for sometime and the hearing returns with a snap. Catarrhal condition with a feeling of stoppage of the ear which is better by swallowing.

NOSE

Silicea is useful in nasal catarrah when ulcers exist on the mucous membrane and the discharge is thin bloody excoriating and there may be annoying dryness of nose. It is useful when the catarrhal process extends backwards and involves the outlets of the eustachian tubes producing intolerable itching and tingling in this locality.

FACE

Pale, waxy, sickly aneamic and tired face. Pustular and vesicular eruptions form over the face, wings of the nose crack and lips fissure easily, crusts form on the margin between the mucous membrane and skin. Indurations form on the skin and they pull off without healing.

Teeth – Break down and loose their enamel (dentine is made of silicate of lime) and surface of the tooth becomes rough, loses its shining appearance and caries set in. This takes place at the margin of the gums. Neuralgic toothache worse in cold air.

Nails – Rough and yellow with white spots on them.

RESPIRATORY SYSTEM

Cold – Chronic tendency for cold to settle in the chest and bring on asthmatic symptoms. Chronic bronchitis, inflammation of lungs with suppuration.

Cough – Cause – early stage of pthisis. Humid asthma, catarrhal cough.

Character of cough – Dry teasing cough with hoarseness, threatening tuberculosis of the larynx, peculiar cracked voice from thickening of laryngeal mucous membrane. Tickling cough as if from suprasternal fossa.

Asthma (Humid Asthma) – with coarse rattling. Chest seems filled with mucus and feels as if he would suffocate. Inveterate cases of catarrah of the chest and asthmatic wheezing and overexertion. Asthma of sycotics or in children of sycotic origin.

Expectoration – profuse, foetid, green purulent.

Modalities – Worse with cold drinks (Rhus tox, Scilla), speaking (Phos, Rumex, Ambra), lying down at night (Rumex, Phos, Lyco).

Pthisis – Silicea is useful in suppurative stage of tuberculosis when the cough is first dry and then becomes loose with the expectoration of offensive mucopus.

Tonsils – Glands suppurate and refuse to heal. Inflammation of extensive tissue of the body going on to suppuration which is sluggish and tends to become chronic. Quinsy with great pain in the tonsils threatening suppuration. Inflammation of parotid, sublingual, submaxillary gland with pain in the neck. Inflammation is better by warmth and worse by cold. In acute inflammations of neck he suffers from flushes of heat, an irregular flushing fever, cold extremities while the upper part of the body is hot, sweat about the head and neck, sensation of heat and suffocation in a warm room (Silicea in chronic manifestation is aggravated by heat but in acute troubles is chilly.)

Silicon is seldom indicated in acute forms because its pace is slow. It comes on after there is a series of cold but still continues to settle in the tonsils or in the glands of neck. There is a catarrhal state in the throat that is roused by taking cold with hoarseness settling back into a chronic state again; chronic catarrah of the pharynx.

GIT

Stomach :

Aversion – fatty food, salt, meat, milk (infant is unable to take any kind of milk). Aversion to hot things. Desires cold things. Chest complaints increase with cold things. Stomach is in a weak state. Old dyspeptics who have been vomiting for a long time especially those who have an aversion to warm food; who cannot take milk and are averse to meat.

Diarrhoea :

Silicea is a good remedy in chronic diarrhoea. Stools are offensive and usually painless and lientric. Child vomits its food. Diarrhoea after vaccination.

Constipation :

The stool escapes from the rectum and then seems to slip back again. There is defective expulsion power on part of the rectum; with a great deal of straining the stool is partly pushed out. When the bearing ceases, it slips back. Straining is violent so that the patient breaks down into pools of sweat.

RHEUMATISM

Chronic hereditary rheumatism. Pains are predominantly in the shoulders and in the joints. Worse at night and by uncovering. (Ledum is opposite – Rheumatism starts from feet and goes upwards. Patient is worse from covering up).

Diseases of hip and knee joint. Discharges are thin and offensive when there are fistulous tracks opening into the joint. (Marked feature – *offensive foot sweat that makes the toes sore and raw.*)

Spine :

Stiff neck that causes headache. This stiffness of neck is neither from cold nor from rheumatism of various muscles but from spinal irritation. Small of the back aches with trembling of the legs. They easily grow weary particularly in the morning. (Loss of animal fluids causes marked aggravation of these symptoms.)

SKIN

Inflammation – Silicea produces extensive inflammation of tissues and this inflammation easily matures into suppuration but suppuration is indolent and sluggish (takes a long time to heal). The pus that Silicea absorbs or let loose is copious, watery, thin and gelatinous; the putrid portion extends to joints, ligaments and tendons (Merc sol – facilitates maturity, Hepar sulp – expels the pus that Merc sol generates; Silicea comes in after all the foreign substances are expelled and promotes steady healing.)

Boils :

Silicea helps dispose cold indurations; boils and abscesses are partially cured and there usually remains a surrounding area of hardness due to secretions of plastic exudate during inflammatory process. Silicea leads to absorption of these substances and establishes normal consistancy of tissues. Silicea absorbs or obliterates connective tissue growths in case of scar tissue.

Mucous membrane – offensive thin, ichorous and corossive discharges from various mucous membranes (Ozeana, pharyngitis, laryngitis and blepharitis.)

Bony Tissue :

Malassimilation of bony tissue with malformation and disfigurement, curvature and necrosis of vertebral column, disfigurement of joints, non closure of cranial bones, disfigurement of ribs and caries of tibia and fibula. Unhealthy skin – slightest scratch suppurates and turns into sore.

Nails :

Becomes brittle and crack easily. Wax like and earthy skin covered with exanthemata, pustules, acne rosacea, herpes.

Ulcers :

Flat and bluish base with high, hard and spongy edges. Worse by warm applications and better by cold application. Sensation of coldness of these ulcers.

Sweat :

Offensive sweat especially about axilla, palm, sole of feet and complaints are caused by suppressed foot sweat. Acrid sweat that chews up the socks (Psor., Sulph.)

NERVOUS SYSTEM

Paralytic weakness due to defective nutrition of nerves, spinal cord and brain. Want of vital warmth even when he takes exercise. Sense of weakness and debility and the patient constantly wants to lie down. There is tremulousness, nervous debility, drowsiness, lassitude, depression.

FEMALE SYMPTOMS

Silicea reduces excessive indurations of cervix, resolves cysts in vagina, cures amenorrhoea and leucorrhoea etc.

Indications are :

- Itching of pudenda.
- Profuse acrid and corroding flow coming out in gushes from vaginal canal.
- Cold feet.
- Discharge of blood between periods.
- Nipples of breasts are disfigured with cracks and rhagades.
- Sharp pain in either breast when the child is nursing.

(Pain in breast while nursing – this symptom has been indicated in several cases of cancer that were cured.)

FEVER

Cause – Suppression of foot sweat.

Chill Stage – Intense shaking chill and slightest movement aggravates chill. The patient keeps his hands and feet nicely covered. Shivering is not relieved by heat of fire. Feet and legs are icy cold.

Heat stage – It causes dark redness of face with strong thirst.

Sweat stage – Profuse sweat which breaks out periodically, offensive, sour and debilitating.

Concomitants – Loss of taste and appetite with marked aversion to warm food. Profuseness of sweat caused by slow suppurative process in the lungs.

General Modalities :

Aggravation – NEW MOON, FULL MOON
COLD, DURING MENSES
WASHING, UNCOVERING.

Amelioration – WARMTH, WRAPPING THE HEAD
AND SUMMER.

Relations :

Complementry – Thuja, Sanicula.

Incompatible – When used before and after Merc sol.

Followed well by – Hepar sulph and Flouric acid.

Important Questions ?

Q.1. Give indications of Silicea in the following :

a) Cold [1986]
b) Skin [1969, 75, 81, 87]
c) Child [1971, 73, 77, 75, 82, 95]
d) Sinusitis [1987]
e) Keynotes [1989, 91]

f) Headache [1973, 74, 75, 82]
g) Marasmus [1974, 75, 76]
h) Fever [1978]
i) Constipation [1976, 77, 79, 82]
j) Indigestion of milk [1977]
k) Teeth decay [1981]
l) Breast [1982]
m) Otorrhoea [1979]

Q.2. Compare Calcarea flour/Silicea in overgrowth. [1994]

CALCAREA FLOUR	SILICEA
• Calcarea flour is found in surface of bones and enamel of teeth. It acts favourably by obliterating osseous growths and suppurations of bones.	• Malassimilation of bony tissue with malformation and disfigurement.
	• Tendency of slightest scratch to suppurate. It produces inflammations about a fibrinous nidus and suppurates it out. It will throw out abscesses in old cicatrices and throw them out. Promotes expulsion of foreign bodies from the tissues by promoting formation of a healthy cicatrix (fish bones, needles, bone splinters).

Q.3. Compare Silicea and Calcarea carb child. [1997]

CALCAREA CARB	SILICEA
• Fair fat and flabby child.	• Malnourished child due to defective assimilation.
• Weak bones.	
• Open fontanelles, large head and delayed dentition.	• Highly psoric and chilly patient with a pot bellied abdomen.
• Chilly patient.	
• Desires eggs and undigestible things	• Offensive foot sweat with various kinds of skin troubles.
• Sweating profusely while sleeping.	
• Coldness of single parts.	• Aversion to mothers milk.

• Discharges smell sour. • Constipation – stools have to be mechanically removed.	• Desires cold things. • Constipation – stool is difficult to evacuate from rectum due to inactivity.

Q.4. Compare Headache of Silicea and Sanguinarea.

SILICEA	SANGUINAREA
• Cause – Mental exertion, vaccination, suppressed foot sweat.	• Cause – Mental exertion.
• Location – Headache goes upto the back of the neck especially to the right side of the head and settles down the right eye.	• Headache begins in the occiput, spreads upwards and settles over the right eye. Headache returns at climacteric.
• Worse – Cold air, mental exertion, noise.	• Worse – Morning and rises during the day.
• Better – Warmth, wrapping up, urination.	• Better – Sleep and lying perfectly quiet.
• Concomitants – Excessive sweating with vertigo.	• Concomitants – Neuralgia of face and pain extends to all directions from upper jaw. Better by kneeling down and pressing the head against the floor.

Q. 5. Lycopodium and Silicea in Mentals. [1987]

LYCOPODIUM	SILICEA
• Person has sense of inadequacy and lack of self confidence mostly in moral and social responsibilities.	• Patient is mild, reserved and yielding. Patients are tired. They lack stamina because they conserve their energies.
• Dread of appearing in public because of a feeling of incompetence.	• Thin, pale and delicate individuals.
• The patient wants to be alone and has a dread of solitude. The patient dreads the presence of new persons or visitors.	• Person has fixed ideas about certain things. General state of weakness with a dread of failure in all states including moral and social.

Q.6. Compare Thuja and Silicea in Constipation. [1986, 88, 89]

THUJA	SILICEA
• Chronic constipation when stool partly goes back after being expelled. Passage of stool produces violent rectal pain which compels the patient to cease the effort. Anus is fissured and painful to touch surrounded by flat warts, moist mucous condylomata. Along with constipation piles may also appear which is painful and swollen. Pain is more severe while sitting.	• Sensation of weakness or paresis which results in obstinate constipation so much so that feaces is retained for a long time in the rectum. Stool passes out with great straining. *Character* – Stool is partly expelled and then recedes back again. Consequently it has to be removed mechanically. Constipation occurs before, during and after menses.

67. SULPHUR

Hahnemann

Common Name – Flowers of Sulphur. Brimstone ('S' an element).

Constitution – *Sulphur* is adapted to people of light complexion who are easily angered although dark complexioned persons also yield to its influence. Suited to persons subject to skin affections particularly those who have a harsh and rough skin. Uncleanliness with offensive odour from the body. Bathing aggravates his complaints. There is a dislike for water. Harsh and coarse hair with craving for alcoholic drinks especially those of coarse type like beer and whisky.

Spare and stoop shouldered person, walks and sits stooping. Standing is the most uncomfortable position for him. Delicate face with long and thin eyelashes.

Sulphur is chronic ofAconite in acute diseases.

Dosage – Doses of Sulphur should not be repeated too frequently as the tendency of Sulphur is to arouse whatever is dormant in the system. It should be given with caution as it may wrongly precipitate a disease which it was desired to cure.

Temperament – Sanguine temperament.

Relation with heat and cold – Hot patient but sensitive to atmospheric changes.

Miasm – King of Antipsoric remedies.

Diathesis – Scrofulous diathesis.

KEYNOTES

1) ***Dirty and filthy stoop shouldered person*** prone to skin affections (Psorinum).
2) ***Itching of skin*** with scratching, feels good to scratch. Scratching causes burning which is ***worse at night*** in the ***heat of the bed*** (Medorrhinum).
3) Skin affections that have been treated by medicated soaps and washes.
4) Complaints that are ***continuously relapsing.*** Patient seems to get almost well when the disease returns again.
5) ***Congestion of single parts*** – eyes, nose, chest, abdomen, ovaries, arms, legs or any organ of the body marking the onset of tumors or malignant growth especially at climacteric. Portal congestion with heamorrhoidal trouble.

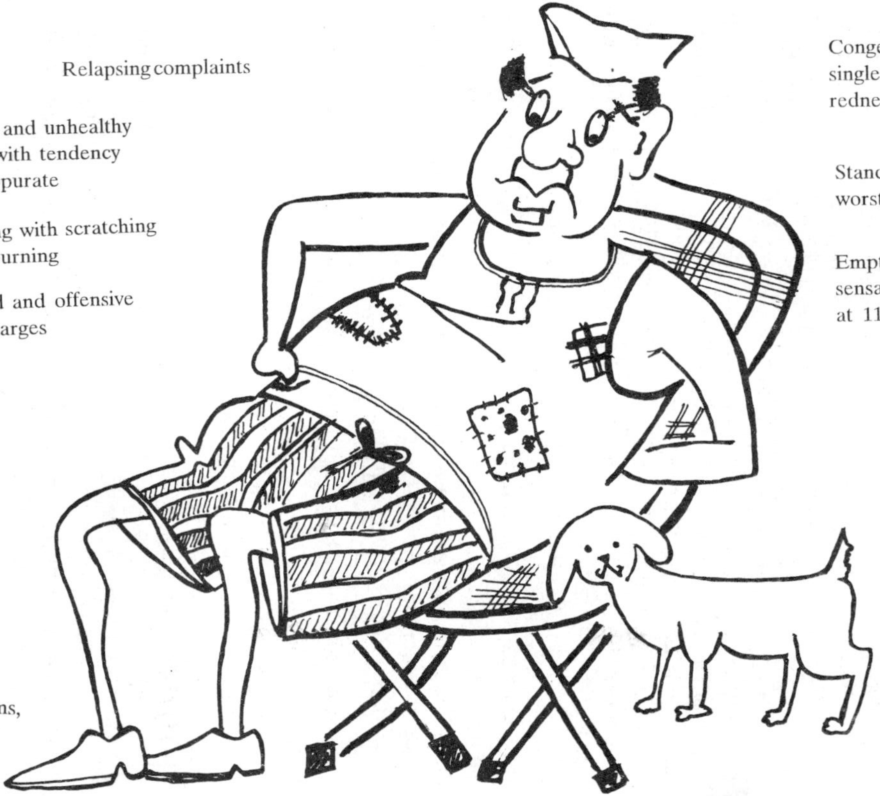

Relapsing complaints

Dirty and unhealthy skin with tendency to suppurate

Itching with scratching and burning

Acrid and offensive discharges

Heat of palms, soles, vertex

Congestion of single parts with redness and burning

Standing is the worst position

Empty all gone sensation in stomach at 11 O'clock

SULPHUR

6) ***Redness of various orifices*** with irregular distribution of blood redness of ear, redness at anus, vulva etc.

7) ***Flushes of heat*** – Sensation of heat on top of the head. Cold feet with sinking feeling at the epigastrium. Cold feet in daytime and hot at night and looks for a cool place at night (Med). ***Burning sensation*** on the vertex and smarting in the eyes, in face, scalding in urine, hot flushes in spots, between scapulae. Patient wants doors and windows open no matter how cold the weather may be. Heat on top of the head, cold feet, palpitation of heart on ascending, pain through the left chest from the nipple to the back are all associated symptoms.

(The above symptoms – 5,6,7 are caused due to *irregular distribution of blood with deranged circulation*. It acts more prominently on the venous circulation producing a sort of plethora. These congestions occur from abdominal troubles especially fullness of the portal system. For eg. piles have suddenly stopped bleeding and fullness of the head, with distended blood vessels, fullness of the liver show that congestion of these parts has resulted. Sulphur eases the congestion and restores the accustomed discharges.

Irregular distribution leads to congestion, redness of orifices, flushes of heat with burning of single parts.

8) Scrofulous, psoric, chronic diseases that results from suppressed emotion.

9) ***Standing is the worst position*** for Sulphur patients; they cannot stand. Every standing position is uncomfortable.

10) Children *cannot bear to be washed* or *bathed* (in cold water – Ant crud). Restless and hot patient who kicks off the clothes at night, have worms, but best selected remedy fails.

11) ***Nightly complaints*** worse in warmth of bed, covering up and washing.

12) ***Weak empty all gone sensation in the stomach at 11 A.M.***, cannot wait for lunch.

13) *Craving for sweets,* acids, fats, alcohol , beer, whisky, aversion to meat and milk.

14) *Periodicity of complaints* – Sulphur has periodicity, eg pains in head every 7 days, every 14 days, discharges every day at 5 a.m. etc.

15) *Boils* – Coming in crops in various parts of the body or a single boil succeeded by another as soon as the first one heals.

16) Sulphur facilitates *absorption of serous* or inflammatory exudates in brain, pleura, lungs, joints when (Bry, Apis, Kali mur) etc fail.

17) *Chronic alcoholism*; dropsy and other ailments of drunkards. They reform but are continuously relapsing.
18) Sensation of *movement of child in abdomen* (Crot., Thuja).
19) *All discharges* – leucorrhoeal discharges etc are *acrid and offensive*.
20) ***Early morning diarrhoea*** – drives the patient out of the bed in the early hours of the morning with a feeling as if his bowels were too weak to retain the contents.

Particulars :

1) MIND
2) CHILD
3) EYE
4) RESPIRATORY SYSTEM
5) DIGESTIVE SYSTEM
6) SEXUAL SYMPTOMS – Male and female.
7) NERVOUS SYSTEM
8) SKIN

MIND

Sulphur patient is a *ragged philosopher*. Every thing looks pretty which the patient takes fancy for. Even rags seem beautiful. He is very forgetful. Forgets recent events and remembers old ones. Everything seems full of beauty. He dresses himself in most tattered rags but considers them the most elegant of decorations. *Unhealthy patient* who smells offensive and is averse to washing. Even washing does not reduce his odour. *Selfish patient* with no regard for others. Sulphur is indifferent and disinclined to work. Nothing appeals to him. *Happy dreams* and wakes up singing.

CHILD

Marasmus of children with three red line symptoms :

a) *hunger at 11 A.M.*
b) *heat on top of the head.*
c) *cold feet.*

Sulphur is the mainstay in scrofula i.e. diseases of lymphatic system. It is useful in the commencement of diseases particularly in patients having temperament of Sulphur.

Dirty nosed children with sore discharging nostrils.

Marked tendency to *eruptions* such as crusta lactea, boils and acne in older children. Head is large in comparison to the body. Fontanelles remain open for too long from defective osseous growths. Tendency to *bone affections*, to caries particularly in early childhood, to rickets and to curvature of spine. Child has a *voracious appetite*. He greedily clutches at all what is offered.

Defective assimilation – glands are so diseased that while sufficient food is taken into the system it is not appropriated to the nourishment of the body so that the child is always hungry and yet emaciated. Child looks *shrivelled and dried up* like an old man and skin hangs in folds and is rather yellowish, wrinkled and flabby. *Dirty and filthy look of the child and yet cannot bear to be washed or bathed.* (Ant crud and Amm. carb). Untidy and unkempt with coarse rebellious hair who takes his own rebellious way. These babies suffer from morning diarrhoea which is painless, involuntary and acrid with redness of anal orifice. Prone to *worm infestation* with intense craving for *sweets*.

EYE

Sulphur is useful in conjunctivitis especially when trouble has resulted from a foreign body in the eye. Red and injected eye with a feeling as of a splinter of glass in the eye. Inflammation is worse in hot weather. Sulphur patient has a tendency to congestion. During winter the child is comparatively free from trouble and is aggravated by heat. It is used in retinitis, cataract, marginal blepharitis.

RESPIRATORY SYSTEM

Nose :

Profuse catarrhal discharges from the nostrils when out of the doors but indoors the patient feels his nostrils blocked up. It has cured freckles and black spots on the nose and face. Chronic catarrah with scabs in the nasal cavity, nose bleeds readily and is swollen. Redness of outlet of nasal cavity.

Laryngitis :

Hoarseness worse in morning. More chronic the case the better is Sulphur indicated.

Bronchitis :

Oppression of the chest with a feeling of hoarseness. Patient feels suffocated and wants the doors and windows open especially at night. Sharp stitching pains through the left lung to the back worse when lying on the back and aggravated by least movement.

Cough :

Dry cough caused by rawness of the larynx and is excited by a sensation of tickling as from a feather. In the evening and night there is no expectoration but in the morning and daytime the patient brings up a sort of darkish bloody sputum. Sometimes it is yellow greenish or milky white mucus. Cough is accompanied by pain in chest as if it would burst to pieces. Peculiar sensation of *coldness in chest* as from a lump of ice. Cough is aggravated by lying in horizontal position and may be so violent as to cause nausea and vomiting. Sulphur sometimes *prevents pneumonia* by relieving the lungs of the hyperemia which necessarily precedes the deposit of plastic matter. If Sulphur is given in the very beginning symptomatically the disease can be prevented. Sulphur can also be used in the stage of exudation with slowness of speech and dryness of tongue. All sorts of rales can be heard with mucopurulent expectoration, increase of blood to chest, dullness on percussion at apex of lungs, diminished respiratory movements in the upper portion of chest. Sulphur will cure by equalising the circulation. It should not be used after tubercles have formed.

Serous Membranes :

Sulphur is indicated in pleurisy. *Sharp stitching pains through the left lung to the back worse by lying on the back* and least motion. Sulphur is useful in cases that refuse to respond to a well chosen remedy.

DIGESTIVE SYSTEM

Tongue :

Coated white with red tip at edges. Sometimes it is full of apthae. (Borax, Merc. sol, Hydrastis).

Stomach :

Sulphur patient is a chronic dyspeptic. Faint weak all gone feeling at 11 A.M. He feels an empty sensation with fainting fits at 11 A.M. He must eat something there and then.

Cravings for sweet, acids, alcohol, beer, whisky and fats.

(Sulphur being a hot patient has strong craving for fats).

Aversion – meat, milk, business.

Dyspepsia from farinaceous food. He vomits a great deal. He cannot take any milk. Vomited matters are apt to be sour and mixed with undigested food (common symptom in drunkards). The patient is hungry at 10-11° clock even after eating a moderate breakfast. Goneness and faintness or gnawing feeling in the epigastrium. When he gets food and relieves his hunger he begins to feel puffed up. He feels heavy and sluggish and low spirited. Sulphur is indicated not so much in the beginning of these affections as Nux vom. When Nux vom only partially relieves Sulphur comes in to complete cure.

Diarrhoea :

Cause – suppression of skin diseases, alcoholism.

Time – Early morning diarrhoea – It drives him out of bed early in the morning (5 a.m.) with a feeling as if bowels were too weak to retain their contents (Bry, Nat sulph, Podo, Rumex, Phos.)

Character of stools – brown, watery fecal, undigested, frothy, sour fetid and corossive offensive odour of stools. There is a feeling of fullness and weight in the rectum and loss of power of sphincter ani.

Concomitants – Diarrhoea alternates with constipation.

Constipation :

Cause – alcoholism, suppression of skin eruptions.

Character of stools – Hard, dry knotty and painful stools as if burnt. Patient is afraid to pass stool on account of pain. Pain compels the patient to give up the effort and the discharge of feaces is painful to parts over which it passes.

Piles :

Sulphur patients suffer from *abdominal plethora or passive congestion of the portal system* as indicated by a sensation of tightness or fullness in the abdomen with a feeling of repletion after partaking of a small quantity of food. Liver is congested, enlarged and sore on pressure. Bowels are constipated with frequent ineffectual urging to stool with heamorrhoids which are direct results of abdominal plethora. Increased congestion of heamorrhoidal vessels. Blind or bleeding piles with violent bearing down pains from small of the back towards the anus. Sensation of fullness of anus. Suppressed heamorrhoids with colic, palpitation, congestion of lungs, back feels stiff as if bruised.

Redness with burning of anal orifice.

FEMALE SEXUAL SYMPTOMS

Great congestion of female sexual parts and consequently she complains of a sense of fullness with bearing down in the pelvis towards the genitals. This pressing down is felt more acutely while she is standing and as a consequence of that posture she is very reluctant to assume. She always wants to sit. Over and above this she suffers from leucorrhoea. Burning in the vagina in association with pruritis and appearance of papules on mons veneris.

Menses :

Sulphur is useful in dysmenorrhoea and menorrhagia.

Time – Too late.

Duration – Short.

Quantity – Scanty and sometimes profuse.

Character of blood – Black thick, dark, acrid; wherever it touches it makes the parts sore.

Concomitants – Menses are preceded by headache if suddenly stopped. With menses there is fullness with bearing down in pelvis towards genitals. Pressing is felt more acutely when she stands up.

MALE SEXUAL SYMPTOMS

Sulphur patient is weak and debilitated with faintness, flushes of heat, cold feet and heat on top of the head. Involuntary emission of semen at night exhausting him the next morning. Seminal flow is thin watery and almost inodourous, has lost all its characteristic properties. The genital organs are relaxed, the scrotum and testicles hang flabbily, penis is cold and erections are few and far. If coitus is attempted, semen escapes too soon almost at the first contact. Patient suffers from backache and weakness of [illegible]bs so that he can scarcely walk.

Sulphur, Nux vom, Calc. carb are trio of remedies of masturbation and excessive venery. Beginning with Nux—there is some improvement in the patient; by and by symptoms of Sulphur start presenting themselves and if Sulphur fails after producing partial relief Calc. carb completes the cure.

Gonorrhoea—Sulphur is indicated in gonorrhoea where there is bright redness of lips of the meatus urinaris.

SKIN

Dirty and filthy people prone to skin infections. Person *cannot bear to be washed or bathed.* Hot patient, emaciated and big bellied, kicks off clothes; have worms. Skin is apt to be harsh, rough, coarse and measly. Little tendency to perspiration or if there is perspiration it is only partial and offensive, sour or musty. Tendency to formation of *acne* principally on the face, hands and arms. Tendency to *intertrigo*; soreness and rawness appear wherever there is a fold of skin on the groin, mammae, axilla or in joints of skin. Itching in the bends of the joints and between the fingers as soon as the patient gets warm in bed. Skin becomes rough and scaly and little vesicles form. As the disease progresses there are little pustules appearing here and there over the eruption. Severe itching and patient goes on scratching. It feels good to scratch but scratching is followed by severe burning, rawness and soreness of parts.

Burning and formication on skin of whole body.

Sulphur has a great tendency to expel everything internal to the surface. Sulphur is indicated on all sorts of skin affections that have been treated by medicated soaps and washes, suppressed by ointments. It is a good drug for suppuration. Every little injury suppurates (Hepar, Graph. Sil.). There are boils and abscesses especially in summer season. Boils come in crops or a single boil is succeeded by another. Suppression of disease causes diarrhoea (Petroleum).

Aggravation—Warmth of bed, night, covering, washing.

Amelioration—Open air, uncovering, putting feet out of bed.

FEVER

Intense perspiration with long continued fever, hot and dry skin with burning, 103-105 °F temperature with little or no remission.

NERVOUS SYSTEM

Sulphur is useful in *spinal congestion* when the trouble results from suppression of a heamorrhoidal flow or suppressed menses. The back is so sensitive that any sudden jarring of the body causes sharp pains along the spine. There is dry heat particularly in the small of the back and this is associated with cold feet.

Paralysis – Sulphur is given when central cause of trouble is not so chronic and alteration in structure of spinal cord is not so profound. Paralysis of both legs with total retention of urine and numbness extending up to umblicus. When urine is drawn by a catheter it is turbid and offensive.

Rheumatism – Sulphur is indicated in acute and chronic rheumatism when inflammatory swellings seem to ascend i.e they begin in the feet and extend up the body. Patient feels *worse at night*. Patient uncovers on account of burning heat of the feet. Sulphur is indicated in acute rheumatism with marked symptoms. Jerking of limbs on falling asleep.

Synovitis – Sulphur produces absorption very rapidly particularly in the *knee*.

General Modalities :

Aggravation – STANDING, AT REST
WARMTH OF BED, WASHING,
BATHING, FROM ALCOHOLIC STIMULANTS
CHANGEABLE WEATHER.

Amelioration – DRY WARM WEATHER
LYING ON RIGHT SIDE.

Relations :

Complementry – Aloes, Psorinum, *Calcarea carb must not be given before Sulphur.* Sulphur is chronic of Aconite especially in acute diseases. When Sulphur fails think of Psorinum and Tuberculinum.

Follows well – Calcarea, Lycopodium, Sarsaparilla, Sepia.

Important Questions ?

Q.1. Give indications of Sulphur in the following :

a) Totalities [1987]
b) Stool modalities [1983, 87, 86]
c) Diarrhoea [1974, 75, 76, 77, 82]
d) Skin [1975, 76, 77, 79, 87, 88, 90, 95]
e) Modalities [1987, 74]
f) Marasmus [1987]
g) Impotence [1987]
h) Drug picture [1974, 73, 77]
i) Eczema [1972, 81]
j) Piles [1974, 77]
k) Generalities [1975, 76]
l) GIT [1981]
m) Intolerance of milk [1981]

n) Respiratory Diseases [1976]
o) Measles [1976]
p) Epilepsy [1977]
q) Cerebro spinal fever [1979]
r) Ascites [1981]

Q.2. Sulphur is called the king of psora. Describe Sulphur patient in details.

[1972, 73, 76, 78]

Q.3. Differentiate :

Skin symptoms of Petroleum/Sulphur/Psorinum

[1983 C, 88C, 91]

PETROLEUM	PSORINUM	SULPHUR
• Very chilly.	• Very chilly patient.	• Hot patient.
• Skin eruptions are worse in winter.	• Extremely chilly and offensive smelling patient.	• Complaints worse at night and heat of bed, bathing, covering.
• Skin is rough, bleeds with numerous cracks and fissures.	• Skin eruptions appear every winter and is thick and dirty looking.	• Skin affections that have been treated by medicated soaps, ointments etc.
• Tendency for every little injury to suppurate. Skin eruptions are dry with violent itch.	• Eczema caused by suppression of skin eruptions. Skin looks unhealthy and dirty even after washing.	• Dirty and filthy skin with offensive odour.
• Foul smelling sweat over the winter.		

• < Winters > Summers	• Intense itching which leads the patient to despair. He scratches until the part becomes raw. Itching is worse in warmth of bed, warm application, covering and open air. Skin is dry and sweats rarely. Sweat relieves suffering.	• Severe itching and scratching is followed by severe burning rawness and soreness. • Good drug for suppuration. Boils in crops. • Suppression of skin eruptions causes diarrhoea

Q.4. Compare mentals of Sulphur and Psorinum – [1977, 90, 88C]

SULPHUR	PSORINUM
• Hypochondriacal patient – Ragged philosopher – Even rags seem beautiful when the patient takes fancy for it. He dresses himself in the most filthy rags but still considers them the most elegant decoration.	• Anxious and melancholic.
• Great weakness of memory, very selfish and has no regard for others, disinclined to work.	• Full of fear. Fears that he would die and fail in business. Feels that he has sinned his days of grace; sees darkness around him. Extremely irritable and wants to be alone.

Q.5. Compare constipation of Sulphur and Bryonia. [1988]

SULPHUR	BRYONIA
• **Cause** – Alcoholism, suppression of skin eruption.	• **Cause** – Dryness of mucous membranes.
• **Character of stools** – Hard dry and knotty stools, dry as if burnt, painful and large. Difficult and painful defeacation.	• **Character of stools** – Dry hard and knotty stools as if burnt.
• **Concomitant** – Constipation alternates with diarrhoea.	**Concomitant** – Headache due to constipation with dry tongue and thirst for large quantities of water.

Q.6. Compare symptoms of Hepar sulph. and Sulphur. [1987]

HEPAR SULPH	SULPHUR
• More suppuration.	• Less suppuration.
• Hypersensitive to touch of even clothes.	• Not so.
• Worse – Uncovering.	• Worse – Covering, heat of bed.
• Better – Hot application, wants covering all the time.	• Better – Uncovering.
• Discharges smell like old cheese.	• Not so
• Profuse sweating without relief.	• Not so
• Splinter like pain.	• Burning every where.

Q.7. Compare skin symptoms of Bovista, Sulphur. [1996]

BOVISTA	SULPHUR
• Unhealthy skin with moist and dry eruption.	• Hot patient – Dirty and filthy person.
• Thick crust formed by very thick, tough, stringly and tenacious discharges from the eruptions.	• Severe itching and scratching followed by burning, rawness and soreness.
• Urticarea on excitement. Itching at tip of coccyx.	• Tendency to suppuration.
	• Boils in crops.
	• Worse – Covering, warmth of bed.

Q.8. Compare Kali Brom. and Sulphur in skin ailments. [1993]

KALI BROM.	SULPHUR
• Great depression and forgetfulness with great melancholy.	• Hypochondriacal and ragged philosopher.
• Great remedy in acne simplex and acne indurata. They appear in young persons with a fleshy and lymphatic constitution and leave unsightly marks thereby causing great mental depression.	• Hot, dirty and filthy patient.
• Removes the tendency to boils that come in successive crops over the face and tongue with much troublesome itching.	• Acne principally on the face. Tendency to intertrigo in folds of skin.
	• Worse heat of bed, warmth, covering and washing.

68. SPONGIA TOSTA

Common Name – Roasted sponge.

Diathesis – Tubercular Diathesis.

Constitution – Adapted to diseases of women and children with light hair and lax fibre.

Spongia is a deep and slow acting remedy.

KEYNOTES

1) ***Swelling and induration of glands.*** Goitre (Brom.). Thyroid glands swollen with suffocative paroxysms at night.
2) *Awakens in fright and feels as if suffocating,* as if he had to breathe through a sponge.
3) Cough is worse after sleep and mental excitement.
4) Sore throat worse on eating sweet things.
5) ***Great dryness of mucous membranes of air passages*** – throat, larynx, trachea and bronchi – "dry as a horn".
6) ***Dry, barking and croupy cough*** with every thing perfectly dry, no mucous rales.

   Worse – Cold drinks, smoking, lying with head low, dry cold winds, reading, singing and talking.

   Better – Eating and drinking warm things.
7) *Croup* – Anxious wheezing with *suffocation at night.* Worse – during inspiration, before midnight.
   (Worse during expiration – *Aconite*)
   (Worse before morning – *Hepar sulph)*
8) *Angina pectoris* – Spongia is a heart remedy with contracting pains, heat, faintness, suffocation, anxiety and sweat. Palpitation with violent pain and gasping respiration. Awakened suddenly after midnight with suffocation and great anxiety.
9) *Orchitis* – with swelling of spermatic cord. Painful testicles with swelling.

Particulars :

1) HEADACHE
2) RESPIRATORY SYSTEM
3) CARDIAC TROUBLE
4) MALE

HEADACHE

Location – Occiput, forehead.

Character of pains – Congestive headaches that are associated with goitre, cardiac affections and asthma. They are due to sluggish circulation in the brain.

RESPIRATORY SYSTEM

Spongia patient has a tubercular diathesis.

Laryngitis :

There is a tendency of the larynx to be involved in pthisical patients. The patient takes an acute cold and it settles in the larynx with hoarseness. Hoarseness with loss of voice and great dryness of larynx from cold. Coryza with sneezing and the whole chest rings, is as dry as a horn. Larynx is sensitive to touch.

Character of expectoration – Scanty expectoration with very little accumulation of mucous. Laryngeal stridor is very common in women. Mucus is tough which is difficult to expectorate and has to be swallowed.

Character of cough – Dry spasmodic cough. Dryness of air passages with whistles and wheezing and seldom rattling. The patient must sit up bent forward.

< Evening, cold air, talking, singing, moving.

> Eating, drinking, warm things.

Concomitants – Dyspnoea is worse on lying down. Larynx is extemely sensitive to touch due to inflamed condition of laryngeal troubles.

Voice :

Hoarse voice with cracked, faint and choking sensation. Feeling of plug in the larynx with sensitiveness. Talking hurts.

Goitre :

Thyroid gland is affected with hypertrophy and inflammation. Large and hard swelling with suffocative spells at night. Awakes out of a sleep from a sense of suffocation with violent and loud cough, great alarm, agitation, anxiety and difficult respiration, sense of suffocation at night.

Croup

Dry and sibilant or sounds like a saw driven through a pine board; each cough corresponding to a thrust of a saw. Worse by exposure to dry cold wind, during sleep.

Tuberculosis :

Solidification of lung tissue with dullness on percussion. Cough is hard and ringing of a metallic character. Weakness and great congestion of chest. Frequent flushes of heat in pthisical patients. Patient experiences chill in the back and shakes even near a warm stove.

HEARTH

Spongia is a great heart remedy. The patient cannot lie flat on the back with low head without bringing on a sense of suffocation. He is frequently aroused from sleep as if smothering. He sits up in the bed with an anxious look, flushed face, rapid and hard breathing. Cardiac diseases develop slowly with actual tissue changes, enlargement of heart, it takes on a steady growth and the valves become changed, do not fit and hence there is blowing and whizzing sounds, regurgitation with mental symptoms. Rheumatic endocarditis with loud blowing with each heart beat. Angina pectoris with contracting pain in chest, heat and suffocation, faintness and anxious sweat.

Worse – Mental lassitude, coughing, lying on the right side, before menses, after lying down, sitting bent forward, smoking, going upstairs.

MALE

Orchitis – (Gels, Puls, Hamemelis, Merc sol.)

Screwing like squeezing pain in the spermatic cords, testicles with hardness.

General Modalities :

Worse – COLD AIR, TALKING
SINGING, EVENING.

Better – EATING, DRINKING
WARM THINGS, WHEEZING.

Relations :

Follows well – Acon, Hepar sulph.

In cough and croup when dryness prevails after Spongia, give Hepar sulph (when mucus commences to rattle).

Important Questions ?

Q.1. Give indications of Spongia in the following :

a) Respiratory symptoms [1986, 89, 90]

b) Cough [1993]

c) Keynotes [1994]

Q.2. Compare – Spongia/Drosera/Sambucus nigra in respiratory system. [1990, 91, 88]

SAMBUCUS N	SPONGIA	DROSERA
• Snuffles of small children.	• Oedematous swellings in various parts of body.	• Nocturnal barking cough worse at night and lying down.
• Dry coryza completely obstructing the nose, the child must breathe through mouth.	• Mucous in bronchi with difficult expectoration.	• Crawling sensation as from a feather in the larynx.
• Dry heat while asleep and profuse sweat when awake.	• Great dryness of respiratory tract.	• Violent tickling in the larynx with spasmodic difficulties of chest and larynx.
• Suffocation at night and sits up in bed turned blue and gasping for breath.	• Dry and sibilant cough which sounds like saw driven through a pine board.	• Burning sensation in chest with copious sweat all over the body.
• Dry and hollow cough with high degree of dyspnoea.	• Sense of suffocation with violent and loud cough, great alarm, agitation anxiety and difficult respiration.	
• Face, lips and hands turn blue and break into profuse sweat.	• Suffocation on going to sleep.	
• Tendency of attacks to reccur.		

69. THUJA OCCIDENTALIS

Hahnemann

Common Name—Tree of Life (White Cedar).

King of Antisycotic drugs

Constitution—*Hydrogenoid constitution.*

(Ant tart, Nat sulph, Medorrhinum), Rain, cold damp weather, vegetable food increases the number of molecules of water in the system. The patient looks like *Ganeshji* with a distended abdomen and a bulky body having lavish growth of various tissues everywhere.

Thuja patient has a waxy shiny face and it looks as if it had been smeared over with grease and is often transparent. He is a sickly looking person and looks as if entering upon some cachexia.

Thuja is the only *efficacious remedy for figwarts and gonorrhoea.* The patients are fleshy having undue and unwanted growth such as warts, tumors, cysts etc. having dark hair and dark complexion, unhealthy oily skin, dirty brownish with white spots.

Temperament—Lymphatic temperament; sluggish in action and perception.

Relation with head and cold—Chilly patient.

Miasm—Sycosis is in the background.

KEYNOTES

1) Ailments from ***bad affects of vaccination*** (Ant tart, Silicea) from suppressed or maltreated gonorrhoea (Med).
2) ***Fixed ideas*** as if a strange person were at his side; as if soul and body are seperated; living animal is in the abdomen; being under the influence of a superpower; limbs are made of glass and they would break easily.
3) *Vertigo—when closing the eyes.*
4) ***Headache***—as if a nail had been driven into the parietal bone or as if a convex button were pressed on the part. Worse from sexual exertion, overheating, tea (Selenium), chronic sycotic or syphilitic origin.
5) Left sided affections—Left ovary affected, left side of head affected etc.
6) *White scaly dandruff* with dry hair and falling out.
7) *Eyes*—Opthalmia Neonatorum—sycotic or syphilitic, large granulation like warts or blisters, better by warmth and covering, if uncovered feels as if a cold stream of air were blowing through them.

8) *Chronic catarrah* after thick exanthemata with green thick mucus, blood and pus (Pulsatilla).
9) *Teeth decay at roots* – crowns remain sound (Mez; on edges – Staph.); crumble and turn yellow (Syph.).
10) On blowing the nose a pressive pain is felt in the hollow of the tooth or at its side.
11) Distending *pain in left ovarian region* when walking or riding, must sit or lie down (Croc.).
12) *Constipation* – Violent pain in the rectum compels cessation of effort; stool recedes after being partly expelled (Sil, Sanicula).
13) *Diarrhoea* – Early morning diarrhoea, stools are expelled forcibly with much flatus (Aloes), gargling as water from a bunghole. Worse – after breakfast, coffee, fat food, vaccination, onions.
14) *Piles swollen* – pain most severe when sitting.
15) *Anus* – fissured and surrounded with flat warts or moist mucous condylomata.
16) ***Skin looks dirty brown with brownish white*** spots here and there, large and pendunculated warts (Staph). *Eruptions only on covered parts* – burn after scratching.
17) Flesh feels as if beaten from the bones (Phyt; as if scraping – Rhus).
18) Sensation as if urinating, as if urine is trickling in the urethra, severe cutting at the close of urination (Sarsaparilla).
19) *Sweat – only on covered parts* or all over except the head (head – Silicea) when he sleeps; sweat stops when he awakes; profuse sour smelling and foetid at night. Perspiration on genitals smells like honey.
20) ***Mucopurulent, copious foul smelling discharges*** from all the mucous membranes of the body.
21) Deformed and brittle nails.

Particulars :

1) MIND
2) HEADACHE
3) EYE
4) EARS
5) GIT
6) RESPIRATORY SYSTEM
7) SEXUAL SYSTEM
8) SKIN
9) NERVOUS SYSTEM

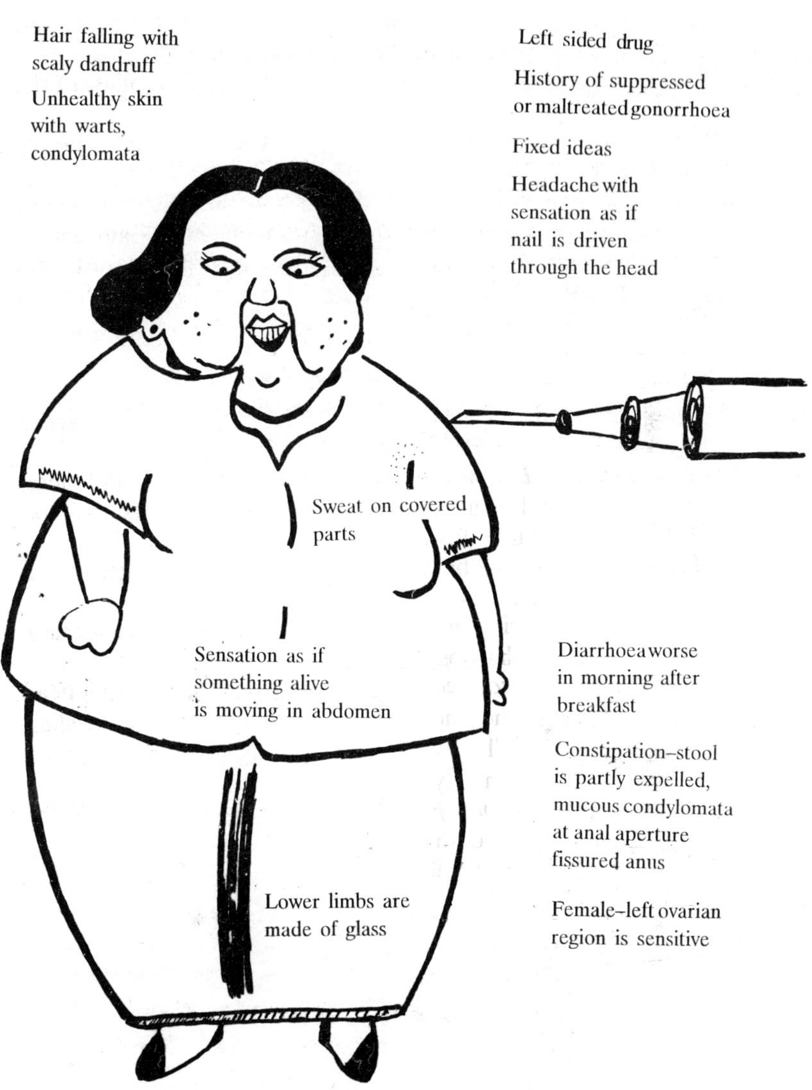
Hair falling with
scaly dandruff
Unhealthy skin
with warts,
condylomata
Left sided drug
History of suppressed
or maltreated gonorrhoea
Fixed ideas
Headache with
sensation as if
nail is driven
through the head
Sweat on covered
parts
Sensation as if
something alive
is moving in abdomen
Diarrhoea worse
in morning after
breakfast
Constipation–stool
is partly expelled,
mucous condylomata
at anal aperture
fissured anus
Lower limbs are
made of glass
Female–left ovarian
region is sensitive

THUJA OCCIDENTALIS

Hydrogenoid constitution

MIND

Deranged nervous state. Patient is constantly in a hurry. When he talks, he talks in rush. Movements are hurried and impatient. The slightest disturbance puts him off his balance. When reading or writing he uses wrong expression and gives one the impression of approaching mental derangement.

Fixed ideas – Sensation as if a strange person was standing at his side; as if soul and body are seperated; as if body is made of glass and that he would break easily, as if an animal were in his abdomen, as if legs were made of wood. He feels he is under the control of a superior power from which he cannot break away.

Extemely quarrelsome and he gets easily angered about trifles. Loathing of life, depression of spirits, sleeplessness and dissatisfaction. He shuns everybody. At time he exhibits a sort of suicidal mania. Speaks slowly as if at a *loss for words*, prolonged thoughtfulness about the merest trifles. Uneasy sleep; dreams of falling from a height, of dead people.

HEADACHE

Cause – Sycotic or syphilitic. Exposure to heat, sunstroke, overeating, sexual excess, tobacco, tea, coffee, suppression of gonorrhoea and syphilis.

Location – Left temple, left parietal bone.

Sensation – As if head was forced and as if pierced by a nail into the parietal bone (Ign. Coffee).

Character – Violent congestion with heaviness in occiput. Headache in the morning. Boring pains in the temples. Screwing in the frontal eminence or temples as if a convex button was pressed upon the part.

Modalities –

Worse – Sexual excesses, overeating, tea, coffee, exposure to heat and sun.

Better – Exercise, open air, looking up, turning the head upwards.

Concomitants – The patient has a syphilitic or sycotic history. Peevish and taciturn patient. Scalp is sensitive to touch. Vertigo when closing the eyes.

EYE

Important remedy in keratitis, syphilitic iritis, opthalmia.

Great photophobia is always present.

Discharge is purulent and the eyelids are agglutinated when fungal tumors make their appearance in orbit. When styes and tarsal tumors complicate Thuja is a deep acting miasmatic remedy. Large granulations like warts or blisters.

EARS

Polyps or condylomatous growths in the ear, chronic otitis exciting profuse purulent acrid and offensive discharges.

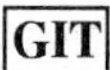

GIT

Teeth :

Teeth decay at the root, the crowns being apparently normal. On blowing the nose there is pain in the hollow of the tooth. Teeth crumble and turn yellow.

Mez. – teeth decay at root.

Merc sol – Crown decay, roots intact.

Staph. – Edges decay.

Kreosote – Teeth decay as soon as they begin to appear.

Abdomen :

Persistent indigestion and loose bowels. Distended abdomen with flatus and rumbling. Croaking and grumbling noise in the abdomen. The movement of the flatus which gives rise to this peculiar noise is so great to resemble the quickening of a child in the gravid uterus. The abdomen protrudes here and there from flatus as though something alive were moving in the abdomen.

Diarrhoea :

Cause – Vaccination, onion, tea, coffee, bread, butter, fatty food, damp air, break fast.

Time – Morning diarrhoea.

Character of stools – Stools are forcibly expelled, copious gurgling like water from the bung hole of a barrel.

Concomitants – Great rumbling as from immense gas in the abdomen. Anus fissured or surrounded with condylomata.

Constipation :

In chronic constipation when stool produces violent rectal pain which ultimately compels the patient to cease the effort. Anus is fissured and painful to touch, surrounded by flat warts or mucous condylomata. Piles may also appear along with constipation which is swollen and painful. Pain is worse when sitting.

RESPIRATORY SYSTEM

Nose :

Discharges are thick and greenish. Pus or scabs are found in it.

Cough :

Time – Daytime, cough hardly comes at night.

Character of cough – Cough is excited by a choking sensation.
Expectoration – Yellow or green lumps.

Worse – Eating.

Asthma :

A peculiar asthmatic condition occurs in sycosis (Ars. and Aloes. are indicated in acute cases) Thuja and Natrum sulph will take up the work and cure.

SEXUAL SYSTEM

Male :

Thuja is the king of sycotic drugs. It is an important remedial agent in gonorrhoea when the dischage is thin and greenish accompanied by scalding pain during urination. Urethra is swollen as a result of which there is always a retention of a few drops of urine which ooze out and soil his clothes sometimes after urination has finished.

Thuja is indicated in maltreated and suppressed gonorrhoea.

Prostatitis, impotence and condylomatous growths are seen everywhere. Penis is disfigured by appearance of these warty excrescences which look like figwarts. Warty growths discharge a sort of a viscid fluid of which the stench is unbearable. It smells like old cheese or herring brine. Patient complains of rawness between the legs and on the sides of the scrotum. This emits a strong sweetish honey like smell and stains the linen yellow.

Female :

In women warts and excrecences appear about the vulva. They render the part extremely sensitive. Condylomata with thick green leucorrhoea corresponding to the thin greenish yellow gleet of the male.

Ovarian pain – Thuja affects glands particularly the left ovary coming on at the time of menses and continuing during the flow, extending down the thighs.

SKIN

Thuja cures moist tubercles, blood boils, bleeding fungal growths, warts, condylomata, pemphigus, impetigo, shingles, ring worm and other varieties of deadlier cutaneous disorders.

Dirty looking skin with dirty brownish discolourations. A net work of fine capillaries visible like the veining of a piece of marble. The *nails* too crumble as they are very *brittle*. They are absolutely devoid of moisture and of the healthy glow to be seen normally.

Sweat on uncovered parts, the covered parts remaining hot and dry.

Tendency of the patient to throw out *warts* like excrecences which are soft and pulpy and very sensitive, burn itch and bleed easily when rubbed by the clothing.

Horny excrecences that form on the hands and split open and crack at the base. Warts of a brownish colour especially on the abdomen, great brown spots like liver spots form upon the abdomen.

Herpes around the chest (Thuja, Rhus, Graph, Kali hydr. Mezerium, Sepia).

Thuja is a strong medicine to *antidote a trace of animal poisoning* in the history as snake bites, small pox, vaccination etc.

Thuja is useful in ulcers that have originated from flat warts, fissures or furrows. These ulcers have a dirty yellow base with hard edges. Thuja has a property of *softening hard tissues*, naturally hard as the nails (It thus reduces the warts by softening them and causes their absorption). Thuja *antidotes bad affects of vaccination* eg – eczema for 20 yrs with a pustular eruption on leg, eruption on chin involving the lower lip, post orbital neuralgia of twenty years standing. Chronic headache of nine years duration.

Cases of glands, hairless patches, habitual influenza, with illhealth and headaches where the patient has been successfully vaccinated 4 times of acne, face, nose, nasal dermatitis after unsuccessful revaccination.

NERVOUS SYMPTOMS

Thuja acts strongly upon the nervous system causing disturbance of circulation which leads to sensation of ebullitions of pulsation particularly in the precordial region.

Thuja affects the nervous system – the patient exhibits a manner which is hurried and impatient. His movements are unnaturally active and hurried. His temper is easily aroused. Even trifles make him angry. Music causes weeping and trembling of feet. The patient has fixed ideas – his mind is made of brittle substance and he would not permit to be approached.

RHEUMATISM

Articular rheumatism after suppressed gonorrhoea. Pains in joints limbs feel as if made of glass and would break easily when walking.

< Heat, warmth of bed.

> Open air, motion, after perspiration.

General Modalities :

Aggravation – NIGHT, FROM HEAT OF BED
3 A.M. AND 3 P.M., FROM COLD
DAMP AIR, NARCOTICS.

Amelioration – OPEN AIR, WARMTH
MOVEMENTS
PRESSURE
RUBBING AND
SCRATCHING.

Relations :

Complementry – Medorrhinum, Sabadilla, Silicea.

Compare – Cannabis sativa, Cantharis, Staphysagria.

Cinnaberis is prefferable for warts on prepuce. Follows well after Med, Nitric acid.

Important Questions ?

Q.1. Give indications of Thuja in the following.

a) Skin [1967, 69, 74, 79, 91, 93]
b) Mind [1972, 73, 74, 77]
c) Asthma [1972, 79]
e) Rheumatic pains [1975, 81]
f) Teeth decay [1981]
g) Headache [1982]
h) Perspiration [1976]
i) Heamorrhoids [1979, 82]
j) Rectal, Anal troubles [1979]

Q.2. Sulphur is called king of Psora and Thuja the king of Sycosis. Discuss. [1974, 76, 79, 82]

Q.3. Compare – Constipation – Silicea/Thuja. [1986, 88, 89]

CONSTIPATION :

SILICEA	THUJA
• Sensation of weakness or paresis which results in obstinate constipation so much so that feaces is retained for a long time in the rectum. Stool passes out with great straining.	• Chronic constipation when stool produces violent rectal pain which ultimately compels the patient to cease the effort.

• Stool is partly expelled and then recedes back (in Thuja due to pain).	• Anus is fissured, painful and surrounded by condylomata, flat warts or mucous condylomata.
• Constipation always occurs before and during menses.	• Piles may also appear along with constipation which is swollen and painful.
• Fistula in ano alternates with chest complaints.	• Constipation alternates with diarrhoea.

Q.4. Compare Sepia/Thuja in mental generals. [1983, 87]

MENTAL GENERALS

SEPIA	THUJA
• The patient is excessively nervous and indifferent.	• The patient has ***fixed ideas.***
• Indifference runs through the whole drug.	• Sensation of a strange person is at his side.
Indifference to one whom she loved the best.	• The soul and body are seperated.
• She cannot narrate her symptoms without weeping (Puls, Med.).	• He is under the control of some super human being.
• Great sadness and weeping.	• Something alive is moving in the abdomen.
• Cannot bear tobacco in any form.	• The body is made of glass and would break easily.
• Consolation aggravates her mental condition.	• A nail had been driven into the parietal bone.
• Depressed, anxious and fearful.	
• Sense of helplessness and susceptibility to excitement and still more to terror. Frequent attacks of weeping and despair of life.	• Music is unbearable. Deranged nervous state as if the patient is always in a hurry.

Q.5. Compare bowel symptoms of Natrum sulph, Thuja, Veratum album [1973]

BOWEL SYMPTOMS :

NATRUM SULPH.	THUJA	VERAT. ALBUM.
• Natrum sulph starts getting his stools after he gets up and moves about.	• Thuja gets an urget call for stools as soon as he drinks his first cup of tea.	• Cause of diarrhoea – fright, eating, drinking, taking fruits.
• Great rumbling as from immense gas in abdomen.	• Constipation alternates with diarrhoea.	• Profuse watery stool mixed with flakes, cold sweat on forehead with great prostration.
• Rumbling in right side of ileo ceacal region.		• Diarrhoea before and during menses.

Q.6. Compare Keynotes of Nitric acid/Thuja. [1990, 91]

NITRIC ACID	THUJA
• Cracks and fissures where the skin and mucous membranes join with splinter like pricking pain.	• Unhealthy skin.
• Heamorrhagic tendency – mouth, nose, bowels, uterus.	• Warts on any parts of the body with a stalk called figwarts, tubular warts, flat warts and condylomata.
• Inflammation and suppuration of glands especially from abuse of mercury in syphilitic people.	• Dirty brownish colour of the skin, brownish white and mottled spots on skin.
• *Desire* – fats, undigestible things, chalk, charcoal, stone.	• White scaly dry eruptions on skin.
• Ulcers with irregular edges, base looks like raw flesh and exuberant granulations.	• Eruptions on covered parts. Only burn violently after scratching.
• Sycotic or syphilitic condylomata that bleed easily on slightest touch.	• *Desire* – Salt, cold food and drinks.
• Moist oozing with offensive discharges with splinter like pain.	

70. VERATRUM ALBUM

Hahnemann

Common Name – White Hellebore.

Constitution – Veratrum album is an acute remedy. For children and old people in extremes of life. Persons who are habitually cold and deficient in vital reaction.

Temperament – Nervous and Sanguine temperament.

Relation with heat and cold – Chilly patient .

Miasm – Psora is in the background.

KEYNOTES

1) Collapse with general ***coldness*** and ***cold sweat,*** especially on forehead; hippocratic face.
2) ***Mania*** with desire to cut and tear things especially clothes with lewdness and lascivious talks, religeous or amorous.
3) Disposed to silence but if irritated gets mad, scolds, calls name and talks of faults of others.
4) ***Profuseness of all discharges*** – Rice watery stools, profuse and exhausting with cramps in calves, coldness and collapse.
5) ***Copiousness of all discharges*** – stools, vomiting, urine, saliva, sweet, craving for acids or refreshing things.
6) Rapid sinking of vital forces, *complete prostration, collapse*.
7) Sensation of a lump of ice on vertex with chilliness as of heat and cold at same time on scalp. ***Icy coldness of face, tip of nose, feet, legs, hands, arms.***
8) *Face* – Pale, blue, collapsed and sunken. Hippocratic face, red while lying and pale while rising.
9) *Thirst – Intense, unquenchable for large quantities of very cold water and acid drinks.*
10) *Violent vomiting with profuse diarrhoea*.
11) *Constipation* with no desire for stools. Large and hard stools from inactive rectum.
12) *Dysmenorrhoea* – with vomiting and purging of exhausting diarrhoea with cold sweat. Patient is so weak that he can scarcely stand for two days at menstrual nisus.
13) Bad affects of fright, opium, tobacco.
14) *Rheumatic affections* – worse in damp weather, drives the patient out of bed.

15) Congestive and pernicious intermittent fever with extreme coldness and collapse of face. Cold and clammy skin with great prostration, cold sweat on forehead and deathly pallor.

Particulars :

1) MIND
2) GIT
3) FEMALE SYMPTOMS
4) RHEUMATISM
5) FEVER

MIND

Mental symptoms are marked by *violence and destructiveness*. Patient wants to destroy or tear something, he tears clothes from the body.

Mania with desire to tear clothes especially lewdness and lasciviousness. *Peurperal mania* with convulsions and violent cerebral congestions, blue and bloated face, protruding eyes with disposition to bite and tear. Loquacity – he talks rapidly during peurperium. The lady is inconsolable over a fancied misfortune, runs into the room howling and screaming.

Despair and hopelessness – The patient attempts to commit suicide. She talks about indecent things, makes impudent gestures. They pass on to a real vehemence of fitful rage. Sensation of lump or ice on vertex. Thinks that she is pregnant.

(Veratrum album has all 3 types of manias – Violent mania of Belladonna, Religeous mania of Stramonium and lascivious mania of Hyoscyamus.

HEADACHE

Congestive headache :

Character of headache – Neuralgic headache with great violence accompanied with coldness, vomiting of bile and blood, great exhaustion and profuse sweat. Vomiting and retching after the stomach is empty. Spasmodic retching and cramping in the stomach. Violent rush of blood to the head with coldness of extremities.

Sensation – Head feels as if packed with ice, feels as if ice lay on vertex and occiput.

GIT

Cholera :

Coldness of discharges, coldness of body.

Appearance – Collapse, rapid sinking of vital forces. Complete prostration with cold sweat and cold breath. Hippocratic face with a pointed nose; whole body is icy cold. Feet and legs are icy cold. Cramps in calves. Blue purple, cold and wrinkled skin. Sensation of lump of ice on

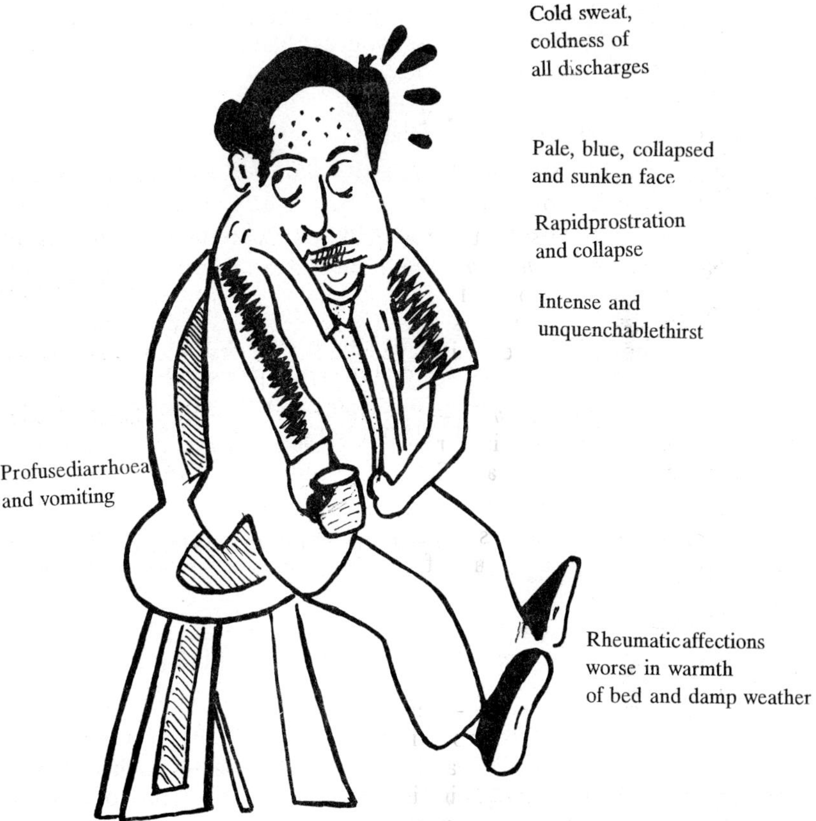
Cold sweat,
coldness of
all discharges
Pale, blue, collapsed
and sunken face
Rapidprostration
and collapse
Intense and
unquenchablethirst
Profusediarrhoea
and vomiting
Rheumaticaffections
worse in warmth
of bed and damp weather

VERATRUM ALBUM

vertex with cold extremities as if dead. Circulation seems to be stopped. Heat is totally absent in all limbs. He tosses frequently and exhibits great anguish.

Character of stools – Profuse sweat with vomiting and diarrhoea. Profuse watery and greenish stools sometimes containing flakes that look like spinach. Rice watery stools.

Vomiting – Huge quantity of painful and frequent evacuations. Vomiting of large quantities of watery blackish, yellowish bilious substance; undigested food particles.

Thirst – Violent thirst for cold water.

Sweat – Cold sweat on forehead.

Cramps – Cramps commencing in hands and feet and running all over the body.

Pains – Severe pains drive the patient to delirium. It is felt near the umblicus and gives the patient a sensation as if the bowels would open up.

Stomach :

Violent diarrhoea with vomiting or constipation. Violence is very striking. Cold feeling in the stomach and cutting pains with sinking feeling in the stomach. Nausea and vomiting just after eating and drinking. Patient craves acids and refreshing juicy things.

Constipation :

Sensation – Desire is felt in the epigastrium.

Character of stools – Dry hard and painful round black balls with much straining that exhausts the patient.

Gastrodynia :

Pain starts in the epigastrium. It is at first dull but it grows almost agonising and subsiding slowly again. Pain radiates from the epigastrium both upward and sideways reaching the back between the lowest points of the scapula. It is accompanied by a shaking cold sensation (Colocynth).

FEMALE SEXUAL SYMPTOMS

Extreme irritation in parts turning them into nymphomaniacs (Veratum album soothens the irritation and removes all abnormal cravings of mind).

Menses :

Time – Too early.

Character of blood – Profuse and very exhausting; makes the patient weak. She can scarcely stand for two days at each menstrual nisus.

Pain – Dysmenorrhoea with cutting pain in abdomen. Faints from least exertion.

Concomitants – Cold sweat on forehead. Collapsed condition with great weakness, cholera like symptoms before and during menses.

RHEUMATISM

Cause – Warmth of bed, during wet weather.

Character of pain – Neuralgia like pain in the extremities. Severe pain that makes the patient jump from bed especially at night.

Worse – Warmth of bed; during wet weather.

Better – By continued motion but continued motion produces heat and this causes further aggravation.

FEVER

Veratrum album is efficacious in pernicious fevers accompanied by general exhaustion, rapid sinking of strength and profuse diarrhoea.

Time of paroxysm – 6 a.m.

Chill stage – Prominent and starts with severity and icy coldness of entire body. Despite great chilliness the patient craves cold and refreshing drinks.

Heat stage – Face gets congested and his brain becomes confused.

Sweat stage – Cold and clammy sweat which bursts over the forehead. Red face turns pale and haggard.

General Modalities :

Worse – HEAT, MOTION, DRINKING
BEFORE AND DURING STOOLS
PERSPIRATION and AFTER FRIGHT.

Better – WALKING AND WARMTH.

Relations :

After – Ars, Arnica, Cinchona, Cup, Ipec.

After Camphor in cholera and cholera morbus.

After Ammonium carb, Carbo veg and Bovista in dysmenorrhoea vomiting and purging.

Important Questions ?

Q.1. Give indications of the following :

a) Cholera [1986]

b) Diarrhoea [1972, 73, 74, 76, 77, 79, 81]

c) Desire and Aversions [1991]

d) Colic [1987]

e) Modalities [1978]

f) Insanity [1973, 75, 81]

g) Perspiration [1976]

Q.2. Compare Cholera of – Arsenic alb/Verat alb/Cuprum met /Camphor. [1990, 94]

VERATRUM ALBUM	ARS. ALB	CAMPHOR	CUP. MET
Profuseness of stools with blueness, coldness and cold sweat on forehead. Desire to eat and drink cold and refreshing things.	Small *offensive* dark stools with sudden and rapid prostration. Diarrhoea worse at *night* between 12-2 A.M. Offensive and rice watery stools. *Burning* in rectum before and after stools.	*Dry cholera*- Coldness, Scanty, sweat vomiting and purging with coldness and blueness. Intense prostration without exhausting discharge.	Convulsive character with extreme coldness and more or less dryness. Profuse vomiting and purging with increased sweat Flexor type of cramps.

VIVA—QUESTIONS

DRUG	AFFECTIONS: LEFT HAND SIDE (L.H.S) OR RIGHT HAND SIDE (R.H.S)	HOT REMEDY OR COLD REMEDY	MIASMS
1. ABROTANUM	–	CHILLY patient	Psora
2. ACONITE	–	–	Psora
3. AESCULUS HIPP	–	–	–
4. AETHUSA CYN.	–	HOT patient	Psora, Sycosis Syphilis
5. ALLIUM CEPA	L.H.S.	HOT patient	Psora
6. ALOE SOCOTRINA	–	HOT patient	Psora
7. AMMONIUM CARB	R.H.S	CHILLY patient	Psora
8. ANTIM CRUM	–	–	Psora and Sycosis
9. ANTIM TART	–	–	Psora and Sycosis
10. APIS MELL	–	HOT patient	Psora
11. ARG. MET	–	–	Syphilis
12. ARG. NIT	–	HOT patient	Psora, Syc, Syph.
13. ARNICA	–	CHILLY patient	Psora

14. ARS. ALB.	–	CHILLY patient	Psora, Syc, Syph.
15. ARUM TRIPH	–	CHILLY patient	–
16. ARUM MET	–	CHILLY patient	Syphilis
17. BAPTISIA T.	–	CHILLY patient	Syphilis, Psora
18. BARYTA C.	–	CHILLY patient	Psora
19. BELLADONNA	R.H.S	CHILLY patient	Psora
20. BERB. VULG.	L.H.S	–	Psora, Sycosis
21. BORAX	–	HOT patient	Psora
22. BRYONIA	–	HOT patient	Psora
23. CALCAREA CARB	–	CHILLY patient	Psora, Sycosis
24. CALCAREA PHOS	–	CHILLY patient	Psora
25. CALCAREA SULPH	–	–	–
26. CALCAREA FLOUR	–	–	–
27. CALENDULA	–	–	–
28. CARBO VEG	–	HOT patient	Psora
29. CAUSTICUM	R.H.S	CHILLY patient	Psora, Sycosis
30. CHAMOMILLA	–	CHILLY patient	Psora
31. CINA	–	–	Psora
32. CINCHONA	–	CHILLY patient	Psora
33. COLCHICUM	–	CHILLY patient	–
34. COLOCYNTH	–	CHILLY patient	Psora
35. DROSERA	–	CHILLY patient	Psora, Sycosis

36. DULCAMARA	–	–	Psora
37. EUPHRASIA	–	–	Psora
38. GELSIMIUM	–	–	Psora
39. GRAPHITES	–	CHILLY patient	Psora
40. HELLEBORUS	–	CHILLY patient	Psora
41. HEPAR. SULPH	–	CHILLY patient	Psora
42. HYOSCYAMUS	–	CHILLY patient	Psora
43. IGNATIA	–	–	Psora
44. IPECAC	–	CHILLY patient	–
45. KALI BICH	–	CHILLY patient	Psora, Sycosis, Syphilis
46. KALI CARB	–	–	Psora
48. KALI PHOS	–	CHILLY patient	Psora
49. KALI SULPH	–	HOT patient	Psora
50. FERRUM PHOS	–	–	Psora
51. LACHESIS	L.H.S	–	Psora
52. LEDUM PAL	–	HOT patient	Psora
53. LYCOPODIUM	R.H.S	CHILLY patient	Psora, Sycosis, Syphilis
54. MAG. PHOS	R.H.S	CHILLY patient	Psora
55. MERC. SOL	–	–	Syphilis
56. MERC. COR	–	–	–
57. NATRUM MUR	–	HOT patient	Psora, Sycosis, Syphilis
58. NATRUM PHOS	–	–	Psora
59. NATRUM SULPH	–	CHILLY patient	Sycosis

60. NITRIC ACID	–	CHILLY patient	Psora, Sycosis, Syphilis
61. NUX VOMICA	–	CHILLY patient	Psora
62. PODOPHYLLUM	–	–	Psora & Syphilis
63. PULSATILLA	–	–	Psora & Syphilis
64. RHUS. TOX	–	CHILLY patient	Psora
65. SECALE COR.	–	HOT patient	Psora
66. SILICEA	–	CHILLY patient	Psora, Sycosis, Syphilis
67. SULPHUR	–	CHILLY patient	Psora
68. SPONGIA	–	–	–
69. THUJA	–	CHILLY patient	Sycosis
70. VERAT ALB	–	CHILLY patient	Psora

TRIOS

1. Trio of restlessness – Arsenic, Aconite, Rhus tox.

2. Trio of pain – Aconite, Coffea, Chamomilla.

3. Trio of flatulence – Carbo veg, China, Lycopodium.

4. Trio of burners – Sulfur, Arsenic alb, Phosphorus.

5. Trio of condylomata – Thuja, Staphysagria, Nitric acid.

6. Trio of offensiveness – Kreosote, Merc. sol, Baptisia.

7. Trio of cholera – V. alb, Arsenic alb, Camphor.

8. Trio of sleepiness – Ant. tart, Gelsimium, Nux mosch.

9. Trio of offensive urine – Benzoic acid, Nitric acid, Sepia.

10. Trio of homoeopathic last aid – Carbo veg, Arsenic, Muriatic Acid.

11. Trio of paralysis – Causticum, Rhus tox, Sepia.

12. Trio of ptosis – Causticum, Gelsimium, Sepia.

13. Trio of prostration – Carbo veg, Ars. alb, Muriatic acid.

14. Trio of excess hyper aesthesia – Plumbum, China, Capsicum.

15. Trio of chronic rheumatism – Causticum, Rhus tox, Sulphur.

16. Trio of warts – Causticum, Thuja, Dulcamara.

17. Trio of delirium – Belladonna; Hyoscyamus, Stramonium.

Other Highlights :

SEPIA – Washerwomen's remedy

ACTEA RACEMOSA – Homoeopathic milk for allopathic babies

PLATINA – Black letter medicine

MERC. SOL – Human Thermometer

SILICEA – Surgeon's Knife

LYCOPODIUM – Vegetable Sulphur

MEZERIUM – Vegetable Mercury

GELSIMIUM – King of Polio

CALENDULA – Homoeopathic Antiseptic

CAMPHOR – Universal Antidote to medicines prepared from vegetable kingdom.

CANTHARIS – Vehement drug for stress and strain.

CARBO VEG – Homoeopathic Last Aid

MAGNESIA CARB – Gregorys Powder, Laxative, Antacid, Sweetens the stomach

NATRUM SULPH – Glaubers Salt

KALI SULPH – Schuzzlers Pulsatilla

NUX VOMICA – Male Counterpart of Pulsatilla and Ignatia

PYROGEN – Homoeopathic Dynamic Antiseptic

COCA – Mountains Remedy.

KING OF ANTI PSORIC REMEDIES – Sulphur

KING OF ANTI SYCOTIC REMEDIES – Thuja

KING OF ANTI SYPHILITIC REMEDIES – Mercurius

- Alumina is chronic of Bryonia.
- Silicea is chronic of Pulsatilla.
- Natrum mur is chronic of Ignatia.
- Calcarea is chronic of Belladonna.
- Sulphur is chronic of Aconite.

- THIRST LESS Remedies – AETHUSA CYNAPIUM, APIS,
  BELLADONNA (during fever)
  GELSIMIUM
  IPECAC
  PULSATILLA
  ANTIM TART

- THIRSTY Remedies – ACONITE
  ARSENIC ALBUM (Thirst for little sips of water.)
  BRYONIA
  VERATRUM ALBUM
  RHUS TOXICODENDRON.
- DESIRE REFRESHING THINGS – *Verat. alb, China.*
- DESIRE SWEETS – *Lycopodium, China, Sulphur, Argentum nit.*
- DESIRES SALT – *Carbo veg, Phos, Nat mur, Arg. nit.*
- ALTERNATE DIARRHOEA AND CONSTIPATION – *Ant. crud, Nux vom, Sulph, Chelidoneum, Verat alb, Ant tart, Podophyllum.*
- MARASMUS – *Iodum, Abrot., Sanicula, Tuber, Aethusa, Nat mur, Silicea, Calc. phos, Sulphur.*
- SLOW ONSET OF SYMPTOMS – *Bryonia, Gelsimium,*
- SUDDEN AND VIOLENT ONSET OF SYMPTOMS – *Aconite, Belladonna.*
- WELL MARKED LINEA NASALIS – *Aethusa cynapium*
- JELLY LIKE MUCUS IN STOOLS – *Kali bi, Podo, Helleborus.*
- CHILDREN DISLIKE WASHING – *Amm carb, Ant. crud, Sulphur.*
- CHOLERA LIKE SYMPTOMS AT ONSET OF MENSES – *Bovista, Verat. album, Amm. carb.*
- CONSTIPATION AT THE ONSET OF MENSES – *Silicea.*
- SYMPTOMS CHANGE THEIR LOCALITY – *Ant. crud, Lac can., Tuberculinum.*
- IRRESISTABLE DESIRE TO SLEEP – *Ant tart, Nux mosch, Aethusa, Gelsimium.*
- WANDERING PAINS FROM ONE PART OF THE BODY TO ANOTHER – *Kali bi, Lac. can, Puls, Apis.*
- EXTREMELY SENSITIVE TO TOUCH – *Apis, Bell, Hepar. sulph, Lachesis, China.*
- OEDEMA – over the eyes – *Kali carb.*
  around the eyes – *Phosphorus.*
  below the eyes – *Apis*

- INVOLUNTARY DIARRHOEA WITH A SENSATION AS IF ANUS IS WIDE OPEN – *Thuja, Apis, Secale cor, Phos.*
- LAUGHING CAUSES COUGH – *Dros, Arg. met, Stannum, Phos.*
- URINE PASSES UNCONCIOUSLY DAY AND NIGHT – *Caust, Arg. nit.*
- NERVOUS DIARRHOEA – *Gels. Arg. nit.*
- OFFENSIVE DISCHARGE WITH CADAVEROUS ODOUR – *Ars. alb.*

  Rotten egg smell – *Sulphur*

  Rotten cheese smell – *Hepar sulph*

  Sour milk – *Calc. carb*

  Like fumes of Sulphur – *Phos.*
- CANNOT BEAR SMELL OR SIGHT OF FOOD – *Colch, Ars alb Sepia, Stann.*
- WORSE BY THINKING ABOUT COMPLAINTS – *Medo, Calc phos, Gels, Baryta carb.*
- VERY SLEEPY BUT CANNOT SLEEP – *Bell, Cham, Stram, Opium.*
- FISTULA ALTERNATES WITH CHEST COMPLAINTS – *Gels, Bryonia.*
- CHILD SCREAMS BEFORE URINATING – *Lyco, Borax.*
- FAIR FAT AND FLABBY CHILD – *Calc. carb.*
- CONSTIPATED – STOOL TO BE REMOVED MECHANICALLY – *Calc carb, Aloes, Sepia, Silicea, Thuja.*
- COLDNESS, SWEAT IN SINGLE PARTS – *Calc. carb.*
- HEAT IN SPOTS – *Sulphur.*
- DESIRE FOR UNDIGESTIBLE THINGS – *Alumina, Nitric acid, Cina, Cicuta, Psorinum, Calc. carb.*
- AVERSION TO MEAT – *Graph, Alumina, Puls, Mur. acid.*
- COMPLAINTS WORSE BY THINKING ABOUT THEM – *Calc. phos, Baryta carb, Gelsimium, Medorrhinum, Helonias, Oxalic, acid.*

- HEADACHE OF SCHOOL GIRLS AT PUBERTY – *Natrum mur, Calc. phos, Psorinum, Tuberculinum.*
- WANTS TO BE FANNED RAPIDLY FROM A CLOSE DISTANCE – *Carbo veg.*
- WANTS TO BE FANNED SLOWLY FROM A DISTANCE – *Lachesis.*
- WORSE IN CLEAR FINE WEATHER AND BETTER IN DAMP WEATHER – *Caust, Hepar. S, Nux. vom, Medo.*
- PARALYSIS OF SINGLE PARTS – *Causticum.*
- ANGER REMEDY – *Chamomilla*
- WORM REMEDY – *Cina*
- APHONIA FROM EXPOSURE TO COLD AIR – *Aconite, Spongia, Phosphorus.*
- PERIODICITY OF COMPLAINTS IS MARKED – *China, Eup. perf, Nat mur, Ars. alb, Ipec.*
- BROKEN DOWN CONSTITUTION – *China.*
- PROFUSE ACRID LACHRYMATION AND BLAND CORYZA – *Euphrasia*
- ACRID CATARRAH AND BLAND LACHRYMATION – *Allium cepa.*
- DAYTIME COUGH – *Euphrasia, Eup. perf, Ferrum met, Staphysagria.*
- HEADACHE RELIEVED BY PROFUSE URINATION – *Gelsimium, Silicea.*
- FAIR FAT AND FLABBY LADY WITH UNHEALTHY SKIN, HABITUAL CONSTIPATION, DELAYED MENSES – *Graphites*
- CONSOLATION AGGRAVATES COMPLAINTS – *Helleborus, Ignatia, Natrum mur, Lilium tig, Sepia, Silicea.*
- CONSOLATION AMELIORATES COMPLAINTS – Pulsatilla.
- HYPERSENSITIVE, HYPERIMPULSIVE, HYPER SWEATING, HOARSENESS, HASTENS SUPPURATION, BETTER BY HEAT, COVERING – *Hepar sulph.*
- SPLINTER SENSATION IN THROAT – *Hepar sulph, Arg. nit, Anacardium*
- EVERY INJURY CAUSES SUPPURATION – *Graphites, Silicea, Merc. sol.*

- DESIRE TO UNCOVER – *Hyoscyamus*
- PAIN IN A SMALL SPOT WHICH CAN BE COVERED WITH THE TIP OF A FINGER – *Ignatia, Kali bich, Lil. tig.*
- COMPLAINTS FROM LONG CONTINUED AND CONCENTRATED GRIEF – *Ignatia.*
- REMEDY OF CONTRA INDICATION – *Ignatia.*
- COLD SWEAT ON FOREHEAD – *Ipec, Verat. alb, Carbo veg.*
- SWEAT, BACKACHE AND WEAKNESS – *Kali carb.*
- ASCENDING RHEUMATISM – *Ledium pal, Arnica.*
- DESCENDING RHEUMATISM – *Kalmia, Cactus.*
- DESPITE COLDNESS SYMPTOMS ARE RELIEVED BY COLD APPLICATION – *Secale cor, Ledum*
- PROFUSE PERSPIRATION WITHOUT RELIEF – *Verat album, Merc. sol, Hepar. sulph.*
- PERSPIRATION GIVES RELIEF – *Nat. mur, Psorinum*
- MOIST TONGUE WITH THIRST AND IMPRINT OF TEETH – *Chelidoneum, Podo, Merc. sol, Rhus tox.*
- DRY TONGUE WITHOUT THIRST – *Pulsatilla, Nux mosh*
- DRY TONGUE WITH MUCH THIRST – *Bry, Ars. alb*
- MAPPED TONGUE WITH RED INSULAR PATCHES – *Nat mur, Ars, Canth, Merc. sol, Nit. acid*
- INVOLUNTARY URINATION WHEN WALKING, LAUGHING OR COUGHING – *Caust, Puls, Lil. tig, Nat mur*
- CANNOT PASS URINE IN PRESENCE OF OTHERS – *Nat mur, Hepar sulph, Mur. acid*
- AILMENTS WORSE DURING THUNDERSTORM – *Petroleum, Phos, Psorinum, Rhus Tox, Rhododendron*
- BAD AFFECTS OF VACCINATION – *Thuja, Ant tart, Crot. horr, Mezerium*

CHARACTERISTIC TONGUE'S

1) *ANTIM CRUD* – Thick milky white coated tongue.
2) *ANTIM TART* – Tongue is covered with thick, white pasty coat, red streaks, small and painful pustules.
3) *APIS* – Fiery red tongue (Crot horr., Ferrum met Pyrogen).
4) *ARS ALB* – Initially during fever the tongue is white coated with red papillae in the middle and later dry cracked and ulcerated.

6) *BELLADONNA* – Tongue is dark red and dry.

7) *BRYONIA* – Dry white coating on tongue with intense thirst.

8) *CINA* – Clean tongue with white papillae raised on edges.

9) *GELSIMIUM* – Thick, yellowish tongue with trembling and paralysis.

10) *HYOSYAMUS* – Leather like paralysed tongue with difficult speech.

11) *LACHESIS* – Bluish or black tongue with trembling.

12) *LYCOPODIUM* – Dryness of mouth with dry and cracked tongue. Sour taste in mouth.

13) *MERC. SOL* – Swollen and flabby tongue that takes imprint of teeth, intense thirst for cold water.

14) *NUX VOMICA* – Anterior half of the tongue is clean and posterior half is coated thick white and yellow.

15) *PULSATILLA* – Yellow or white tongue. Dry tongue without thirst.

16) *PHYTOLACCA* – Foul tongue with imprint of teeth with thirst for large quantities of water.

17) *RHUS TOX* – Triangular red tipped tongue with imprint of teeth and bitter taste in mouth.

CHARACTERISITC PAINS

1) CRAMPING PAIN – Cuprum, Colocynth, Mag phos.

2) BURNING PAINS – Ars, Cantharis, Phosphorus, Capsicum, Sulphur.

3) COLDNESS (Sensation) – Calcarea carb, Ars alb, Cistus.

4) COLDNESS (Objective) – Camphor, Secale, Verat alb, Heloderma.

5) FULLNESS (Sensation) – Aesculus, China, Lyco.

6) EMPTINESS (Sensation) – Co cculus, Phosphorus, Sepia.

7) BEARING DOWN – Bell, Lilium tig, Sepia.

8) BRUISED SORENESS – Arnica, Baptisia, Eup perf, Pyrogen, Ruta.

9) CONSTRICTION – Cactus, Colocynth, Anacardium.

10) PROSTRATION/WEARINESS – Gelsimium, Picric acid, Acid phos.

11) NUMBNESS – Aconite, Cham, Platina, Rhus tox.

12) ERRATIC PAINS – Lac. can, Puls, Tuberculinum, Kali bich..

13) SENSITIVENESS TO PAIN – Aconite, Chamomilla, Coffea.

14) SENSITIVENESS TO TOUCH – China, Hepar sulph, Lachesis.

15) BONE PAINS – Aurum, Asafoetida, Eup. perf, Merc sol.

16) STITCHING PAINS – Bryonia, Kali carb, Squilla.

17) STINGING PAINS – Apis.

18) PULSATING OR TROBBING PAINS – Belladonna, Glonoine, Melilotus.